Rhesus haemolytic disease

Rhesus haemolytic disease

Selected papers and extracts

Commentaries by

Professor Sir Cyril A. Clarke,
KBE, MD, PRCP, FRS

Nuffield Research Fellow, Department of Genetics, and Emeritus Professor of Medicine,
University of Liverpool

MTP Medical and Technical Publishing Co. Ltd.

Published by
MTP
Medical and Technical Publishing Co. Ltd.,
St. Leonard's House, St. Leonardgate,
Lancaster, England.

ISBN-13: 978-94-011-6140-4   e-ISBN-13: 978-94-011-6138-1
DOI: 10.1007/978-94-011-6138-1

Acknowledgements

I am extremely grateful to Dr R. R. Race, FRS, and Dr Ruth Sanger, FRS, for their valuable advice over the commentaries and the general lay-out of the book.

I am also greatly indebted to my wife for much hard work and help—not only did she help with the selection of papers but provided first drafts for many of the commentaries.

Mr L. M. Payne and his staff at the library of the Royal College of Physicians have been most helpful in obtaining original papers.

I am also grateful to Dr A. S. Wiener for the interest he has taken and for permission to reproduce Papers 3, 4, 8, 13, 14.

Dr. Wiener felt, however, that papers dealing with nomenclature were inappropriate in a book of this type, and that instead of them the papers listed below should have been included as being a better representation of his other more important work, being among those included in his book, Rh-Hr Blood Types, pp763, Grune and Stratton, New york (1954).

1. Landsteiner, K. and Wiener, A. S. (1941). Studies on an agglutinogen (Rh) of Human Blood Reacting with Anti-Rhesus Sera and Human Isoagglutinins. *J. Exp. Med.*, **74**, 309-320

2. Wiener, A. S. (1945). Conglutination Test for Rh Sensitization. *J. Lab. and Clin. Med.*, **30**, 662-7

3. Wiener, A. S. (1945). Competition of Antigens in Isoimmunization by Pregnancy. *Proc. Soc. Exp. Biol. and Med.*, **58**, 133-5

4. Wiener, A. S. and Wexler, I. B. (1946). The Use of Heparin when Performing Exchange Blood Transfusions in Newborn Infants. *J. Lab. and Clin. Med.*, **31**, 1016-9

5. Wiener, A. S., Wexler, I. B., and Gamrin, E. (1944). Hemolytic Disease of the Fetus and Newborn Infant, with Special Reference to Transfusion Therapy and the Use of the Biological Test for Detecting Rh Sensitization. *Amer. J. Dis.Child.*, **68**, 317-323

6. Wiener, A. S. and Sonn-Gordon, F. B. (1947). Simple Method of Preparing Anti-Rh Serum in Normal Male Donors. *Amer. J. Clin. Path.*, **17**, 67-70

7. Wiener, A. S. (1943). Genetic Theory of the Rh Blood Types. *Proc. Soc. Exp. Biol. and Med.*, **54**, 316-9

8. Wiener, A.S., Sonn, E. B. and Belkin, R. B.(1943). Heredity and Distribution of the Rh Blood Types. *Proc. Soc. Exp. Biol. and Med.*, **54**, 238-40

9. Wiener, A. S. (1945). Rh Factors in Clinical Medicine, *J. Lab. Clin. Med.*, **30**, 957-76.

My thanks are also due to Dr. Philip Levine and to Dr. F. Stratton for advice at various stages of the book.

Introduction

Jaundice of newborn infants was described by several authors in the 17th century. The condition, however, was usually thought of as being similar to adult jaundice and due to occlusion of the bile ducts by 'glutinous humours'. On the other hand, some writers reported on the fact that more than one consecutive baby was often affected, and there is a classic example of the disease in twins written by Louyse Bourgeois, the midwife of Marie de Medici, in 1609.

It was not until early in the 20th century that it was realised that the common link between these familial cases was anaemia, and later still that this was of the haemolytic type.

The breakthrough, in terms of an idea, came in 1938, when Darrow postulated that the baby's red cells were destroyed by an immune reaction on the part of the mother, the result of immunisation by paternal factors in the fetus. Shortly afterwards Wiener discovered an entirely new blood group system, 'Rh', and it was found that it was incompatibility within this system that was responsible for the vast majority of cases of haemolytic disease of the newborn.

When the gene and phenotype frequencies of the new system had been worked out it became apparent that the disease occured much less frequently than might have been expected. With a total birth rate in the United Kingdom of about 700,000 per annum, one might have expected about 60,000 Rhesus babies a year since 15% of the population is Rh-negative. In fact, because of various naturally occurring protective factors, the figure is actually only about $\frac{1}{20}$ of this. Nevertheless, for a small number of families Rhesus disease is a great tragedy.

It has been the aim in this book to collect and discuss many of the most important basic papers and extracts on the subject and the material falls naturally into three sections; the discovery of the system, the methods of treating the established disease, and the way in which prophylaxis can be effected. Because it has been the chief interest of the editor, the preventive aspect has been dealt with in considerably more detail than the other two sections.

The papers exemplify what Bruce Chown wrote in 1967: 'In less than 30 years our understanding of Rhesus haemolytic disease of the newborn has run full cycle from hypothesis to prevention'.

Rhesus haemolytic disease provides an excellent model for investigating 'at risk' factors and highlights a fundamental principle in medicine—namely that it is just as important to determine why some people do not get a particular disorder as why some do.

Contents

CONTENTS

CONTENTS

Section I

Discovery of the Rh blood group system and related matters

Paper 1

1.   Darrow, Ruth. (1938). Icterus gravis (erythroblastosis) neonatorum. *Arch. Pathol.*, *25*, 378-417.

Commentary

Though this paper strictly speaking has nothing to do with the Rhesus blood groups, yet it is included because it provides an excellent introduction.

Ruth Darrow not only gives a full clinical description of what in 1938 was known as icterus gravis neonatorum, but she examines in detail the theories of causation which were current at that time. Having dismissed them all, she proposes a hypothesis based on an antigen-antibody reaction between mother and fetus. She puts forward the view that fetal haemoglobin may be immunologically different from adult, and that if it gains access to the maternal circulation the mother may become sensitised and the resulting antibody cross the placenta, destroying the fetal erythrocytes.

She thus discovers the principle, but misses by a hair's breadth the actual mechanism, discounting the possibility of a difference in blood group between mother and child because of a previous report (see page 33).

From R. R. Darrow (1938). Arch. Pathol., 25, 378–417. Copyright (1938), by kind permission of the author and the American Medical Association

General Review

ICTERUS GRAVIS (ERYTHROBLASTOSIS) NEONATORUM

AN EXAMINATION OF ETIOLOGIC CONSIDERATIONS

RUTH RENTER DARROW, M.D.

CHICAGO

The etiology of icterus gravis neonatorum is still a subject of speculation. The purpose of this study is (1) to evaluate on the basis of a set of criteria formulated from case histories certain of the theories as to the origin of this condition and (2) to examine the evidence as to the fundamental pathologic processes which give rise to the clinical symptoms and to the organic changes found at necropsy. In view of the wide divergence in the opinions of writers on the subject, such an evaluation seems a necessary preliminary to any further investigation concerning the underlying cause or causes of this disease and those related to it. Although adequate accounts of this malady have been given in numerous recent papers (Hawksley and Lightwood [1] and others to be cited), it will be well, before considering the theories of etiology, to summarize the facts regarding the clinical course, the laboratory findings, the pathologic changes found after death, and other common or unique observations which may have a bearing on, or require an explanation in, an acceptable theory of etiology.

CLINICAL OBSERVATIONS

Icterus gravis neonatorum is characterized by marked jaundice, occasionally present at birth, but more often appearing within the first day or two of life. The jaundice usually becomes intense, the color deepening oftentimes to deep bronze. The liver and spleen are usually enlarged, and the spleen may increase further in size during the period of intense jaundice. There may be a low grade fever, or the entire course may be afebrile. There may or may not be petechiae or purpuric spots on the body, and there may occasionally be slight edema, usually in the extremities, eyelids or scrotum. The urine yields urobilin in excess, and often bilirubin and bile salts as well. Albuminuria is exceptional, and oliguria occurs only in rare cases. The stools are not usually acholic, containing varying amounts of urobilin. The icteric index may be elevated to an extreme degree. The indirect van den Bergh test is always positive and the direct reaction variable; a biphasic reaction is most commonly reported. The child at birth may be covered with golden yellow vernix caseosa, and the amniotic fluid may be colored yellow to orange or brown, although this is not invariable. The placenta on gross examination may appear normal or somewhat enlarged.

Another outstanding feature is found in the blood picture. If a

---

From the Women and Children's Hospital.

1. Hawksley, J. C., and Lightwood, R.: Quart. J. Med. 27:155, 1934.

blood count is taken soon after birth the number of red cells is usually found lowered to an extent varying from slight to marked as compared with the number found in normal new-born infants, and the hemoglobin, to a relatively less extent. Smears often reveal greatly increased proportions of young and immature red cells—reticulocytes, normoblasts and erythroblasts. Nucleated red cells in excess of 5,000 per cubic millimeter of blood at birth are considered abnormal,[1] and in this condition numbers over 100,000 per cubic millimeter have been reported. Commonly associated with this immaturity of the erythrocytes are anisocytosis, poikilocytosis and polychromatophilia. Leukocytosis is likewise found almost invariably, with a definite shift to the left shown by the hemogram, and often there is an absolute as well as a relative increase in eosinophils and monocytes. The platelets are reduced in number in some cases, while the bleeding time may be normal, slightly prolonged or markedly prolonged, with a normal or increased coagulation time. However, the increased bleeding and coagulation time seem not to be related consistently to the decrease in the platelet count. Fragility tests usually show normal, occasionally slightly increased or decreased, resistance to hypotonic saline concentrations. A normal albumin-globulin ratio was found by Ross and Waugh[2] in a case in which edema was present in the lower extremities.

I. A. Abt[3] stated that "most of these children are strong, robust, and mature at birth." In many cases, however, icterus and enlargement of the liver and spleen may be detected shortly after birth. Cardiac hypertrophy may also be found, and a systolic murmur is sometimes present. The clinical course of the malady in the untreated infant tends most frequently toward a fatal outcome. The stools may become frequent and catarrhal in character, and occasionally vomiting occurs, often projectile in type. As the disease progresses, hemorrhages from the mucous surfaces and into the skin, as well as oozing from the umbilicus, may take place. There may be evidence of gastro-intestinal distress. The cry becomes feeble and whining, respiration may become labored and grunting, and spells of cyanosis may develop. The infant appears "drowsy and toxic, difficult to arouse, and refuses or is unable to take the breast or bottle."[4] In contrast to this somnolence and flaccidity, clonic contractures, opisthotonos or even generalized convulsions may occur. Death, following collapse, usually occurs within the first week or two, unless treatment is instituted early and vigorously. Only occasionally has spontaneous recovery been reported (Hawksley and Lightwood;[1] Abt[3]).

The observation of Hawksley and Lightwood[1] should be reiterated at this point. These authors pointed out that in some instances after early treatment with one or more transfusions recovery may seem to be well on the way when more or less suddenly a relapse occurs, indicated by reappearance of symptoms. There may be recurrence of the hemorrhagic tendency, projectile vomiting, evidence of gastro-intestinal distress with frequent stools, cyanosis and labored respirations, and a rise,

2. Ross, S. G., and Waugh, T. R.: Am. J. Dis. Child. 51:1059, 1936.
3. Abt, I. A.: Am. J. Dis. Child. 13:231, 1917.
4. Abt, A. F.: J. Pediat. 3:7, 1933.

or in some cases a marked fall, from the normal in temperature, while the cry again becomes high pitched and weak. Such relapses tend to occur most frequently from the third or fourth to the sixth week and have been reported as late as the tenth week. More than one such recurrence may take place. Prompt amelioration usually follows one or more additional transfusions.

Although some of these infants may be premature, the majority are born at term, with usually a normal and frequently a short and easy delivery. There is no evidence of asphyxia at birth. The parents are healthy. The Wassermann and Kahn tests of the parents as well as of the baby are negative. Tuberculin tests of the infant are also negative. The mother usually has had an uneventful pregnancy, and age, dietary deficiencies and anemia in the mother cannot be ascribed as causative factors; nor can infection of the infant in its passage through the birth canal. Wanstrom,[5] for example, reported the condition in the infant of a 17 year old girl, and A. F. Abt[4] cited Smyth's case of an Australian mother who had given birth to 9 children; the first 2 were normal, the third was premature and stillborn, while in the next 6 icterus gravis neonatorum developed and all died in from three to eleven days after birth. During the entire course of her tenth pregnancy the mother was hospitalized under extremely careful supervision and with regulation of her diet, and she had an entirely normal pregnancy. Seven days before labor was due a cesarean section was performed and an apparently normal child delivered. The infant remained normal for twenty-four hours; then it became drowsy and increasingly icteric, and died seventy hours after birth.

There is no direct evidence that a hereditary factor determines this condition. Hilgenberg's case, cited by A. F. Abt,[4] of a mother who had had several normal children by a first marriage and who following a second marriage gave birth to a number of babies that died of icterus gravis neonatorum does not prove that the second father was biologically implicated, since the same sequence might have occurred with the first husband as father. Gierke's case, also cited by Abt, in which a man with a normal child by a first wife had, in a second marriage, children in whom icterus gravis neonatorum developed does not allow the presumption of a hereditary taint in the second wife. Hoffmann and Hausmann[6] stated that the parents in one of their affected families (family B) were related, but the possibility of familial acholuric jaundice was not ruled out in this case, in which the erythrocytes showed decidedly increased fragility. Hampson[7] noted that this hereditary malady, while it does not usually affect severely the new-born infant, may cause death during the first few weeks of life from progressively increasing jaundice. This occurred in all the children in three families known to him, the mother in each case showing diminished resistance of the red cells to hypotonic saline solutions. Hawksley and Lightwood[1] included in their series a case in which the parents were cousins and there was a history of fatal neonatal jaundice in the preceding generation (case 18), but it is

5. Wanstrom, R. C.: Am. J. Path. **9**:623, 1933.
6. Hoffmann, W., and Hausmann, M.: Monatschr. f. Kinderh. **33**:193, 1926.
7. Hampson, A. C.: Lancet **1**:429, 1929.
8. Clifford, S. H., and Hertig, A.: New England J. Med. **207**:105, 1932.

questionable whether the infant in this case had the grave type of jaundice, since jaundice did not appear until the third day, there was no enlargement of the liver or spleen, there were no nucleated red cells in the blood smear, no leukocytosis was present and the infant recovered uneventfully. Hoffmann and Hausmann,[6] however, reported another case (family X) in which the affected infant was the grandchild of a woman whose sister lost 2 babies with severe jaundice on the fourth day of life. Examples reported in early series of cases, on the other hand, before an accurate diagnosis of syphilis was possible, must be considered as questionable. Further evidence purporting to relate this disease to certain genes or, less specifically, to a defect in the germ plasm, will be considered later.

While in most cases of this disease there is nothing in the family history suggestive of a hereditary influence, there is, on the other hand, a definite familial incidence. The term "familial" is used in this connection to designate the tendency for the disease to recur in children of subsequent pregnancies of a mother who has already given birth to a child either with this malady or with one of the apparently related conditons, congenital edema or congenital anemia of the new-born. Clifford and Hertig[8] stated that the first child is usually spared and that this occurs so frequently as to seem significant. A number of authors, however, have reported cases of the condition in first-born infants, among them May, cited by I. A. Abt,[3] Buhrman and Sanford[9] and Andrews and Miller.[10] In addition to the familiar instances of this malady, sporadic cases seem also to occur, but the ratio of the incidence of the sporadic to that of the familial type has apparently not been determined, nor has it been demonstrated that the etiology of the sporadic is or must be identical with that of the familial form of the disease.

That this disease is not extremely uncommon is shown by the statistics of Clifford and Hertig,[8] who in 1932 reported 7 proved cases of icterus gravis neonatorum associated with erythroblastosis in 2,400 new-born infants in nine months, an incidence of 1 in 340. Andrews and Miller[10] reported 4 cases in 1,958 new-born infants, a rate of 1 in 490. These figures do not include congenital edema, which is of less frequent occurrence, reported as observed once in 2,000 and once in 3,000 new-born infants by Stoeckel and Döderlein[11] and once in 1,200 new-born infants by Clifford and Hertig.[8] The disease has been reported in many countries. Ku and Li[12] reported it in a child of Chinese parentage, and Andrews and Miller[10] found it in 2 Negro infants.

PATHOLOGIC OBSERVATIONS

Necropsy of infants with this condition reveals, aside from the deep yellow-green staining of all the internal viscera, mucous and serous membranes, skin, scleras and fat tissues, little gross change other than enlargement of the liver and spleen. Pallor, however, is

9. Buhrman, W. L., and Sanford, H. N.: Am. J. Dis. Child. 41:225, 1931.
10. Andrews, H. S., and Miller, A. J.: Am. J. Dis. Child. 50:673, 1935.
11. Stoeckel and Döderlein, cited by Clifford and Hertig.[8]
12. Ku, D. Y., and Li, Y.: Virchows Arch. f. path. Anat. 283:62, 1932.

usually noted to a varying degree in spite of the jaundice, and petechial and small ecchymotic hemorrhages are frequently found in the skin and in the mucous and serous membranes.

The brain is usually pale, but in a certain relatively small number of cases, according to Schmorl,[13] the brain substance takes on a more or less intense coloration, appearing as if inbibition of the yellow pigment had taken place. On microscopic examination the whole tissue appears colored uniform pale yellow, while bilirubin crystals may be found in the blood vessels and in the spinal fluid. It cannot be demonstrated that this color is bound to any special structural elements. In this diffuse icterus of the brain there are foci of fat granules, appearing as opaque yellow flecks, distributed symmetrically in the medullary layers of the hemispheres, lateralward from the central ganglions. They are localized, occurring outside of this region only exceptionally, and are more numerous in the more posterior sections. In microscopic sections these foci appear as areas of softening. In addition to the fat granules there are occasional red blood cells and more or less numerous intracellular and extracellular pigment granules and bilirubin crystals. Occasionally a nest of fat granules shows peripherally an infiltration of round cells. These foci stand in close relation to the blood vessels. Frequently, in the region of a focus, the walls of the blood vessels reveal hyaline degeneration, with thrombi in the lumens, which appear partly as homogeneous shining masses containing leukocytes in the process of destruction and partly as fibrin in the meshes of which white blood cells and platelets are held. It is not known whether the thrombi are constant nor whether they stand in a pathologic relation to the foci. These foci of fat granules, however, are associated with icterus, since they occur only simultaneously. Although some authors attributed them to sepsis of the spinal cord on an embolic basis, Schmorl was not inclined to do so, since he had not especially observed sepsis of the cord in icteric children on whom he had performed necropsies. and he could demonstrate bacteria in the regions of the foci neither through culture nor through staining.

In addition to this diffuse icterus of the brain there is a second type in the new-born in which the yellow coloring is circumscribed, being limited entirely to those areas of the brain where larger groups of ganglion cells are found, that is, to the nuclear areas. This type Schmorl designated as *Kernikterus*. The cortex of the cerebrum and cerebellum, the head of the striate body, the caudate nucleus and the optic thalamus are free from pigment, according to Schmorl. Zimmerman and Yannet,[14] on the other hand, found that the structures most commonly affected are the caudate, lenticulate, subthalamic and dentate nuclei, the thalami, the mamillary bodies, the cornua ammonis, the nuclei of the cranial nerves, the olives and even parts of the cerebellar cortex, as well as the anterior and posterior horns of the spinal cord. Many of the colored ganglion cells show necrotic changes, and the axis cylinders are especially intensely colored. Schmorl felt that the sharp demarcation of the pigmentation shows that this yellow coloration is

13. Schmorl, G.: Verhandl. d. deutsch. path. Gesellsch. **6**:109, 1904.
14. Zimmerman, H. M., and Yannet, H.: Am. J. Dis. Child. **45**:740, 1933.

not related to simple imbibition of bile pigment but is bound to definite structural elements. He found, furthermore, that when this nuclear icterus was noted the yellow pigment in the ganglion cells did not turn to the green of oxidized bilirubin in formaldehyde and mercuric chloride solutions. This was likewise true in regard to all the organs, including the liver, which became yellow-brown, although in the fresh specimens they had not differed in appearance from the organs of other icteric infants who did not show this nuclear staining in the brain. Furthermore, the pigment in these nuclear elements reacted only faintly or not at all to nitric acid (Gmelin test). Schmorl felt, therefore, that this yellow color was not due to the ordinary bilirubin but possibly to a modified bile pigment. Schmorl found this condition in 6 of 120 necropsies in cases of jaundice of the new-born.

Much more frequent than nuclear icterus, however, may be spontaneous intracranial hemorrhage, which was found in 6 of 18 cases reported by Hawksley and Lightwood.[1]

The liver, which may be enlarged to two or three times the normal size, presents very often a pathologic picture which has given rise to considerable speculation regarding the underlying cause of this disease. Frequently outstanding in this organ on microscopic examination are large numbers of what appear to be hematopoietic masses, usually predominantly erythropoietic, scattered in the periportal spaces and within the hepatic sinusoids. These islands of blood cell formation may be so numerous as to compress and narrow the cords of hepatic cells, sometimes distorting greatly the general architecture of the liver. This marked extramedullary hematopoiesis is most commonly found in the apparently related condition designated as universal edema of the fetus (fetal hydrops). In icterus gravis neonatorum, on the other hand, it is sometimes only moderate and occasionally almost entirely absent. This fact is remarked by Hawksley and Lightwood.[1] It is demonstrated in the first case of Zimmerman and Yannet,[14] in which were found "but few islands of blood formation," and even more clearly in a case recorded by de Lange,[15] in which the liver of a twin who died revealed "an entirely isolated small focus of hematopoiesis in one capillary loop . . . and a single red blood cell showing amitotic nuclear division in a sinusoid, certainly no more than in normal new-born infants of this age." In a few cases the extramedullary islands of blood formation have seemed to consist mostly of cells of the leukocytic rather than of the erythrocytic series, as in the case of "leukoblastosis" described by Gierke;[16] in others neutrophilic leukocytes share more or less equally with the red cells in the extramedullary hematopoiesis, as in the cases of "erythroleukoblastosis" described by Salomonsen,[17] Wanstrom[5] and others.

The liver cells themselves may appear unchanged,[18] or they may show damage varying from cloudy swelling and fatty degeneration to outright diffuse necrosis and disintegration as seen in Klemperer's first

15. de Lange, C.: Jahrb. f. Kinderh. **145**:273, 1935.

16. von Gierke, E.: Virchows Arch. f. path. Anat. **275**:330, 1930.

17. Salomonsen, L.: Ztschr. f. Kinderh. **51**:181, 1931.

18. de Lange, C., and Arntzenius, A. K. W.: Jahrb. f. Kinderh. **124**:1, 1929.

case.[19] The biliary canaliculi may be distended with bile, presenting the so-called bile thrombi, although these are not invariably found; Diamond, Blackfan and Baty, for example, found them absent in 2 of 4 cases at necropsy.[20] The central veins and the blood capillaries may be dilated, as observed in several instances by de Lange and Arntzenius [18] and in MacClure's case.[21] Many of the liver cells contain bile pigment as well as numerous granules which on proper staining prove to be hemosiderin. A case was reported by de Lange and Arntzenius in which occasional granules of iron pigment lay free in the blood spaces. The Kupffer cells may be increased in number and are often distended with bile and iron pigment. They may become loosened and lie free in the sinusoids. Frequently they exhibit erythrophagocytosis, and de Lange and Arntzenius [18] and MacClure [21] found erythrorrhexis and erythrocytolysis. Eosinophils may be numerous in the periportal spaces and are sometimes found associated with the islands of blood formation. In 7 of 9 cases in which the period of survival was five weeks or longer Hawksley and Lightwood [1] observed a fine fibrosis among the polygonal cells of the atrophic areas and near the portal tracts.

The spleen is greatly enlarged and engorged with blood. The malpighian bodies may be hardly visible. Microscopically, the germinal centers appear to be decreased in size and number and more widely separated than in the normal spleen. Many red cells are engulfed in phagocytes, and numerous macrophages contain bile and in some cases iron pigment also. Here, likewise, masses of hematopoietic cells may be found.

The heart is frequently larger than normal. There are usually no septal defects. Petechial hemorrhages are often visible on the epicardium. In an occasional case edema of the muscle bundles has been observed.[20]

The lungs in many of the reported cases have shown hemorrhages varying from subpleural petechiae and small dark brown ecchymotic areas to fairly extensive hemorrhages involving a portion of a lobe. Areas of "bronchopneumonia" have also been reported, while in one case Diamond, Blackfan and Baty [20] found edema of the interstitial tissue, and in another, nucleated red cells in groups within the alveolar walls.

The kidneys, pancreas, thymus, thyroid, adrenals and lymph glands have also been reported as having foci of hematopoiesis. Ross and Waugh [2] described a case in which myeloid elements were present in the adventitia of large blood channels in the thymus, lungs, kidney and adrenals and in the tissue surrounding the hypogastric vessels. The kidney may reveal siderosis, and bile casts may be found in the tubules. Parenchymatous degeneration in this organ is infrequently but occasionally reported.

The bone marrow reveals active hematopoiesis, often in excess of normal, in some cases causing overcrowding of the marrow spaces.

19. Klemperer, P.: Am. J. Dis. Child. 28:212, 1924.
20. Diamond, L. K.; Blackfan, K. D., and Baty, J. M.: J. Pediat. 1:269, 1932.
21. MacClure: Ztschr. f. Kinderh. 51:86, 1931.

Buhrman and Sanford[9] reported numerous megakaryocytes in a case, although occasionally a diminution in their number has been observed.

This picture of unusual and occasionally extreme extramedullary blood cell formation is regarded as abnormal for a full term infant. The condition is that usually found in a 5 month fetus. Although slight to severe anemia exists in these children, there is an increased output of young and often quite immature red cells, not only from the bone marrow but presumably also from the numerous erythropoietic foci in many visceral organs. This is the origin of the descriptive term "erythroblastosis." It is associated with enlargement of the liver and spleen, pallor of the tissues and in some cases jaundice or edema or both, although Ferguson,[22] Salomonsen[17] and de Lange[23] have each reported cases in which marked erythroblastosis was found on necropsy with neither hydrops nor jaundice.

FAMILIAL ASSOCIATIONS

On the basis of these facts one may now consider a possible relationship between icterus gravis neonatorum and congenital edema of the new-born (fetal hydrops), on the one hand, as pointed out by Gierke[16] and Eichelbaum and concurred in by Salomonsen,[17] de Lange[23] and others, and icterus gravis and the so-called idiopathic anemia of the new-born, on the other hand, as noted by Grulee and by Diamond, Blackfan and Baty.[20] Pathologic examination reveals a much more fulminating process at work in congenital edema than in icterus gravis neonatorum. There are, however, definite points of similarity. Edema, which is marked in hydrops, is sometimes seen in icterus gravis, although when present it is usually slight and localized. Jaundice is more pronounced in icterus gravis but often present in hydrops. The liver and spleen are enlarged in both conditions. The placenta is usually greatly enlarged in universal edema and may be slightly enlarged in grave jaundice. Anemia is found in both disorders, and extramedullary hematopoiesis and circulating immature red blood cells may be a feature in hydrops as in icterus gravis. Both conditions likewise reveal a familial tendency and have been reported by a number of authors as occurring in siblings. Salomonsen,[17] among others, reported the case of a family in which healthy parents had 4 children, the first of whom was living and well, while the second had icterus gravis, the third hydrops with erythroblastosis and the fourth icterus gravis. De Lange[23] reported the case of twins, one of whom was born with fetal hydrops, while the other presented icterus gravis soon after birth. In a recent study by Macklin,[24] both conditions were found in 14 families reported on in the literature. Such a familial association of two conditions in which the pathologic changes differ in degree rather than in kind is difficult to explain except on the basis of an identical etiology.

The evidence in regard to a close association between icterus gravis and congenital (idiopathic) anemia of the new-born is also suggestive.

22. Ferguson, J. A.: Am. J. Path. 7:277, 1931.
23. de Lange, C.: Acta pædiat. 13:292, 1932.
24. Macklin, M. T.: Am. J. Dis. Child. 53:1245, 1937.

The latter condition, as defined by A. F. Abt,[25] is "a severe anemia manifesting itself usually within the first two weeks of life in an infant in whom may be excluded the accepted causes of secondary anemia, namely sepsis, syphilis and hemorrhagic disorders." Erythroblasts may be present in the circulating blood. Mild icterus, enlargement of the liver and spleen, and extramedullary hematopoiesis are frequent. Stransky [26] expressed the belief that there are two types of primary anemia of the new-born. The first and more frequent type is characterized by a nonregenerative blood picture, with no true shift to the left and no embryonal cells, which he ascribed to a constitutional insufficiency of the bone marrow. The second type, which is more rare, shows an embryonal blood picture, with areas of hematopoiesis in the liver, spleen and lymph glands. That these two types represent differing individual responses to a similar etiologic factor is indicated by the appearance of both types in children of the same parents. Abbott and Abbott,[27] for example, reported a case in which the family history revealed such a relationship:

The first child in this family exhibited a yellowish tinge of the skin at birth. Slight fever developed on the second day, and cough and bleeding from the nose on the fifth day, when he died. Necropsy revealed in the lungs "a hemorrhagic bronchopneumonia" and in the liver a number of fetal blood islands in the lobules and nucleated red cells in the capillaries. The spleen, kidneys and peribronchial lymph nodes were normal, and bacteriologic examination of the spleen and bone marrow gave negative results. The second child gradually became pale and took food less well, dying on the eighth day. On necropsy numerous blood islands were found in the liver, but they were of myeloblastic and myelocytic elements, with nucleated red cells conspicuously few. A heavy infiltration of eosinophils and myelocytes was found in the portal spaces The spleen was enlarged, with the malpighian corpuscles inconspicuous. All other organs were essentially without change. The third pregnancy ended in a spontaneous abortion. The fourth child was the one reported. The mother's pregnancy had been supervised with great care and was entirely uneventful. The child at birth appeared well nourished, cried lustily and was of a normal, ruddy appearance. A blood count on the first day revealed only an occasional normoblast, with red cells 4,136,000, leukocytes 13,600 and hemoglobin (Sahli) 82. A differential count according to percentage showed polymorphonuclear neutrophils 55 (segmented forms 42, stab cells 11, juvenile forms 2), lymphocytes 37, monocytes 6, eosinophils and basophils 0. On the fifteenth day pallor was noted. There was no jaundice, no hemorrhagic manifestation, no bile in the urine, and the stools were normal. The liver was slightly enlarged, the spleen palpable and the inguinal and axillary lymph nodes slightly enlarged, but no demonstrable focus of infection could be found. Hemograms showed "marked primary anemia," which grew progressively worse in spite of the administration of blood intramuscularly and of liver extract. On the twenty-third day the red cell count was 1,664,000, the leukocyte count 10,200 and the hemoglobin (Sahli) 36. There were no normoblasts, no reticulocytes and no myelocytes. On the twenty-ninth day the anemia was less marked, there was 1 normoblast per hundred white cells, and the reticulocytes were designated 3 +. From this time on recovery was progressive until complete.

Here one has a definitely nonregenerative congenital anemia associated familially, on the one hand, with a congenital anemia exhibiting erythroblastosis and, on the other, with one presenting the pathologic picture designated as "leucoblastosis" by Gierke. Diamond, Blackfan

---

25. Abt, A. F.: Am. J. Dis. Child. **43**:337, 1932.
26. Stransky, E.: Ztschr. f. Kinderh. **51**:239, 1931.
27. Abbott, K. H., and Abbott, F. F.: Am. J. Dis. Child. **49**:724, 1935.

and Baty[20] likewise presented an interesting family series, the first 4 children being normal, the next 3 showing congenital anemia of the regenerative type, and the eighth exhibiting all the clinical symptoms of icterus gravis neonatorum. These authors have called attention to the fact that congenital anemia presents a clinical picture identical with that found in an infant with icterus gravis in whom treatment has brought about disappearance of the jaundice. Finally, Pasachoff and Wilson[28] presented a report showing the extraordinary combination of congenital anemia of the new-born and fetal hydrops in offspring of the same parents, and it is noteworthy that erythroblastosis was not present in either child.

The association between edema, icterus gravis and anemia of the new-born was postulated by Diamond, Blackfan and Baty[20] on the basis of what they considered the common underlying pathologic condition, erythroblastosis. There have, however, been cases reported of each of the three disorders in which there has been little evidence of abnormal erythroblastic activity.[29] Furthermore, as Pasachoff and Wilson[28] pointed out, erythroblastosis is by no means pathognomonic of this group of disorders, for it occurs in other conditions as well, notably in congenital syphilis and in sepsis of the new-born. It seems rather that it is the familial association of these three conditions which constitutes the most convincing evidence for an etiologic relationship, and this association must be taken into consideration in the evaluation of theories as to etiology.

THEORIES AS TO ETIOLOGY

The foregoing consideration of the symptoms, clinical course and pathologic changes found in icterus gravis neonatorum, together with its familial association with the apparently related diseases, fetal hydrops and idiopathic anemia of the new-born, may now constitute a foundation for a critical evaluation of some of the theories as to its etiology. It may be stated that any attempted explanation of its cause must allow for the following observations: (1) the apparent absence of any hereditary factor; (2) the fact that birth of healthy, normal children may precede that of the child in whom the condition first manifests itself in a family; (3) the frequent familial tendency; (4) the apparent health of the parents; (5) the apparent absence of significant factors in the prenatal history in the large majority of cases; (6) the presumptive association of edema, grave jaundice and anemia of the new-born; (7) the clinical symptoms; (8) the observations at necropsy, and (9) the erythroblastosis.

The theories as to etiology which have been proposed in the literature fall into two groups, (1) those implicating the mother primarily and (2) those finding the cause solely within the child.

28. Pasachoff, H. D., and Wilson, L.: Am. J. Dis. Child. 49: 411, 1935.

29. Zimmerman and Yannet.[14] de Lange.[15] Abbott and Abbott.[27] Pasachoff and Wilson.[28]

Theories Involving the Mother.—Under this heading one finds ascribed as possible causative factors:

1. Nutritional disturbances in the mother, brought about either by dietary deficiencies or by frequent gestations and lactations. Parsons,[30] for example, holds that maternal anemia resulting from a long-deficient diet is the most probable cause of congenital anemia in the offspring, and other authors have recommended the administration of liver or iron or both to the mother before birth of the child and to the infant after birth. In the large majority of cases, however, the mother presents a normal blood picture, and since a close supervision of the diet has been exercised in numerous cases,[31] one can consider neither anemia nor nutritional disturbances in the mother as primarily operative in the causation of icterus gravis neonatorum or of the presumably related conditions.

2. Disease in the mother. Some of the earlier writers, attempting to assign a cause for icterus gravis neonatorum, failed to differentiate this disease from a similar condition found in syphilitic infants and ascribed it to syphilis. Syphilis, however, has been repeatedly ruled out, not only by the negative serologic tests of the parents' and of the child's blood, but by the entire absence of spirochetes in sections of organs stained by the Levaditi method. Tuberculin tests of the infant have likewise been consistently negative, and there is no pathologic evidence of tuberculosis on necropsy. Acute infection in the mother, on the other hand, might be a factor in the sporadic case, but it does not account for the frequent familial tendency.

3. Toxemias of pregnancy. Toxemia has been manifested in a certain proportion of cases and has been considered as the causal factor by Rolleston,[32] Hoffmann and Hausmann[6] and others. Among the symptoms reported in the mother during the pregnancy from which an affected child was born may be listed edema, usually of the lower extremities, as noted by de Lange, jaundice, reported by Rolleston in 15 of 130 collected cases, nephritis, observed in 2 cases by Gierke,[16] severe pain, reported by MacClure,[21] and frequent attacks of faintness together with marked weakness, as in Zimmerman and Yannet's[14] second case. In the case reported by Bullard and Plaut[33] the mother, after giving birth to 1 normal child and 2 in whom icterus gravis neonatorum developed, all 3 pregnancies being uneventful, suffered during her fourth pregnancy three attacks diagnosed as "Ménière's disease, classical and unmistakable" and was troubled with edema of the feet and with constant nausea and insomnia, but with no ocular symptoms and no headaches. The blood pressure, urine and blood picture were normal. She finally delivered prematurely a stillborn hydropic fetus. The mother of 4 children whose cases were reported by Diamond, Blackfan and Baty[20] felt marked lessening of fetal movements before the birth of each of these children, although this had not occurred with the first 4 of her offspring, who were unaffected. In 2 cases known to me

30. Parsons, L. G.: Acta pædiat. **13**:378, 1932.
31. Smyth's case, cited by Abt.[4] Abbott and Abbott.[27]
32. Rolleston, H.: Brit. M. J. **1**:864, 1910; Practitioner **104**:1, 1920.
33. Bullard, E. A., and Plaut, A.: Arch. Pediat. **43**:292, 1926.

abnormal spotting occurred at 4 and 4½ months, respectively. It seems that such incidents may have an explanation other than as mere accidents. On the other hand, by far the largest number of reports describe the mother's pregnancy in these cases as normal and uneventful. Hampson,[7] accordingly, suggested that the mother's symptoms may be secondary, resulting from carrying an anomalous fetus.

Theories That Locate the Cause in the Child.—Woolley[34] and Oberndorfer[35] each reported a case of fetal hydrops involving twins. Since it has been shown that this condition appears to be related etiologically to icterus gravis neonatorum, their observations are of interest. In each instance an edematous twin, manifesting fetal hydrops with erythroblastosis, was accompanied by an apparently normal twin. Oberndorfer felt that such an occurrence speaks against maternal influence in the causation of erythroblastosis and that the cause must in truth be sought in the fetus. His argument appears to be strengthened by the fact that in a still later pregnancy the edema which the mother of the twins whose case he reported invariably experienced from the fourth month in each pregnancy in which the fetus was affected disappeared in the fifth month with the cessation of fetal movements, and was followed two months later by the delivery of a macerated fetus, apparently long dead. It must be considered, however, that in neither Woolley's nor Oberndorfer's case was the apparently normal twin examined at necropsy, although in Woolley's case the infant was stillborn, and presumably Oberndorfer's "normal" twin, which was premature (7 months), likewise did not survive. Since de Lange[23] reported a case in which one twin was born with fetal hydrops and the other presented icterus gravis after birth, it is entirely possible that the supposedly normal twins in the cases reported by Woolley and Oberndorfer would, had they lived, have manifested the latter condition. Macklin[24] found in the literature 7 cases of twins in 5 of which both twins were affected with icterus gravis; in the sixth case one twin was icteric and the other hydropic, and in the seventh case icterus gravis developed in one twin, while the other died at birth. With respect to congenital edema, however, she found one twin affected and the other normal in 8 of 9 cases. Whether the unaffected twin in each case was born living and remained alive and normal is not stated, nor were the sources of these statistics tabulated.

The search for the cause of icterus gravis may now tentatively be shifted from the mother to the offspring, and indeed there is a predominance of theories based on some presumed anomaly in the child:

1. Some of the older theories of jaundice in the new-born were based on the conception set forth by Eppinger that the bile pigment was elaborated by the liver cells and that the jaundice was the result of obstruction either in the extrahepatic ducts or within the liver, where blocking of the canaliculi was thought to be caused by the formation of bile thrombi by inspissated bile. It is now known that the pigment bilirubin is formed outside of the hepatic epithelial cells, probably by the reticulo-endothelial cells, especially those in the liver,

34. Woolley, P. G.: J. Lab. & Clin. Med. **1**:347, 1916.
35. Oberndorfer, S.: Zentralbl. f. Gynäk. **51**:1830, 1927.

spleen and bone marrow, from hemoglobin, and that jaundice may result from an abnormally rapid breakdown. When this occurs in the absence of obstruction or of actual necrosis within the liver the direct van den Bergh reaction of the serum is negative while the indirect reaction is positive. Rich[36] stated that "no form of jaundice is known which results from a purely functional depression of the excretory power of the liver, that is, without actual loss of cells through necrosis, when the production of bilirubin is in normal amounts." Hence one must infer that when only the indirect or, delayed, reaction is found strongly positive one is dealing with excessive production of bilirubin or, in other words, with increased destruction of erythrocytes. This explanation is accepted generally for icterus simplex neonatorum. Since the positive indirect van den Bergh reaction is likewise constant (to a degree greater than normal) in the malady under discussion, while the direct reaction has in some instances been reported negative, as in Buhrman and Sanford's[9] cases, one can for the same reason no longer ascribe the jaundice in icterus gravis neonatorum to obstruction only, but must here also recognize increased destruction of red cells as an important factor. Such a conclusion, moreover, is substantiated by the observation of increased erythrophagocytosis, erythrorrhexis and even erythrolysis[37] in the liver and in the spleen, as well as of hemosiderosis in these organs, and by the significant observation of A. F. Abt[4] in one of his cases that the amount of hemoglobin as calculated from the blood iron was greater than the amount of hemoglobin actually found by the Newcomer method, a finding confirmed as abnormal by Sobel.[38] Pfannenstiel[39] held that icterus gravis neonatorum is simply an intensification of the physiologic jaundice of the new-born, but it seems that the jaundice in icterus gravis neonatorum is the result of a pathologic process of a different character from that resulting in icterus simplex, as indicated not only by the higher icteric index and the frequently positive direct van den Bergh reaction but also by the production of anemia, in some cases extremely severe, even in the presence of greatly increased hematopoiesis. Furthermore, in icterus gravis neonatorum there is frequently evidence of injury to various organs, especially to the liver. That this injury to the liver is not secondary to obstruction alone is suggested by the much less rapidly devastating, although ultimately fatal, course of the jaundice due to congenital atresia of the bile ducts, as pointed out by Yllpö,[40] an observation confirmed recently in a case reported by Kass and Osgood,[41] in which an infant lived to the age of 11 months and 29 days with complete obliteration of the cystic, hepatic and common ducts and a nonfunctioning gallbladder.

2. Gierke[16] considered as the cause of both fetal hydrops and icterus gravis neonatorum a "primary constitutional (familial or hereditary) anlage defect of the hematapoietic system." Salomonsen[17] was inclined to agree with him, and in this country Clifford and Hertig[8]

36. Rich, A. R.: Bull. Johns Hopkins Hosp. **47**:338, 1930.
37. de Lange and Arntzenius.[18] MacClure.[21]
38. Sobel, I. P.: Am. J. Dis. Child. **51**:104, 1936.
39. Pfannenstiel, J.: München. med. Wchnschr. **55**:2169 and 2233, 1908.
40. Yllpö, A.: Ztschr. f. Kinderh. **17**:334, 1918.
41. Kass, I. H., and Osgood, F. P.: J. Pediat. **9**:91, 1936.

felt that such a defect is the most likely cause, stating that "an unknown stimulus manifests itself in late uterine life as a pathologic prolongation of, or reversal to, the embryonic system of blood formation. As a result abnormally young forms of red cells appear in the circulating blood. Concomitant with this abnormal production there is an increased destruction of the red cells." A. F. Abt,[4] likewise, bases his theory of "embryonal hematopoietic persistence" in the familial type of case on a defective anlage or a defect in the germ plasm.

It is reasonable to assume a defect in the germ plasm in these related diseases since such a defect provides an explanation for their appearance in subsequent children of the same family. It is therefore necessary to examine this hypothesis in some detail. In considering this explanation it is important to remember, as Clifford and Hertig pointed out, that the first child is usually spared. This is frequently true of the second as well, and Diamond, Blackfan and Baty,[20] indeed, recorded a case in which 4 unaffected children preceded the first child with congenital anemia, who was followed by two more with the same condition and an eighth child, in whom icterus gravis neonatorum developed. There is no history of infection, exposure to roentgen rays, evidence of endocrine dysfunction or other baleful influence on the germ plasm in the mother to account for the appearance of the malady in later children. Hawksley and Lightwood[1] suggested the possibility of a mendelian recessive characteristic as responsible, but the incidence of the condition in a large family or in a series of families is too large, as Macklin[24] pointed out. This author recently undertook a statistical study of these diseases and came to the conclusion that they are inherited rather as a dominant mutation. By including with the hydropic infants all miscarriages, stillborn infants and infants showing erythroblastosis in the families furnishing the data on fetal hydrops and eliminating from her group with icterus gravis neonatorum all miscarriages, stillborn infants, infants with hydrops and icteric babies who recovered, she found the incidence of each of these maladies in a large group of families to be approximately 50 per cent, the incidence required theoretically, she stated, if these diseases are due to a dominant mutation. She suggested further that the diseases accompanied by erythroblastosis are probably the result of an adjunction of multiple allelomorphs to the normal gene or genes for the formation of blood in the fetus. The following considerations, however, tend to invalidate such conclusions:

(*a*) Macklin apparently did not distinguish between idiopathic anemia of the new-born with erythroblastosis and Cooley's erythroblastosis; nor is it clear that she differentiated hereditary acholuric jaundice from familial icterus gravis of the new-born, since she included in her discussion Hichens'[42] cases of 2 children who, with their mother and other siblings, seem to have suffered from hereditary hemolytic icterus.

(*b*) The premise that the gene or genes for blood formation in the fetus are involved in these diseases is open to question, since there are cases on record, as already pointed out, in which abnormal extramedullary hematopoiesis was demonstrable neither by the finding of

---

42. Hichens, P. S.: Proc. Roy. Soc. Med. (pt. 1) **6**:197, 1913.

erythroblastemia during life nor by the observation of erythroblastosis at necropsy, while on the other hand, erythroblastosis is not uncommonly found in infants with congenital syphilis.

(c) If these diseases were dependent on a dominant mutation occurring in the germ plasm of one of the parents, they would be distributed at random among the offspring, since it would be largely a matter of chance whether any one child inherited the modified gene or not. In the familial conditions under discussion, however, the distribution is not random. The normal children are born first, while following the birth of the first affected child one or another of these conditions occurs in every child born subsequently by the same mother. The severity of the condition may vary somewhat, and occasionally the manifestation of the disease may be so mild that spontaneous recovery is possible, as remarked by Hawksley and Lightwood,[1] but a palpable liver and spleen and anemia, however benign, may still indicate the familial abnormality.[27]

(d) The deductions and additions with which Macklin weights her data bring the incidence of each of the related disorders fairly close to 50 per cent, but on critical examination such procedures seem unjustifiable. As various authors have pointed out,[28] it is probable that many of the miscarriages and stillbirths in families with familial icterus gravis neonatorum, as well as in those affected with fetal hydrops, have an etiology identical with that of the condition affecting the infants who survive birth or longer. When aborted fetuses and stillborn infants are included with the infants manifesting one or the other of these conditions, the incidence of the respective diseases in affected families is increased, according to Macklin's own figures, as shown in the following tabulation:

	Incidence with Exclusion of Abortions and Stillbirths	Incidence with Inclusion of Abortions and Stillbirths
Fetal hydrops	30.1%	55.3%
Icterus gravis neonatorum.......	58.1%	70.0%

Furthermore, it must be considered that fetal hydrops may be manifested in a family affected with icterus gravis neonatorum, and icterus gravis may be seen in a child of a family usually affected with congenital anemia of the new-born, as in Diamond, Blackfan and Baty's case, cited; or, rarely, anemia and hydrops may occur in the same family. Thus, while one or another of these conditions does predominate in any one family, the incidence of affected children in a family cannot be computed on the basis of one only of these three diseases.

(e) The extent to which the afflicted parents may have limited their offspring when they became aware of the repetition of the malady in each new child may be only speculated on. The effect of such limitation, however, may be estimated from Macklin's data: In 17 families of 3 children each there were 26 affected children, an incidence of 50 per cent; but in 2 families of 15 children each there were 27 affected children, an incidence of 90 per cent. This difference suggests that the potential incidence in affected families might well be given more consideration in formulating hypotheses as to the inheritance of these diseases.

(f) The assumption that inheritance of a dominant mutation is indicated by an incidence of 50 per cent in affected families and the conclusions from her data as interpreted by Macklin may be questioned further. Dr. Dorothy Adkins, of the University of Chicago, has supplied a critical evaluation of Macklin's statistical treatment of her data and the conclusions therefrom.[43] She has pointed out that if a mutation involves the germ cell ancestral to all subsequently formed germ cells (by division) in one of the parents, the incidence of affected offspring would approximate 50 per cent, as postulated by Macklin. Such a mutation involving blood formation, however, would be extremely rare. If, on the other hand, mutation occurs in a gene in a germ cell formed by later divisions of the ancestral cell, as is much more frequently the case, the incidence of affected offspring would be something less than 50 per cent, approaching low values in some instances, according to the division at which the mutation occurred.[44] It is obvious, therefore, that the incidence of icterus gravis neonatorum at least, in a series of affected families, is far too high for a mutation in a germ cell in one parent to be responsible. This is especially true if stillborn infants, aborted fetuses and siblings manifesting fetal hydrops or congenital idiopathic anemia are included, an inclusion which seems not only justifiable but required. She has pointed out further that if a formula is used which disregards hereditary transmission and is based only on two arbitrary assumptions, namely, (1) that once a child is born with one of these conditions (icterus gravis neonatorum, for example) all subsequent children in that family will be affected, and (2) that each child in a family of affected children is equally likely to be the first child affected, the predicted number of affected children in a large number of families agrees more closely with the actual number of affected children than does Macklin's prediction based on the postulation of a dominant mutation.[45]

43. Personal communication to the author.

44. This opinion was corroborated by Dr. Sewall Wright in a personal communication on the subject to Dr. Adkins.

45. Thus, for example, utilizing Macklin's statistics on icterus gravis neonatorum (table 1) and applying the formula $\frac{n(n+1)}{2n^2}$ or $\frac{n+1}{2n}$ one has:

Children in Family*	Families	Total Number of Children	Total Number of Children Affected	Children Affected, R† $\frac{1}{4}$ $1-(\frac{3}{4})^n$	Children Affected, D‡ $\frac{1}{2}$ $1-(\frac{1}{2})^n$	Children Affected, Calc. (Adkins) $\frac{n+1}{2n}$
1	7	7	7	7.0	7.0	7.0
2	25	50	32	28.5	33.3	37.5
3	17	51	26	22.0	29.1	34.0
4	23	92	58	33.6	49.0	57.5
5	20	100	62	32.7	51.6	60.0
6	13	78	37	23.7	39.6	45.5
7	4	28	15	8.0	14.1	16.0
8	8	64	36	17.7	32.1	36.0
9	9	81	46	21.8	40.5	45.0
10	4	40	30	10.6	20.0	22.0
11	1	11	10	2.8	5.5	6.0
15	2	30	27	7.5	15.0	16.0
16	1	16	8	4.0	8.0	8.5
	134	648	394	219.9	344.8	391.0

* All miscarriages and stillbirths were omitted when the number of children in the family was computed, and all children in whom severe jaundice developed were included with the affected children.

† R indicates the theoretical number of affected children if the condition is inherited and dependent on a single recessive gene substitution.

‡ D indicates the theoretical number of affected children if the condition is inherited and dependent on a dominant mutation in the germ plasm of one of the parents.

This greater agreement with the actual incidence (391 calculated, compared with 394 actually affected) is obtained with no assumption as to a hereditary mode of transmission. Thus Macklin's thesis of a dominant mutation does not derive necessarily from her statistics. On the contrary, the relatively high incidence of these related conditions in the children of affected families suggests that the conditions are inherited neither as a recessive characteristic nor as a dominant mutation.

It may be maintained that in these disorders the defective anlage is responsible not so much for a fetal maldevelopment as for a delay in maturation which precludes adequate function of certain organs, chiefly, for example, the liver, thereby rendering the infant at birth unfit for extra-uterine life. If this is the case, one has no explanation of those cases of anemia of the new-born in which the anemia comes on suddenly from seven to fifteen days after birth and in which the symptoms of toxicity or abnormality appear only with the onset of the marked pallor. Segar and Stoeffler,[46] for example, reported the case of a child whose blood counts up to the seventh day showed a fall in hemoglobin and red cells "which was scarcely appreciable." Two transfusions on the eleventh and seventeenth days were followed by a remission of symptoms, but during the fourth week the anemia increased, projectile vomiting recurred, and two more transfusions were necessary. Why, it may be asked, was the liver apparently adequate for the first seven days after birth, to become inadequate until after the fourth week? This delayed appearance of symptoms in a disorder which seems to be intimately related etiologically to icterus gravis neonatorum simulates rather a sort of "incubation period." Moreover, the livers both of full term and premature normal infants may be frequently considered inadequate, as indicated by dye excretion tests, probably by reason of a certain immaturity,[36] yet such immaturity is by no means incompatible with life, even when there is resulting jaundice (physiologic). The symptoms in these diseases of the new-born characterized by erythroblastosis seem to resemble closely those of severe intoxication. Just how a defect of the germ plasm, whether it is manifested in excessive extramedullary hematopoiesis or in hepatic immaturity, is responsible for such symptoms remains obscure. As the theory stands, the strongest and practically the only argument in its favor is the fact of the familial repetition, and this can be more fully accounted for by a different mechanism. Furthermore, as de Lange[23] pointed out, "in those cases of icterus gravis neonatorum in which recovery occurs there is no further evidence of a defective anlage of the hematopoietic system."

3. Diamond, Blackfan and Baty[20] were also impressed by the pronounced extramedullary erythropoiesis and have set forth the view that a metabolic disturbance of the hematopoietic system is the underlying cause of the conditions found in the three associated diseases, edema, icterus gravis and anemia of the new-born, resulting directly in the increased extramedullary hematopoiesis, which in turn gives rise to an overgrowth of immature erythrocytes. This increased extramedullary activity is not called forth, in their opinion, by increased hemolysis,

---

46. Segar, L. H., and Stoeffler, W.: J. Pediat. **1**:485, 1932.

since it is greatest in a condition in which hemolysis is less in evidence, namely, in universal edema of the fetus. The increased destruction of erythrocytes also results from this metabolic disturbance, the edema resulting from the concomitant anemia. Nervous manifestations and respiratory distress are associated with the nuclear icterus in the brain. No explanation of the nature or cause of the metabolic disturbance is attempted. Actually there is no evidence that the specific antianemic factor is lacking, the absence of which causes an arrest of development at the megaloblast stage, according to Haden,[47] since most of the immature cells have gone beyond the megaloblast stage to the erythroblast and normoblast and even to the reticulocyte stage, nor has the administration of liver extract been of demonstrable value.[27] It is likewise obvious that iron is not lacking. Hence the nature of this disturbance in metabolism is quite obscure. Furthermore, while the jaundice is explained, although the condition in which the greatest hemolysis is presumed (icterus gravis) is not that in which the greatest erythroblastic activity is usually seen (fetal hydrops), it is hardly justifiable to base the appearance of edema on anoxemia due to the anemia alone, since edema is practically never seen in the relatively benign idiopathic anemia of the aregenerative type, in which the diminution of red cells is often marked. The symptoms of nervous and gastro-intestinal irritation and of respiratory distress, moreover, are only occasionally associated with nuclear icterus. The diffuse necrosis sometimes found in the liver,[19] the edema, hemorrhage and cellular infiltration in the lungs, the nuclear pathologic change in the brain which when present is associated with an icteric pigmentation differing chemically from that of ordinary bilirubin are likewise not adequately accounted for by this theory. And finally, there is no explanation for the occurrence of the same or a related condition in siblings of subsequent birth.

4. A. F. Abt[4] elaborated a theory, also based on the presence of erythroblastosis, which he termed "embryonal hematopoietic persistence." The persistence of extramedullary hematopoiesis beyond the fetal stage he ascribed to a defect in the anlage or in the germ plasm in the familial cases and to a toxic influence early in pregnancy in the sporadic case. According to his statement, "hematopoietic foci are specific for, and outstandingly characteristic of, fetal liver." These foci give rise to an overwhelming number of immature red cells, which, by reason of their immaturity, reduce the oxygen-carrying power of the blood and cause damage in the liver from anoxemia. This anoxemia may also cause the enlargement of the placenta. Since these immature cells are more fragile, they are destroyed more easily and rapidly, bringing about anemia and the formation of larger amounts of bilirubin and hemosiderin than normal. This excessive production of bilirubin, which, he stated, is merely an intensification of the destruction of hemoglobin which normally occurs in the new-born period, causes the formation of bile thrombi in the biliary capillaries, with resulting diffusion of the bile first into the lymph and then into the blood. This regurgitation of bile increases the jaundice already present from the retention of bilirubin due to hemolysis and explains the positive direct, in addition to

47. Haden, R. L.: J. A. M. A. **104**:706, 1935.

the positive indirect, van den Bergh reaction. The bile is then excreted through the kidneys, giving rise to the "beer-brown" amniotic fluid and to the golden yellow vernix caseosa. This explanation, according to Abt, does not need "to assume a primary metabolic disturbance of the entire hematopoietic system, or a compensatory origin of the extra-medullary islands." He stated, however, that further theoretic consid-erations "must commence with the cause for the persistence of the embryonal type of blood formation."

While this hypothesis has the merit of being explicit, one of its weaknesses is the assumption of premises on which there is no universal agreement. The assumed greater destructibility of immature erythro-cytes within the body is in point. Another assumption which must be questioned is that relating to the dilated, bile-filled canaliculi, which are interpreted as "bile thrombi." As Rich [36] stated:

There are, undoubtedly, instances of febrile infections associated with increased red-cell destruction in which one finds many canaliculi distended with bile at autopsy, but one cannot at once accept these distended canaliculi as being plugged with bile thrombi. It is interesting that such distended canaliculi are ordinarily found in the central part of the lobule about the efferent vein, a fact which suggests a relationship to a zonal damage of liver cells rather than to obstruction because of a general inspissation of the bile. It is possible, it seems to me, that the accumulation of bile in these centrally situated canaliculi may be merely a result of the depression of function of the central cells to the point that they are unable to excrete and force the bile under pressure through the canaliculi. . . . As a matter of fact just this over-filling of the central canaliculi can often be seen in cases in which a poison or chronic passive congestion has damaged specifically the central cells.

The distention of the biliary capillaries with bile, therefore, might justifiably be construed as an effect due to the same process which causes injury to the parenchymatous cells. Furthermore, dilated bile canaliculi are not invariably observed in histologic sections of the liver in erythroblastosis. Diamond, Blackfan and Baty,[20] for example, reported their absence in 2 cases, and de Lange [28] likewise noted their absence in a case of hers. It is possible that a backing up of bile due to sluggish excretion is a factor in the production of a positive direct van den Bergh reaction, but the fact must not be ignored that necrosis of liver cells is frequently observed histologically, and such injury must be considered as a further and perhaps more important reason for the positive direct van den Bergh reaction. Abt's explanation of this injury of the liver as due to the anoxemia resulting from the inade-quate oxygen-carrying power of immature erythrocytes will be con-sidered later. The symptoms of cerebral and gastro-intestinal irritation, however, are adequately explained, and, as Abt himself says, the erythroblastosis is still unaccounted for.

A further criticism of the view that erythroblastosis is responsible for the clinical and pathologic manifestations in edema, icterus gravis and anemia of the new-born, was expressed by Parsons, Hawksley and Gittens.[48] They pointed out that "in some cases of fetal hydrops such foci (erythroblastosis) are present only to a very limited extent or may be absent," as noted in the case studied by them, "thus providing strong

48. Parsons, L. G.; Hawksley, J. C., and Gittens, R.: Arch. Dis. Childhood 8:159, 1933.

evidence that they do not represent the origin of these disorders." They felt that the erythroblastosis is only "a concomitant feature or response . . . to an increased call for erythropoiesis" and that "this response is therefore a symptom and not a cause of the disease." The even greater inconstancy in degree, in fact occasionally the almost entire absence, of extramedullary hematopoiesis or erythroblastemia in icterus gravis and in congenital anemia of the new-born suggests strongly that erythroblastosis, while it usually accompanies, is by no means the fundamental cause of, this group of familially related diseases.

5. Knoepfelmacher,[49] Beneke [50] and Pfältzer,[51] among others, were convinced on the basis of their positive bacteriologic findings that icterus gravis neonatorum is essentially a septicemia. Pfältzer suspected Bacillus coli or organisms closely resembling it, as the most likely agents, since he found clumps of such bacilli between fibers of skeletal muscles. Both the umbilical stump and the erosions of the digestive tract known as "stigmata ventriculi" have been suggested as possible portals of entry. Zimmerman and Yannet,[14] on the basis of Dunham's [52] studies of jaundice and sepsis in the new-born, declared unequivocally for sepsis as the underlying etiologic factor in icterus gravis neonatorum. Grulee [53] felt likewise that "in all probability icterus gravis neonatorum is associated with infection, at least in the vast majority of cases." I. A. Abt,[3] however, was satisfied both from clinical observation and from bacteriologic study that in his cases the condition was not due to sepsis, and Hawksley and Lightwood [1] felt also that the evidence did not point that way. Yllpö,[40] because of negative blood cultures for both aerobic and anaerobic organisms, his extraordinary care to preserve asepsis, the early appearance of the jaundice (one and a half hours after birth), the increased bilirubin content in blood from the cord at birth and the absence of bacteria in histologic sections of the various organs, asserted that postnatal infection cannot be presumed to be responsible. Palm [54] stated likewise "that a new-born infant who . . . having come into the world under all aseptic precautions, sickens a few hours later with a jaundice becoming ever more intense hour by hour . . . dies without clinical as well as without pathologic or bacteriologic evidence on necropsy of the slightest trace of infection either of the navel or of the gastro-intestinal tract renders it unlikely that sepsis is being dealt with." Klemperer,[19] too, considered that the diffuse necrosis to be noted in his first case, in particular, spoke against infection in which the necrosis is usually focal. Dunham's studies certainly indicate the necessity for extremely careful and thorough investigation of all cases of jaundice in the new-born, but they do not enlighten one as to the cause of the familial type of icterus gravis of the new-born in cases in which healthy parents, a negative prenatal history and entirely negative bacteriologic findings fail to justify the

49. Knoepfelmacher, W.: Ergebn. d. inn. Med. u. Kinderh. **5**:205, 1910.

50. Beneke: München. med. Wchnschr. **59**:387, 1912.

51. Pfältzer, B.: Ztschr. f. Geburtsh. u. Gynäk. **76**:685, 1914-1915.

52. Dunham, E.: (*a*) Am. J. Dis. Child. **40**:671, 1930; (*b*) **45**:229, 1933.

53. Grulee, C. G., and Bonar, B. E.: The Newborn: Physiology and Care, New York, D. Appleton and Company, 1926, vol. 2.

54. Palm, H.: Monatschr. f. Geburtsh. u. Gynäk. **49**:264, 1919.

assumption of infection. Severe jaundice secondary to sepsis must not be placed in the same category with the disease under discussion, and a careful differentiation must be made between those cases in which an infection is superimposed on the primary pathologic process and those ⸱in which the infection itself is primary. It seems to be rightly conceded that sepsis, although its symptoms may exactly simulate those of icterus gravis neonatorum, may be excluded as a fundamental etiologic factor in this disease. This opinion is strengthened by the fact that much of the bacteriologic work done in this condition has yielded negative results.[55]

6. Hampson,[7] in considering possible factors causing physiologic jaundice of the new-born, formulated two tentative explanations for the increase in blood bilirubin after birth: 1. Before birth bilirubin may be excreted through the placenta into the maternal blood stream; after birth the liver may be some time in assuming its full excretory function, and hence bilirubin may accumulate in the infant's blood. 2. Some maternal influence may be assumed, possibly hormonic, which may restrain hemolysis; after birth, if this factor is temporarily absent or deficient in the child, hemolysis, owing to alterations in oxygen tension, may become excessive, with the production of jaundice. Hampson held that icterus gravis neonatorum closely resembles physiologic jaundice of the new-born and can be explained by presuming an even greater delay in the assumption of hepatic function than in the latter condition. He stated, however, that "whether the delay in assumption be one of excretion, or in the production of an internal secretion, it seems probable that it is one in which the liver is largely concerned." Hampson felt that his record of 17 recoveries in 18 infants who were treated with small intramuscular injections (5 to 15 cc.) of mother's serum daily tended to substantiate his second hypothesis. Hawksley and Lightwood,[1] however, called attention to the fact that anemia frequently continues to develop rapidly even after transfusions, a procedure which would introduce several times as much serum into the vein as Hampson injected into the muscles. Furthermore, they found intramuscular injections of whole blood of no benefit in the infants with erythroblastemia and used human blood serum without success. They felt "that the transfused blood acts by substitution and not by supplying any hypothetical anti-hemolytic substance." On the other hand, their implied explanation of Hampson's success as due to spontaneous recovery is not warranted by the statistical evidence of 80 per cent mortality in untreated patients. It seems that small amounts of the serum of the child's mother must have some value when the disease is mild, but it also seems obvious that the explanation is not that set forth by Hampson. His alternative hypothesis, however, that bilirubin may increase in the infant's blood after birth because of hepatic insufficiency, while before birth the excess pigment is excreted through the placenta, seems to be borne out by Yllpö's observation of an elevated icteric index in blood from the cord, although the jaundice did not become apparent until one and a half hours after birth.

Hampson further suggested that the products of the abnormal hemolysis of red cells may be toxic and give rise to the symptoms of the

55. Abt.[8]   Diamond and others.[20]   Yllpö.[40]   Palm.[54]

disease. But the destruction of erythrocytes must itself be secondary to a more primary process still unknown; nor is the familial tendency in these diseases explained by such an assumption.

7. Parsons, Hawksley and Gittens,[48] among others, felt that some toxic factor must be the responsible agent in this disease. De Lange and Arntzenius [18] expressed this possibility as follows:

> There are observations of liver-cell necrosis in the literature . . . and such findings show a certain agreement with acute or subacute yellow atrophy of the liver, the occurrence of which is generally associated with the action of a chemical poison. Chemical poisons produced by the mother or by the child itself can cause hemolysis in the child during pregnancy. This destruction of blood gives rise to increased formation of blood . . . which finds its anatomic expression in the changes described in the organs.

This theory appeals by reason of its simplicity. It explains both the symptoms and the pathologic changes. It is easily conceivable that a toxic, influence is at work for some time before birth (there seems to be evidence for this in fetal hydrops) and that the mother's circulation is the mechanism by which the child is spared in utero. When the cord is severed and this avenue for the elimination of toxic substances is cut off, the poisonous products may accumulate, causing increased destruction of erythrocytes, and jaundice, if not already present, may appear. This would explain why the child may appear vigorous at birth and yet suffer a subsequent rapidly fatal decline. The same mechanism may operate to prevent an accumulation of bilirubin in the child in utero, as suggested by Hampson. If in utero the pathologic process becomes fulminating, the toxic substances may not be removed rapidly enough, and edema, jaundice and numerous toxic changes in the organs may result, as in fetal hydrops, or they may even cause the intra-uterine death of the fetus. This is essentially the very plausible explanation offered by Palm.[54]

But an impasse is reached when an explanation of the nature or the source of such a toxic influence is attempted. It is true that in cases too numerous for the observation to be ascribed to chance alone the mother may have various abnormal symptoms, and for this reason Hoffmann and Hausmann [6] and others felt that toxic substances resulting from the pregnancy may affect the fetus adversely. They pointed out that in cases in which the mother is free from symptoms the intoxication may be insufficient to affect the mother clinically, while the more sensitive fetus is affected harmfully. The fact must be reiterated, however, that in the majority of cases of icterus gravis neonatorum the mother reveals no symptoms which might give a clue to the source within herself of a possible toxic substance. The blood pressure of the mother during pregnancy in most of these cases is low rather than high; evidence of renal injury is slight or entirely lacking, and carefully supervised prenatal observation and care, as in Smyth's [31] and in Abbott and Abbott's [27] cases, may reveal nothing abnormal. On the other hand, the incidence of maternal symptoms is much more frequent when the pregnancy results in a child with fetal hydrops. As may be noted in the report of Bullard and Plaut [33] cited, the mother had no symptoms during her second and third pregnancies, although the infants presented icterus gravis neonatorum, but during the fourth pregnancy the symptoms were severe, and the infant was born hydropic. There appears to be some interrelationship, therefore, between the condition of the mother and that of the fetus, at least while the fetus is alive,[35] with the suggestion of a parallel in the severity of the symptoms in each, but it 'is impossible with the evidence at hand to be certain whether the condition of the mother or that of the child is primarily responsible. The fact that the mother is the outstanding constant factor in the manifestation of the disease in a series of offspring, however, must be borne in mind.

Von Reuss [56] suggested that possibly toxic substances derived from the intestinal tract, formed as the result of bacterial decompositon, might be responsible for the symptoms of intoxication in the icteric infant. This possibility, however, seems remote when one considers Yllpö's [40] case, in which the infant became icteric one and a half hours after birth though every aseptic precaution was taken and though nothing had been allowed to enter the infant by mouth. Nor would such toxic substances explain a stillborn edematous fetus.

Hoffmann and Hausmann [6] presented the idea that a food allergy, although not the fundamental cause, might be the ground for exacerbation of the disease after birth. They reported the case of an infant in whom marked gastro-intestinal symptoms developed when it was given its own mother's milk, although it could take a strange woman's milk with impunity. A slightly older normal infant was likewise affected when given this mother's milk. This mother had had several children afflicted presumably with familial icterus gravis neonatorum. The child she did not suckle had only slight jaundice. This recalls Rolleston's [32] admonition to adhere to Auden's policy of not permitting affected infants to take their own mothers' milk. The possibility that the milk of the mother of an affected child might be responsible for the exacerbations following remissions, such as were noted in the case reported by Segar and Stoeffler [46] cited, has not been seriously considered, since there are no outstanding data to verify such an assumption, nor is there as yet a rational explanation for any such effect. Nevertheless, in view of the interesting observation of Hoffmann and Hausmann in this connection, such a possibility might well be investigated.

A number of observers have with considerable justification ascribed many of the symptoms and pathologic changes found in this disease to liver dysfunction.[57] These symptoms, apart from those referable to the blood cells, show a striking similarity to those resulting from poisoning by alkaloids affecting the parasympathetic system. Other substances having the same effect are those resulting from tissue breakdown, such as choline, histamine, guanidine, the proteoses and peptones. Such substances may well be derived from the injured liver of the child itself. Excreted into the maternal circulation through the placenta in sufficient amounts, as might occur in fetal hydrops, for example, the fetus may become a *Giftquelle* for the mother, as suggested by Palm.[54] The maternal symptoms might then indeed be such as have been noted here

---

56. von Reuss, A.: Die Krankheiten des Neugeborenen, Berlin, Julius Springer, 1914.
57. Hoffmann and Hausmann.[6] Pfannenstiel.[39] Palm.[54]

from the literature. Further evidence implicating the fetal liver will be considered later. That toxic substances resulting from such dysfunction or injury in this organ must in turn be explained by a more fundamental pathologic process, however, is obvious, and again the familial tendency must still be accounted for.

A further question may be raised as to whether the anemia or the destruction of blood really gives rise to compensatory regeneration so extensive as that found in erythroblastosis. Certainly this is not the case in congenital anemia of the nonregenerative type.[27] Furthermore, as Gierke[16] pointed out, the anemia in icterus gravis neonatorum may in occasional cases be slight or absent, while the erythroblastosis in such cases may be marked. It seems, therefore, that as a compensatory effort secondary to destruction of blood or to anemia alone the erythroblastosis is inadequately explained.

8. Woolley[34] speculated on the erythroblastosis found in congenital edema (hydrops), and since the evidence is in favor of an etiologic relationship between this condition and icterus gravis neonatorum it may be well, for the sake of completeness, to consider it in this study. He suggested that there was "something of an analogy between erythroblastosis and leucemia" and that erythroblastosis might also be looked on as belonging to the group of tumors, in this case the erythroblastic tissue being involved. Salomonsen[17] also tentatively considered this possibility. This hypothesis was set forth by Woolley in 1916, before the familial association between fetal hydrops and icterus gravis neonatorum was recognized. Since it has been found that icterus gravis neonatorum, even in cases in which there is marked erythroblastemia, responds in a fair number of instances to early and adequate blood transfusions with eventual and lasting recovery, erythroblastosis neonatorum can scarcely be conceived as a type of new growth of erythroblastic tissue comparable to that involving leukoblastic tissue in leukemia.

It appears that no theory has yet been presented which accounts for icterus gravis neonatorum and the apparently allied conditions in an entirely adequate fashion. The erythroblastosis has greatly intrigued those studying these diseases, but the variability of this factor suggests that its importance as a primary etiologic influence has been overemphasized. It seems more probable that it is rather a symptom, in the sense in which the jaundice, the leukocytosis and the hemorrhagic tendency are symptoms, of a more fundamental underlying pathologic process which has not yet been determined. The frequency of its appearance in those cases which come to necropsy suggests that it is associated with the more severe forms of that pathologic process.

The familial association of edema, icterus gravis and idiopathic anemia of the new-born, however, permits one to draw certain tentative conclusions which might not otherwise be justifiable. If, for example, one assumes that these three conditions are etiologically related, one cannot ascribe the evidence of greater injury in the liver, brain and other organs in icterus gravis neonatorum to anemia alone, since in congenital anemia, especially of the nonregenerative type, the anemia is often far more intense, while the evidence of injury to the organs is less outstanding and spontaneous recovery relatively frequent. Furthermore, if, as A. F. Abt[4] postulated, the immaturity of the red cells is the cause of the damage in the liver, owing to the fact that immature erythrocytes are less effective carriers of oxygen than mature cells, it is not apparent why, in those cases of idiopathic anemia of the newborn in which erythroblastemia is not evident in the beginning, the appearance of young red cells is coincident with the onset of definite recovery, as in the case of Abbott and Abbott [27] cited. The observations of Rich and Resnik as to the effects of oxygen deficiency on the liver parenchyma caused Snell [58] to investigate the question whether anoxemia is ever found in patients with clinical hepatic disease, and as a result it was found that anoxemia of the anoxic variety was a fairly constant accompaniment of advanced parenchymal hepatic disease, with some evidence to show that the degree of oxygen unsaturation of the arterial blood in general reflected to some extent the degree of hepatic insufficiency. One must therefore consider that the damage of the liver may not be so much a result of anoxemia as a cause of it in the conditions under analysis. It is true, however, as Judd, Snell and Hoerner [58] pointed out, that while it is difficult to determine definitely the true cause of the anoxemia sometimes observed in cases of hepatic disease, it is quite likely that it in turn has some effect on the progress of the hepatic lesion. It may be seen that one can be easily confused as to what is cause and what is effect. Are the bile thrombi the primary cause of the regurgitation jaundice, or are they, as Rich's statement suggests, the result of damage to the parenchyma? Is the damage in the liver entirely the result of anoxemia of either the anoxic or the anemic type, or is the anoxemia due, at least in part, to hepatic insufficiency? Judd, Snell and Hoerner felt that possibly the low percentage of oxygenation of the arterial blood in patients whose livers have been damaged may be attributable to some change in the pulmonary alveoli causing deficient oxygenation of the reduced hemoglobin, since inhalation of oxygen materially increases the oxygen saturation of the arterial blood. They called attention to the work of Rühl, who observed minute changes in the alveolar walls in experimental animals after shock due to histamine. It seems to be obvious that the answers to the stated questions and the solution of the problems implied are of definite importance for the more complete understanding of icterus gravis neonatorum.

It must be repeated that some observers have found no necrosis in the histologic sections of livers from infants dying of this disease.[59] Is one to assume that in such cases hepatic insufficiency plays no part? The answer must be sought in the clinical manifestations of the disease. It has been thought that the jaundice plays a prominent role in the tendency to hemorrhage.[2] But the assumption that bile pigment is itself capable of causing hemorrhage has been disputed. Scott [60] stated that there is no relation between the degree of jaundice and the tendency to bleed. He reported operating on a baby with an icteric index of 320 and finding no tendency to hemorrhage from either the muscle or the

---

58. Judd, E. S.; Snell, A. M., and Hoerner, M. T.: J. A. M. A. **105**:1653, 1935.

59. Huwer, G.: Ztschr. f. Geburtsh. u. Gynäk. **94**:150, 1929. de Lange and Arntzenius.[18]

60. Scott, J. M., in discussion on Judd, Snell and Hoerner.[58]

bed of the spleen. Kass and Osgood [41] also found no tendency to bleed in an infant receiving a diet high in carbohydrate to sustain the liver, who lived almost a year with complete obliteration of the extrahepatic bile ducts. Furthermore, in hereditary hemolytic icterus there is slight, if any, tendency to bleed. Judd and his collaborators stated that bleeding attributable to hepatic diseases has been known to take place in the absence of clinical jaundice. They suggested that the degree of injury to the hepatic parenchyma may be the most important factor in the production of hemorrhage in cases of hepatic disease. Ottenberg [61] likewise held that "the tendency to bleed depends rather on the extent of liver parenchyma damage than on the jaundice itself." It is entirely reasonable to assume, therefore, that injury of the liver may play a dominant part in the production of the "hemorrhagic diathesis" found in the conditions characterized by erythroblastosis, since it is in those conditions that the purpuric manifestations may occur. In the case of the fifth child of family B, reported by de Lange and Arntzenius,[18] there were hemorrhages in the skin and a conjunctival hemorrhage in the right eye, but in microscopic examination of the liver on necropsy only slight fatty changes were found, with no necrosis. It may not be assumed unquestioningly that absence of histologic evidence of necrosis in the liver necessarily rules out injury of the liver. That this organ is fundamentally involved in icterus gravis neonatorum is not a new concept, of course. I. A. Abt,[62] for example, definitely expressed the belief that "an anatomic inferiority of the liver" is responsible for the symptoms of the disease.

Gierke's [16] report likewise gave interesting corroboration to the view that hepatic damage is a factor in these conditions. He sent a sample of the red-brown serum from the bloody effusion found in the peritoneal cavity in his case, which reacted negatively to the Gmelin test, to Thannhauser, who reported as follows:

The serum contains bilirubin, and the indirect diazo reaction is stronger than the direct. In addition to bilirubin, the pigment designated by us as xantorubin, which we have found in dogs after extirpation of the liver, is also demonstrable spectroscopically. . . . I believe that this finding indicates a severe insufficiency of the liver.

In this case occasional atrophy of the liver cells, in addition to the presence of pigment, was the only observation made regarding the hepatic parenchyma itself.

Gierke felt that this finding was of especial interest in view of the fact that the nuclear staining in nuclear icterus seems to be brought about by a pigment other than bilirubin, as pointed out by Schmorl,[18] since in solution of formaldehyde and solutions of mercuric chloride it does not show the green color characteristic of the oxidized bilirubin. The nuclear staining with necrosis of the ganglion cells found in the brain in some cases of this disease has been related to hepatic injury by a number of observers. Hoffmann and Hausmann,[6] for example, expressed the belief that these changes are due not to an excess of bile pigment, since cerebral symptoms are never met with in the severe cholemia which accompanies congenital atresia of the bile ducts, but to some substance or substances, possibly lipolytic, produced by the necrosis of hepatic tissue. They

61. Ottenberg, R.: J. A. M. A. **104**:1681, 1935.
62. Abt, I. A., in discussion on Dunham.[52a]

pointed out that cerebral necrosis does not occur without hepatitis in those diseases in which the liver and brain are both affected. Wilson [63] himself was impressed by the analogy between icterus gravis neonatorum showing nuclear changes and the disease of young adults associated with cirrhosis of the liver described by him under the term "progressive lenticular degeneration." Crandall and Weil,[64] furthermore, showed experimentally that changes in the brain may be related to injury of the liver. They demonstrated in the serum of dogs, as early as the fourth day following ligation of the common bile duct, toxic substances which still exerted their destructive effects on the spinal cords of rats in vitro after being maintained at 62 C. for thirty minutes and after removal of the proteins by coagulation with acetic acid and boiling. They found also that these toxic substances are not identical with the lipases, which are increased simultaneously. The insult to the liver was followed both in dogs and in rats by spongy necrosis of nerve tissue in the brain, active proliferation of glia and a diffuse disease of nerve cells with predilection for the deep cortical layers and the striate body. In rats vascular changes were more marked than in dogs, and the degeneration of nerve cells was more pronounced in the basal ganglion, the midbrain and the cerebellar nuclei and less in the cortical cells. All the experimental animals, on histologic examination of the liver, revealed severe degenerative changes of the hepatic cells.

Judd, Snell and Hoerner [58] emphasized the value of repeated transfusions of blood, as well as of the use of oxygen in the treatment of hepatic disease to relieve the anoxemia whether of the anoxic or of the anemic variety, and stated that more benefit is apparently received from a transfusion than can be attributed to the amount of hemoglobin alone. The great value of intravenous transfusions of sufficient quantities of blood in the treatment of icterus gravis neonatorum is demonstrated in numerous case histories in the literature. The often dramatic recovery of some of the infants after repeated transfusions, with no subsequent evidence of developmental anomaly provided the brain has not been unalterably injured, suggests that the liver is probably the chief beneficiary, strengthening the impression arrived at by observation and analysis of the clinical and pathologic manifestations that a pathologic insufficiency does exist in the liver, not due to a "constitutional perversion" but to a definite injury or diseased state. It also renders untenable the theory that this condition of the liver is due to a defective anlage or to defective germ plasm.

It is now profitable to consider these conditions of the new-born, in which injury of the liver may be presumed to be indicated and in which one very often observes erythroblastosis, in contrast to a condition in which no such indications are found. If damage to the liver is slight or has not occurred and abnormal destruction of erythrocytes takes place alone, there may presumably be only slight transient jaundice or none, since the undamaged liver could excrete the excess of bilirubin. Edema and the tendency to bleed will also be absent, and although the anemia may become extremely severe, the process will be relatively benign and spontaneous recovery relatively frequent. This seems to

63. Wilson, S. A. K.: Brain **34**:296, 1912.
64. Crandall, L. A., and Weil, A.: Arch. Neurol. & Psychiat. **29**:1066, 1933.

explain the clinical manifestations of congenital anemia of the non-regenerative type. The relative freedom of the liver from damage in this condition is further suggested by Rich's [36] statement, that "whether or not jaundice will occur in any case depends upon the balance between the amount of bilirubin delivered to the liver for excretion and the capacity of the liver to excrete the pigment . . . with very rare exceptions the development of jaundice, even in the absence of obstruction, depends at least partly upon a lowering of the excretory ability of the liver."

In nonregenerative congenital anemia, then, one has reason to suspect that the liver is implicated only slightly or not at all, while in the diseases in which erythroblastosis is a feature, which are frequently fatal when untreated, the clinical evidence of hepatic dysfunction is strong. Whether the erythroblastosis is a response to the anoxic anoxemia resulting from injury to the liver, since no such response occurs in the aregenerative anemia of the new-born in which the anemia may be severe, remains a question, but there is good evidence for it. De Lange [18] felt that transfusions are not indicated as long as severe jaundice and marked regeneration of blood are still apparent, that only the succeeding anemia justifies this treatment. But in their baby "G," who received 40 cc. plus a further indefinite amount of the father's blood through the longitudinal sinus on the fourth day, the normoblasts and megaloblasts, which had numbered 124 per hundred white blood cells, disappeared quickly, the jaundice decreased, the spleen became no longer palpable and the liver of normal size, although the anemia continued to increase in severity. It is difficult to escape the conviction that in all probability it was the hepatic parenchyma rather than the bone marrow which benefited from the therapy and that the diminution of the erythroblastic activity resulted from the improvement in hepatic function. "Embryonal hematopoietic persistence" may thus quite possibly depend on the liver, not because the liver retains its fetal characteristics by reason of a defective anlage or defective germ plasm, but because injury to this organ has resulted in an increase of anoxemia of the anoxic type. Indeed, the resulting inadequacy of oxygenation may thus give rise to the "metabolic disturbance of erythropoiesis" postulated by Diamond, Blackfan and Baty as the cause of erythroblastosis. This idea was likewise expressed by Hoffmann and Hausmann: [6]

It is not inconceivable that, as phosphorus through attachment to oxygen interferes with the oxidative processes in the body and thereby leads to acid intoxication, similar interferences with metabolism in fetal life could be responsible for icterus gravis neonatorum. The increase in nucleated erythrocytes and the persistence of extramedullary foci of hematopoiesis would then be conceived of as compensatory phenomena.

Eastman [65] showed that the mean capillary unsaturation for oxygen in normal fetal blood at birth is three times that of adult blood and that in utero it is twice as great. This affords an explanation of Lippman's [66] studies in which normoblasts and other young forms of blood cells were found almost invariably during the first day of life, disappearing

65. Eastman, N. J.: Bull. Johns Hopkins Hosp. 47:221, 1930.
66. Lippman, H. S.: Am. J. Dis. Child. 27:473, 1924.

rapidly until no longer present toward the end of the first week. This view appears to be further substantiated by the fact that Barcroft [67] found a considerable increase in reticulocytes in adults subjected to a rarefied atmosphere. The fact that nucleated forms of red cells are not usually found in adults under conditions of low oxygen tension is no proof that they may not occur, along with extramedullary hematopoiesis, as a response to an abnormal degree of anoxemia in the fetal and new-born period, when the lability of the hematopoietic system is marked. Suffice it to say, however, that in the aregenerative form of congenital idiopathic anemia the primary cause of the malady cannot be related to erythroblastosis.

From this review of case histories and etiologic concepts found in the literature, analyzed with reference to recent studies on jaundice particularly, the following conception regarding these related disorders emerges: Aregenerative idiopathic anemia of the new-born represents the mildest manifestation of a pathologic condition characterized by a rapid and often marked decrease in the red cells of the circulating blood. This form, although relatively benign, is nevertheless fundamentally related to those more severe forms of the malady associated with erythroblastosis. In the latter, edema, jaundice, cyanosis, hemorrhagic manifestations, gastro-intestinal and nervous irritability, and collapse are found to varying degrees. These symptoms are least evident in idiopathic anemia of the new-born, more pronounced in icterus gravis neonatorum and extreme in universal edema of the fetus; in universal edema, however, the development of marked jaundice is usually precluded by death. These symptoms, leading frequently to a fatal outcome, result from injury to the liver. Roughly proportional to the extent and severity of this injury, there is abnormal diminution in the oxygen content of the arterial blood in the affected child, a condition which gives rise to compensatory erythroblastemia and associated erythroblastosis.

In accordance with this conception, two pathologic processes are postulated as responsible, to varying degrees, for the symptoms and changes in the affected child. These are (1) abnormal destruction of erythrocytes and (2) injury of the liver. While the mother may be affected secondarily by the condition occurring in the fetus, she seems to be the primary source of the influence which gives rise to one or both of these abnormal processes in the fetus and new-born infant, since she is the one constant factor to be found when this pathologic state appears in a series of offspring. If this is the case, one must examine more closely the possible nature of such an influence and the modes of transmission by which it may pass from mother to fetus. The argument that the transmission occurs by way of the germ plasm appears definitely unsupported. There remains only one other means of transfer, namely, the placenta. That a toxic substance generated in the mother is transmitted through the placenta to the fetus seems unlikely in the absence of symptoms in the mother in most cases; the reverse might conceivably be taking place when such symptoms occur. Furthermore, the infant affected by the aregenerative form of congenital anemia exhibits no symptoms of intoxication, but marked

67. Barcroft, J., and others: Proc. Roy. Soc. Med. **16**:58, 1922-1923.

\nemia only. In this form of the malady the erythrocytes alone seem
\o be concerned. If, now, the possible mechanisms giving rise to
destruction of erythrocytes are reviewed,[68] it is found that all may
be eliminated from consideration save one, the destruction of red cells
by some form of immune reaction. If the destruction of red cells by
the action of specific immune bodies is tentatively considered to represent the pathologic mechanism underlying this disease, one may recon-
struct the etiologic events as follows: The mother is actively
immunized against fetal red cells or some component of them. The
immunization may conceivably occur as the result of an accident within
the placenta whereby the fetal cells or their hemoglobin gain entrance
to the maternal blood sinuses. The antibodies formed in the maternal
organism may then pass to the child through the placenta or possibly
to an even greater extent through the colostrum and milk, since the
diminution of red cells in congenital anemia appears to be most acute
following birth. The time elapsing before such antibodies are present
in the infant in sufficient concentration to produce a marked effect may
correspond to the delay in the appearance of symptoms noted in most
cases of congenital anemia.[69] Such a transfer of immune bodies from
an actively immunized mother to the fetus or new-born child sets up
in the offspring a state of passive immunity. Such an immunity is relatively short lived and would eventually disappear completely, leaving
no trace to be passed on to a succeeding generation. Furthermore, each
child born and suckled subsequent to this active immunization in the
mother would possess to a greater or less degree a passive immunity
to the specific antigen, while any children born before the immunization
of the mother would be entirely unaffected. These facts were demonstrated in guinea pigs by Anderson,[70] who showed that after active
immunization of the mother a displacental transfer of specific antibodies
took place in 4 successive litters; this passive immunity in the offspring,
moreover, was not transmitted to the following generation. This conception of possible events leads to the formulation of a hypothesis which
thus explains adequately not only the familial tendency in this disease
but likewise its definite and distinctive distribution among the children
of an affected family. In the operation of such a mechanism the mother
would show no symptoms, yet she would transmit a destructive influence to successive offspring through the placenta and through her milk.
This mechanism, incidentally, bears no relation to a difference in blood
groups in mother and child; nor is such a difference a factor in this
group of diseases.[20]

If one now reexamines the findings which are frequently encountered in so-called erythroblastosis, one finds, in addition to jaundice
and erythroblastemia, (1) increased capillary permeability, manifested
by edema and the "hemorrhagic diathesis;" (2) increased bleeding and
coagulation times; (3) gastro-intestinal irritability, indicated by frequent stools and vomiting, suggesting vagal stimulation; (4) other
effects on the central nervous system, evidenced by somnolence and

68. Wells, H. G.: Chemical Pathology, ed. 5, Philadelphia, W. B. Saunders
Company, 1925.

69. Abt.[25] Abbott and Abbott.[27] Segar and Stoeffler.[46]

70. Anderson, J. F.: J. M. Research **15**:241 and 259, 1906.

flaccidity, twitchings and occasionally convulsions; (5) respiratory distress, indicated by cyanosis and "grunting" expiration, and occurrence of respiratory failure long before cessation of the heart beat, as noted by Huwer.[59] These symptoms, as suggested earlier, resemble closely those following stimulation of the parasympathetic division of the autonomic nervous system by certain drugs. Sollmann [71] included in his discussion of substances having such an action not only certain alkaloids and the toxic products of tissue autolysis mentioned previously but also a process which produces effects remarkably similar to those described here: anaphylaxis.[72] That anaphylaxis may frequently result in marked changes in the liver has been demonstrated for dogs by R. Weil,[73] particularly, and by Dean and Webb.[74] Webb [75] studied also the effects on the blood cells resulting from anaphylactic shock and found marked increase both in the nucleated forms of red cells and in the immature cells of the leukocytic series. He concluded that these were called forth from the bone marrow by the extreme anoxemia. Furthermore, while there was in these dogs immediate intense leukopenia, apparently due to extravascular migration of polymorphonuclear leukocytes, especially in the lungs—an observation which brings to mind the "bronchopneumonia" reported on necropsy in 2 cases of Diamond, Blackfan and Baty [20] and the "hemorrhagic bronchopneumonia" found in the first sibling in Abbott and Abbott's [27] first case—this was succeeded within a half hour following shock by pronounced leukocytosis with a definite shift to the left. The livers in the experimental animals of Dean and Webb were markedly congested and the sinusoids dilated. In the early stages following shock and in those dogs which recovered quickly the liver cells showed cloudy swelling. Later in the more severely affected animals there were all degrees of necrosis, with practically complete disorganization of the hepatic cells in one of the animals that died. The condition of the liver in this animal, as described by the observers, was almost identical with that in the infant with fetal hydrops reported by Parsons, Hawksley and Gittens.[48] In those dogs that recovered and were later put to death, the livers were practically normal within twenty-four hours except for the increased deposits of iron pigment in all the shocked animals. Petechiae were found in the organs of many animals, and in a number hemorrhage from the gastrointestinal tract had occurred.

Without carrying the analogy further, it may be recognized that in anaphylaxis one has a mechanism which is closely related to that tentatively considered for aregenative anemia of the new-born. In erythroblastosis, however, sensitization rather than immunization seems most adequately to explain the observations. The mechanism of its transmission through the placenta and later through the milk is the same. Fetal hydrops and icterus gravis neonatorum would be accounted

71. Sollmann, T. H.: A Manual of Pharmacology and Its Applications to Therapeutics and Toxicology, ed. 5, Philadelphia, W. B. Saunders Company, 1936.

72. Darrow, R. R.: Abstr., Bull. West Side Br., Chicago M. Soc. 1:3, 1936.

73. Weil, R.: J. Immunol. 2:525 and 571, 1917.

74. Dean, H. R., and Webb, R. A.: J. Path. & Bact. 27:51 and 65, 1924.

75. Webb, R. A.: J. Path. & Bact. 27:79, 1924.

for by placental transmission, while the exacerbations after partial recovery noted in icterus gravis and in congenital anemia are sufficiently explained by transmission of additional sensitizing factors through the colostrum and milk. Such a hypothesis is of further interest in that it appears to explain also certain details in case histories which seem otherwise incomprehensible. Among these is Hampson's success with small amounts of the infant's own mother's serum, administered daily by intramuscular injection. If this therapy is considered as a possible desensitization of the infant, the reason for its success is evident. Wells[76] stated that antiamboceptors may be obtained by immunizing an animal with a serum which contains amboceptors, and Opie and Furth[77] found that after injecting an antigen, for example horse serum, into their animals, the animals could be desensitized to the action of antihorse serum by repeated injections of antihorse serum in quantities insufficient to cause symptoms. Rolleston's counsel to withhold the mother's milk from an affected child gains new support from this concept, and Hoffmann and Hausmann's observation on the reaction of their infant to his own mother's milk can be understood.

There is, however, one further assumption which must be made. The antigen giving rise to such amboceptors must be a protein foreign to the blood of the mother in whom the reaction occurs. The observation of Hawksley and Lightwood[1] and the work of Trought[78] and of Barcroft[79] suggest that fetal hemoglobin may differ in its molecular structure from adult hemoglobin of the same species. If this is the case, fetal hemoglobin might be antigenic if it gained access to the maternal circulation, since Wells and Osborne[80] have demonstrated that it is the chemical character of a protein which determines its specificity rather than its biologic source. That hemoglobins are capable of acting as specific precipitinogens has, furthermore, been confirmed by Hektoen and Schulhof.[81] The assumption that fetal hemoglobin may be immunologically different from adult hemoglobin, and thus, possibly, the antigen involved, amplifies and completes the hypothesis that an antigen-antibody reaction is responsible not only for one but for all forms of this malady.

In conclusion, then, it may be proposed that in icterus gravis neonatorum and in those related diseases in which the symptoms indicate injury of the liver passive sensitization to the hemoglobin of his own red cells has been transmitted to the fetus from the mother, primarily through the placenta while the infant was in utero and through her milk after birth. In the aregenerative form of congenital anemia, on the other hand, it is likely that immunization rather than sensitization has taken place in the mother and has been transmitted as such to the child, or that, in some cases, desensitization or possibly mitigation of the sensitization reaction has in some way been accomplished.

---

76. Wells, H. G.: Chemical Aspects of Immunity, ed. 2, New York, Chemical Catalog Company, Inc., 1929.

77. Opie, E. L., and Furth, J.: J. Exper. Med. **43**:469, 1926.

78. Trought, H.: Arch. Dis. Childhood **7**:259, 1932.

79. Barcroft, J.: Lancet **2**:1021, 1933.

80. Wells, H. G., and Osborne, T. B.: J. Infect. Dis. **19**:183, 1916. Wells.[76]

81. Hektoen, L., and Schulhof, K.: J. Infect. Dis. **31**:32, 1922; **33**:224, 1923.

This hypothesis is offered with due reservations, since it is based on theoretical considerations. It has been formulated as the result of a critical analysis of many case histories, with the aid of experimental studies in other fields which appeared to throw light on the pathogenesis of the disorder. It has seemed important in this review to call attention to such studies, as well as to discuss various extant hypotheses regarding the etiology of the disease, especially since they offer experimental material from which a suitable concept seems logically to develop. The proposed hypothesis differs from others considered in this paper in that it meets the criteria which were set up for their evaluation, and likewise in that it is susceptible of confirmation or refutation.

SUMMARY

Icterus gravis neonatorum is a severe disease of the new-born, characterized by jaundice appearing soon after birth, with enlargement of the liver and spleen and with clinical symptoms which may include to varying degrees any or combinations of the following: somnolence, listlessness and flaccidity, or muscular twitchings, opisthotonos and occasionally convulsions; vomiting and diarrhea; petechiae, ecchymoses and bleeding from mucous surfaces; increased bleeding and coagulation times; edema; cyanosis and respiratory difficulty; collapse. In addition are found a marked increase in the number of circulating immature red blood cells, relative anemia, and leukocytosis, with frequently eosinophilia or monocytosis or both. The child may appear strong and vigorous at birth, but the appearance of symptoms is rapid, the illness ending in death within a few hours or days, occasionally in the second or third week, in the untreated case.

At necropsy, jaundice and pallor of the tissues, bile-tinged fluid in the serous cavities and minute or more extensive hemorrhages in the lungs, brain and mucous and serous membranes may be noted. There are enlargement and congestion of the liver and spleen, and frequently extramedullary hematopoiesis in the liver, spleen, lungs, kidneys, thyroid, thymus and lymph glands. Changes in the liver cells are reported as slight or not any in a few cases, while in most instances cloudy swelling and slight atrophy to extensive diffuse necrosis may be found, together with bile and iron pigment and "bile thrombi." Abnormal phagocytosis of the red blood cells by macrophages in the liver and spleen is demonstrable. Edema of the alveolar walls, leukocytic infiltration and small to fair-sized hemorrhages may be noted in the lungs. In a few cases yellow staining and necrosis of the ganglion cells in certain of the nuclear areas of the brain may be found.

While definite evidence of a hereditary transmission of this disease is lacking, its frequent familial occurrence is unquestionable. Healthy parents, normal pregnancies and short, easy deliveries are the rule, with normal healthy children frequently preceding the first affected child in birth.

The occurrence of universal edema of the fetus (fetal hydrops) or of idiopathic anemia of the new-born in siblings of the infant affected with icterus gravis neonatorum, together with suggestive similarities in the clinical and pathologic pictures, constitutes strong evidence for an identical etiology in these three disorders of the new-born.

Measured by criteria based on the foregoing observations concerning this disease, most of the existing theories of etiology are found insufficient in their explanations as to the probable or possible cause or causes.

The clinical symptoms suggest injury of the liver in those cases in which the disease is associated with erythroblastosis. Since an increased oxygen unsaturation of the arterial blood has been found associated with disease or injury of the liver, it seems probable that the erythroblastosis is secondary to anoxemia resulting from damage to this organ, since diminution in hematopoietic activity is found to be coincident both with improvement in hepatic function in an affected infant and with increased oxygenation of the blood following birth in a normal child.

Considerable evidence permits the assumption of two fundamental pathologic processes as responsible for the symptoms and changes in this disease and in the related disorders usually associated with erythroblastosis: (1) abnormal destruction of erythrocytes and (2) hepatic dysfunction due to injury. In aregenerative congenital anemia abnormal destruction of erythrocytes by itself seems sufficient in most cases to explain the course of the disease. The primary influence giving rise to these pathologic processes in a series of offspring in the same family must be traced to the mother. The placenta seems to be the means of transmission of the destructive influence from mother to fetus.

An antigen-antibody reaction seems to explain best all aspects of these related disorders.

Paper 2

2.   Levine, P. and Stetson, R. E. (1939). An unusual case of intra-group agglutination. *J. Amer, Med. Ass., 113,*126-7.

Commentary

This is an account of a woman who had considerable loss of blood associated with the delivery of her second baby. The three blood transfusions which she was given were all from her husband and were compatible on the ABO system, he and she both being group O. Nevertheless, the woman developed a severe transfusion reaction with oliguria and bloody urine, and after this occurred it was found, using a delicate technique, that her serum agglutinated her husband's cells. In addition, it agglutinated about 80% of 104 other group O bloods, but failed to do so in the remainder.

The case was reported as an example of an unexpected blood group incompatibility and before the animal work in Paper 3 was published. The authors pointed out that the new abnormal agglutinin (the antibody) resembled the known agglutinins in animals which result from repeated transfusions in that the agglutinins occurred both at warm (37°C) and cold (20°C) temperatures. This is in contrast to atypical agglutinins (now known as autoantibodies) which are sometimes found in normal people and which then only operate in the cold.

The authors suggested that it was an immunising property in the fetus, deriving from the father and lacking in the mother, which conceivably might have been responsible for the production of the antibody.

From P. Levine and R. E. Stetson (1939), J.A.M.A., 113, 126-7. Copyright (1939), by kind permission of the authors and the American Medical Association

AN UNUSUAL CASE OF INTRA-GROUP AGGLUTINATION

Philip Levine, M.D., Newark, N. J., and Rufus E. Stetson, M.D.,
New York

This report deals with a rare property in the blood of a patient whose serum showed an iso-agglutinin of moderate activity, which agglutinated about 80 per cent of the bloods of her own group. In view of the fact that this agglutinin tended to disappear after an interval of several months and the fact that this agglutinin gave an equally strong reaction at 37 and 20 C., it would seem to resemble agglutinins resulting from iso-immunization following repeated transfusions. This phenomenon is readily reproduced in some species (cattle, chickens, rabbits), by several repeated transfusions, but in the case of man only two clearcut instances of such iso-immunization to cellular elements are described in the literature.[1] The case to be described differs from these in that the immune iso-agglutinin must have been stimulated by a factor other than repeated transfusion. The nature of this factor becomes evident from a summary of the case history.

REPORT OF CASE

M. S., a woman aged 25, a secundipara, was registered in the antepartum clinic of Bellevue Hospital July 12, 1937, at which time she showed some pretibial edema and a blood pressure of 130 systolic, 90 diastolic. (The expected date of delivery was in the last week of October.) Two weeks later the blood pressure was 154 systolic, 106 diastolic, and there was a faint trace of albumin in the urine. Hospitalization and rest in bed resulted in subsidence of all symptoms. The fetal heart sounds were not heard, but there were no x-ray signs of fetal death.

Labor pains and vaginal bleeding started on September 8 (the thirty-third week of the gestation), and at midnight September 9 the patient was admitted to the hospital, at which time labor pains lasting one minute occurred every five minutes. There was considerable bleeding before the membranes were ruptured, and a macerated stillborn fetus weighing only 1 pound 5 ounces (595 Gm.) was delivered. After the placenta was expelled, bleeding was finally controlled and the patient (group O) was given her first transfusion of 500 cc. of whole blood from her husband (group O). Ten minutes after she received the blood a chill developed and she complained of pains in her legs and head. About twelve hours later a piece of membrane was passed and this was followed by more bleeding. At 4 p. m. a second transfusion of 750 cc. of whole blood was given, apparently without any reactions. In view of the renewed bleeding, hysterectomy was performed, followed by a third transfusion of 800 cc. of whole blood with no reaction.

Nineteen hours after the first transfusion and eight hours after the hysterectomy the patient voided 8 ounces (240 cc.) of bloody and dusky urine. At this time tests done with a more delicate technic revealed that, although the patient and her husband—the first donor whose blood caused a reaction—were in group O, the patient's serum nevertheless agglutinated distinctly her husband's cells and, indeed, the cells of most group O donors. Subsequently the patient received six more uneventful transfusions from compatible professional donors very carefully selected by the Blood Transfusion Betterment Association.

Subsequent intensive treatment—diathermy over the kidneys, forced fluids by vein, rectum and mouth, the repeated transfusions mentioned and high hot colonic irrigations—resulted in gradual recovery of kidney function.

From the Department of Laboratories, Newark Beth Israel Hospital, Newark, N. J., and the Blood Transfusion Betterment Association of New York City.

Dr. William E. Studdiford, director, and Dr. John S. Labate, resident, of the Obstetrical and Gynecological Service at Bellevue Hospital, gave the authors permission to study this case.

1. Landsteiner, Karl; Levine, Philip, and Janes, M. L.: Proc. Soc. Exper. Biol. & Med. 25: 672 (May) 1928. Neter, Erwin: J. Immunol. 30: 255 (March) 1936.

COMMENT

The blood was referred to us during the patient's convalescence, October 9, a month after the hysterectomy. Tests previously performed at the Donor Bureau of the Blood Transfusion Betterment Association showed that only eight of fifty group O donors did not react with the patient's serum and hence were compatible. In our series of fifty-four bloods of group O, thirteen failed to react with the patient's serum. Thus, of a total of 104 group O bloods twenty-one were compatible.

It could be readily shown that these reactions differ from those due to so-called atypical agglutinins occasionally found in the serums of normal persons. The former reactions were just as active at 37 as at 20 C., while reactions of the latter variety as a rule do not occur at 37 C. or else are considerably diminished. In other words, identical results were obtained when tests with serums of the patient were kept either at 20 or at 37 C. or were read after centrifuging and resuspending the sedimented cells.

The reactions were found to be independent of the M, N or P blood factors. Owing to the lack of suitable quantities of the blood, it was not possible to perform absorption experiments in order to supply data on the incidence of the reactions in bloods of groups A, B and AB.

Another specimen drawn two months later, December 3, still exhibited the agglutinin, which however gave far weaker reactions. Here again the reactions at 37 C. were just as intense as those at room temperature or lower. It was not possible to examine the serum of this patient until a year later, when all traces of reactions had disappeared.

In several respects this iso-agglutinin, as already mentioned, resembles the iso-agglutinins described by Landsteiner, Levine and Janes and that of Neter, namely (1) reactions within the same group equally active at room temperature and at 37 C. and (2) the temporary character of the agglutinin. In both of these cases the agglutinin was not demonstrable until an interval of several weeks had elapsed following repeated transfusions. In the present case, however, it is evident that the unusual iso-agglutinin must have been present at the time the patient was given her first transfusion with the blood of her husband, which subsequently was shown to be sensitive. Furthermore, this first transfusion was not uneventful in view of the resulting chills, pains in the legs and intense headache.

It is well established that in instances of iso-immunization in animals the iso-agglutinin serves as a reagent to detect dominant hereditary blood factors in the red blood cells and presumably also in the tissue cells. In view of the fact that this patient harbored a dead fetus for a period of several months, one may assume that the products of the disintegrating fetus were responsible not only for the toxic symptoms of the patient but also for the iso-immunization. Presumably the immunizing property in the blood and/or tissues of the fetus must have been inherited from the father. Since this dominant property was not present in the mother, specific immunization conceivably could occur.

No data are available as to the relationship to one another of the immune iso-agglutinin in the two previously reported cases and in the present case. Judging from the frequency of positive and negative reactions, it is evident that the iso-agglutinin in this case is distinct from the other two; i. e., 20 per cent nonreacting bloods in contrast with 75 per cent in the case of Neter and 60 per cent in that of Landsteiner, Levine and Janes.

Agglutinins of this sort can rarely be investigated thoroughly because of their tendency to diminish in activity and eventually to disappear. Consequently attempts were made to produce a hetero-immune agglutinin of identical or similar specificity by repeated injections of sensitive blood into a series of rabbits. These experiments met with failure, since suitable absorption tests with such serums failed to reveal the presence of the desired agglutinin.

201 Lyons Avenue, Newark—48 East Sixty-Fourth Street, New York.

Paper 3

3.   Landsteiner, K. and Wiener, A. S. (1940). An agglutinable factor in human blood recognised by immune sera for Rhesus blood. *Soc. Exp. Biol. NY.*, *43, 223.*

Commentary

For some years Landsteiner and Wiener had been raising immune sera in animals by the injection of red cells from other species, and investigating the capacity of these sera to agglutinate the red cells of still other species. Thus in 1937 and 1939 it had been shown that rabbits injected with the blood of Rhesus monkeys formed antibodies which agglutinated cells carrying the human M antigen.

The present paper describes another antigen of human blood detected by the same antiserum. The discovery was made when it was found that when the anti-M had been absorbed, the serum still agglutinated most human bloods, independently of their MN type. There was therefore a hitherto unidentified human blood group antigen present, and the authors (very naturally) designated this 'Rh'.

It still remained, however, for someone to connect the case of Levine and Stetson (Paper 2) with the findings reported here, and this is done in Paper 4.

It is now known that the clinically important Rhesus antigen is not identical with the one described in Rhesus monkeys. The latter is designated LW (after Landsteiner and Wiener), and Paper 48 should be consulted for more details and for its possible medical relevance.

From K. Landsteiner and A. S. Wiener (1940). Soc. Exp. Biol. NY., 43, 223. Copyright (1940), by kind permission of A. S. Wiener and the Society for Experimental Biology, New York

223

11151

An Agglutinable Factor in Human Blood Recognized by Immune Sera for Rhesus Blood.

Karl Landsteiner and Alexander S. Wiener.

From the Rockefeller Institute for Medical Research and the Office of the Chief Medical Examiner of New York City.

The capacity possessed by some rabbit immune sera produced with blood of Rhesus monkeys, of reacting with human bloods that contain the agglutinogen M has been reported previously.[1,2] Subsequently it has been found that another individual property of human blood (which may be designated as Rh) can be detected by certain of these sera.

Upon exhaustion of such a serum with selected bloods, for instance OM, the absorbed serum still agglutinated the majority (39 out of 45) of other human bloods, independently of the group or the M,N type; moreover, reactions took place with bloods lacking the property P. An example of the reactions is given in Table I.

TABLE I.

	Bloods (all group 0)									
	Type M				Type N			Type M,N		
	1	2	3	4	5	6	7	8	9	10
Absorbed immune serum	+	+	+	0	0	+	+	+	0	+

Technic: Immune serum for Rhesus blood diluted 1:10, absorbed with half volume of sediment of blood 4. One drop each of absorbed serum, cell-suspension (2%) and saline used. Readings after 2 hours at room temperature. Positive agglutination designated by + sign.

The results are of some interest in that they suggest a way of finding individual properties in human blood, namely, with the aid of immune sera against the blood of animals. As an analogy may be cited the demonstration of differences in sheep erythrocytes with immune sera for human A blood.[3] The reactions described, although of moderate intensity only, were obtained with immune sera produced at different times. Whether these observations may possibly lead to a method suitable for routine work is still under investigation.

[1] Landsteiner K., and Wiener, A. S., *J. Immunol.*, 1937, **33**, 19.

[2] Wheeler, K. M., and Stuart, C. A., *J. Immunol.*, 1939, **37**, 169.

[3] Andersen, J., *Z. f. Rassenphysiol.*, 1938, **10**, 104.

Paper 4

4. Wiener, A. S. and Peters, H. R. (1940). Hemolytic reactions following transfusions of blood of the homologous group, with three cases in which the same agglutinogen was responsible. *Annals. Int. Med., 13*, 2306-2322.

Commentary

The authors start by pointing out that though the discovery of the ABO groups by Landsteiner made blood transfusion immeasurably safer than previously, yet from time to time reactions occurred even when the donor and patient belong to the same ABO group. Details of three cases are described.

In the first, the patient was group O and had in all five transfusions of group O blood, and the standard cross-matching technique was always satisfactory. However, using a special technique where the test was done in the cold (page 57) it could be shown that clumping occurred, i.e. the bloods were incompatible in spite of both being group O. The new antibody was then used to test blood samples from a number of individuals, and remarkably (page 46) *'the reactions coincided with those given by certain anti-Rhesus immune rabbit sera recently described by Landsteiner and Wiener which define an agglutinable property of human blood designated as Rh' (editor's italics)*. (See Paper 3).

This then was the major discovery, and it was reasonably easy thereafter to put forward the principles underlying the reactions in the three patients.

It was presumed that patient no. 1 was group O Rh-negative, that the blood he was given was Rh-positive, and that the repeated transfusions had stimulated the production of high-titre Rh antibodies which were responsible for his death.

In the second case, the explanation for the clinical events was as follows:

The patient was group A Rh-negative and was given transfusions from two donors, both of whom were group A but one of whom was Rh-positive and one Rh-negative. The first (Rh incompatible) transfusion sensitised the patient, the second two (Rh compatible) had no deleterious effect, and the fourth (Rh incompatible) caused antibodies to appear in the patient's plasma. These were not demonstrable immediately after the transfusion because they had been completely absorbed by the transfused red cells, but they appeared shortly afterwards.

The third case (with others quoted from the literature) showed that not all hitherto unexplained transfusion reactions could be traced to the formation of Rh-positive antibodies in an Rh-negative individual.

The authors refer to the Levine and Stetson patient (Paper 2) and note that the percentage of bloods agglutinable by their patient's serum was about 80% which was not significantly different from the frequency of Rh-positive individuals in the population (85%). However, Wiener and Peters point out that Levine and Stetson's patient's antibodies gave just as marked reactions at warm temperatures as at low, in contradistinction to their own findings. Nevertheless, they note that Levine and Stetson suggest 'that the fetus inherited an antigenic substance from the father which was lacking in the mother, and the latter became immunised to the antigen after carrying the fetus for a long time after it had died *in utero'*.

Wiener and Peters anticipated much later work when they suggested that one reason why Rh incompatibility does not give rise to symptoms more often was probably because not all Rh-negative individuals were capable of producing anti-Rh antibodies.

From the clinical point of view Paper 4 is much the most important since it brings together the animal and the human work and foreshadows all that is to come. Its emphasis however is on transfusion reactions rather than on Rh haemolytic disease of the newborn. This is the subject of the next paper (Paper 5).

From.A. S. Wiener and H. R. Peters (1940). Ann. Int. Med., 13, 2306-2322. Copyright (1940), by kind permission of the authors and the American College of Physicians

HEMOLYTIC REACTIONS FOLLOWING TRANS-FUSIONS OF BLOOD OF THE HOMOLOGOUS GROUP, WITH THREE * CASES IN WHICH THE SAME AGGLUTINOGEN WAS RESPONSIBLE †

By ALEXANDER S. WIENER, M.D., *Brooklyn, N. Y.*, and H. RAYMOND PETERS, M.D., F.A.C.P., *Baltimore, Maryland*

THE discovery [16, 17] in 1900 of the isoagglutination reaction was one of the most important steps in the history of blood transfusion, since when donors of the same blood group as the patient are used, transfusions are practically free from danger. Even after this discovery was generally adopted and applied, however, occasional hemolytic reactions continued to occur. In the earlier days, practically all of these reactions could be traced to mistakes in blood grouping (Bordley [4]) of the patient, donor or both, and even at the present time such unnecessary errors are made too frequently.‡ Besides the hemolytic reactions caused by the transfusion of blood of the improper group, others have resulted from the indiscriminate use of " universal " donors.[21, 5, 8, 11] In addition, hemolytic reactions have recently been encountered following transfusions in which patient and donor belonged to the same blood group. Evidently such cases are rare, since only about a dozen definitely established instances of this sort have been reported in the literature to date. (For a review of the literature see reference 37.) The hemolytic transfusion reactions belonging to this last category, namely, those due to " intragroup " incompatibility, are the subject of the present paper.

Case 1. The patient was a 52 year old woman, admitted to the surgical service of the Mercy Hospital on August 13, 1939, with the complaint of vomiting, fever and bilateral abdominal pain of eight hours' duration. At the operation, performed on the day of admission, a ruptured solitary ulcer of the ileum § and peritonitis were found. Resection of the ileum with anastomosis and appendectomy was performed.

The patient belonged to group O. The day after the operation (the second day in the hospital) the patient was given a transfusion of 500 c.c. of fresh citrated blood of group O. Later the same day a second transfusion of 300 c.c. of group O blood was given. A third transfusion of 250 c.c. of blood was given on the third day; a fourth transfusion of 500 c.c. on the eighth day; the fifth and last transfusion of 500 c.c. of blood on the thirteenth day. All of the transfusions were from different group O blood donors. Preliminary to each transfusion the bloods of the patient and prospective donor were cross-matched.

* Including case cited in addendum.
† Received for publication March 11, 1940.
Aided by a grant from the Committee on Scientific Research of the American Medical Association.
From the Transfusion Division of the Department of Laboratories of the Jewish Hospital of Brooklyn, N. Y. and the Department of Medicine of the University of Maryland, Baltimore, Md.
‡ With regard to suitable technic of grouping and cross-matching, cf. [38]
§ Separate report in press (Robinson, D. R.: Surg., Gynec. and Obst.).

2306

HEMOLYTIC REACTIONS FOLLOWING TRANSFUSIONS OF BLOOD 2307

There were no febrile reactions whatever to the first four transfusions. However, during the week following the operation the patient had a continuous temperature of 103° F., which might possibly have masked the symptoms of a mild reaction. Of significance is the observation that while the hemoglobin concentration rose from 60 per cent on the day of the operation to 82 per cent after the third transfusion, it soon dropped back to 65 per cent and continued to fall after the fourth transfusion. Fifteen minutes after the completion of the fifth and last transfusion there was a severe chill lasting about half an hour, accompanied by a rise in temperature to 104° F. By the next day the patient had hemoglobinuria and marked oliguria, and became noticeably jaundiced (van den Bergh—direct, immediate positive 2.0 units; icteric index 19). The blood urea concentration rose from normal before the transfusion to 163 mg. per cent. The hemoglobin continued to fall, reaching as low as 46 per cent, and despite alkalinization the patient died four days after the onset of the transfusion reaction. At the postmortem examination, microscopic sections of the kidneys showed lesions considered characteristic of hemolytic transfusion reactions, namely, the typical degenerative changes of the tubular epithelium and the presence in the lumens of the collecting tubules of casts of brownish, pigmented hematin material.

Before the last transfusion, two cross-matching tests (hanging drop method at 37° C.) were reported by the technician and intern as showing no clumping even for periods up to several hours. Unfortunately, the specimens taken before the transfusion had been discarded inadvertently, and these observations could not be rechecked. Blood obtained from the patient after the transfusion and also after death and a fresh sample of blood drawn from the donor for the last transfusion were tested by one of us (W.). It was possible to confirm the fact that both patient and donor belonged to group O. In the cross-match test, however, while no agglutination was observed in the mixture of donor's serum with patient's cells, by a special technic * (vide infra) it could be shown that clumping occurred when the patient's serum was added to the donor's cells. Evidently, therefore, the patient's serum contained a special agglutinin, unrelated to the common isoagglutinins, α and β. That we were not dealing with an autoagglutinin was established by the absence of agglutination in mixtures of the patient's serum with her own cells. With the technics commonly used the abnormal reactions would probably not have been detected.

The properties of the special agglutinin and the corresponding agglutinable property in human blood were then investigated. First of all it was noticed that the reactions were considerably weaker than the common isoagglutination reactions. Moreover, the reactions were most pronounced at low temperatures, no noticeable reaction at all occurring at 37° C. Hemolysis could not be elicited in vitro at any temperature, even after the addition of fresh guinea-pig complement. These properties of the antibody in the patient's serum are somewhat surprising, considering the fact that it was capable of causing a fatal hemolytic reaction (see below). The reactions were best elicited by mixing a drop of a 2 per cent suspension of sensitive cells with two drops of serum in a small test tube (inside diameter 7 mm.) and allowing the mixtures to stand for two hours in the refrigerator. An

* With the common slide technic the reactions were indefinite.

2308   ALEXANDER S. WIENER AND H. RAYMOND PETERS

alternative suitable technic was to chill the mixture for a few minutes, then centrifuge. After gentle shaking, the sediments immediately broke up into a homogeneous suspension in the case of negative bloods, while rather large clumps easily visible to the naked eye persisted with positively reacting bloods. The reactions could easily be reversed by warming the tubes to 37° C.; on chilling, the reactions reappeared.

Blood samples from a number of different individuals have been tested with the patient's serum. Only bloods of group O were selected, on account of the presence in the serum of the isoagglutinins α and β, which precluded direct tests on bloods of the other groups. It was found that the great majority of bloods were agglutinated by the antibody in question. The agglutinable property involved proved to be unrelated to any of the agglutinogens M, N or P, as well as the agglutinogens A and B. Remarkably, however, the reactions coincided with those given by certain anti-rhesus immune rabbit sera, recently described by Landsteiner and Wiener [20] which define an agglutinable property of human blood designated as Rh.

As will be seen from table 1, in which are given some representative reactions, 14 bloods have been tested with both the patient's serum and the reagent prepared from anti-rhesus immune serum. The chance that the reactions of the two reagents should agree in every instance merely by accident is 1 in 2^{14} or about one in sixteen thousand. It is reasonable to conclude, therefore, that the agglutinable property demonstrated with the patient's serum is identical with Rh.

It is now possible to offer an explanation for the hemolytic reaction. The patient belonged to group O (Rh—). Since Rh+ bloods are about 6 or 7 times as common as Rh— bloods, most if not all the donors were probably of group O (Rh+). Apparently, to begin with, the patient had a weak anti-Rh hemolysin in his serum, undetectable by any of the common in vitro tests. This assumption would account for the short period of survival of the transfused blood cells, as indicated by the temporary nature of the rise in hemoglobin after the first few transfusions. While one may assume that the blood received in these transfusions was hemolysed too slowly to produce noticeable symptoms, the repeated injections of Rh+ blood served to stimulate the production of anti-Rh antibodies of higher titer, particularly after the fourth transfusion. Accordingly, the fifth transfusion of Rh+ blood gave rise to an acute hemolytic reaction.

Two questions are raised in connection with the above interpretation. The first is why such reactions are not encountered more frequently, as many patients, of whom about one-seventh would be Rh negative, are given repeated transfusions. The probable answer is that not all Rh— individuals are capable of producing Rh antibodies. Some special constitutional factor may be required—possibly the presence of preformed antibodies. In addition, the interval between transfusions must be long enough to permit an adequate rise in titer of the antibody. The second question is how it is possible for an antibody which in vitro produces agglutination only at low

TABLE I

Comparison of Reactions Obtained with Serum of Patient (Case 1) and with an Anti-Rhesus Immune Rabbit Serum

Bloods all group O Tests made with	Type M				Type N					Type MN				
	1	2	3	4	5	6	7	8	9	10	11	12	13	14
Serum of patient	+++± pos.	+++± pos.	- neg.	+++± pos.	++ pos.	- neg.	+++± pos.	+++± pos.	+++ pos.	- neg.	++ pos.	+++± pos	+++ pos.	- neg.
Anti-rhesus immune serum, diluted 10× and absorbed with half volume of packed sediment of blood No. 14														

The strength of the agglutinations is indicated by the number of plus signs, +++ representing the maximum possible reaction, namely, the formation of a single large clump.

2310   ALEXANDER S. WIENER AND H. RAYMOND PETERS

temperatures and of low titer to give rise to a fatal hemolytic reaction. Possibly the agglutinin found in the patient's serum is only an indicator of some supplementary, more subtle mechanism which is brought into play in the body before hemolysis can occur.

Shortly after the above study was completed, a second case, almost an exact counterpart of the first one, was seen at the Mercy Hospital.

Case 2. In January 1937, the patient was operated on for a perforated gastric ulcer at another hospital. The postoperative course was complicated by pneumonia and neutropenia, the total white count dropping as low as 3000. A transfusion was given and the white count rose. The patient was discharged after 43 days in the hospital. About six months later, the patient began to have attacks of headache, pain in the lower back and in the legs, these symptoms being accompanied by fever and leukopenia. During the six months before the present admission, the attacks became more frequent and more severe, and the patient had chills occurring at all hours of the day. The temperature ranged from subnormal up to 104° F. and the patient became subject to upper respiratory infections. On November 9, 1939, the patient's tonsils and adenoids were removed; he was discharged on November 11.

On November 22, 1939, the patient was readmitted to the Mercy Hospital on the service of Dr. Pincoffs, because of recurrence of chills and fever three days previously. On November 25, the patient, who belongs to group A, was given a transfusion of 200 c.c. of fresh citrated group A blood. About one hour after this transfusion he had a chill which was slightly more severe than those he had had on the previous few days. However, there was no history of hemoglobinuria. The temperature dropped to a subnormal level 12 hours later and remained subnormal for a week. The patient was given two other transfusions of 250 c.c. each on November 27 and November 30, respectively, both from the same group A donor, but not the donor who gave the blood on November 22. There were no untoward symptoms following these transfusions. The patient had no more chills and felt well until his discharge on December 7.

Two days later the patient was readmitted with the same complaints as formerly, namely chills, fever, headache, etc. On December 12, he was given a transfusion of 200 c.c. of citrated blood from the donor who had given the first transfusion on November 22 (21 days previously). Twenty minutes after this transfusion was completed, the patient presented the symptoms of a severe hemolytic reaction. Hemoglobinemia and hemoglobinuria were present. Almost immediately there was complete suppression of urine, and rather persistent vomiting, at times bloody, ensued. The bleeding and coagulation times were prolonged. The blood urea rose as high as 250 mg. per cent and the creatinine to 14 mg. per cent. After complete anuria for one week there was an output of only 50 c.c. on the eighth day and anuria again on the ninth day. Up to this point the patient had been treated with intravenous glucose, sorbital and diathermy On the tenth day, following splanchnic block (separate report by Pincoffs and Peters [30]) there was an immediate outpouring of urine and the blood urea dropped to 45 mg. per cent; the creatinine to 1.9 mg. per cent. Thereafter the patient improved progressively.

Previous to each transfusion the bloods of the patient and the prospective donor were cross-matched by the hanging drop and centrifuge methods. After the hemolytic reaction occurred, blood samples taken from the patient and donor before and after the last transfusion were examined by one of us; also the blood of the donor who gave the second and third transfusion was tested. It was found that both donors belonged to group A, subgroup A₁ type M. On the other hand, the patient's blood belonged to group A, subgroup A_2, type N. The idea that the difference in the subgroups or in the M–N types was responsible for the reaction could be eliminated at once. Careful analysis of the reactions of the patient's blood revealed that before the fourth transfusion it actually consisted of a mixture of two sorts of blood; namely, about 90 per cent A_2N blood and about 10 per cent A_1M blood.* This indicated that some of the blood from the previous three transfusions was still present in the patient's circulation, which would hardly be possible if either of the agglutinogens A_1 or M had anything to do with the transfusion reaction. Moreover, the proportion of foreign A_1M cells did not increase after the transfusion given on December 12, which showed that the blood injected on that day must have been completely destroyed.

TABLE II

Cross-Matching Tests of the Serum of the Patient (Case 2) with the Bloods of His Two Donors

Serum Separated From Patient's Blood Drawn	Patient's Own Blood	Tested Against Blood of Donor for 1st and 4th Trans. (Donor No. 1)	Blood of Donor for 2d and 3rd Trans. (Donor No. 2)
Before transfusion	Q.N.S.	±	Q.N.S.
2 days after transfusion	−	−	−
3 days after transfusion	−	−	−
4 days after transfusion	−	+ + ±	−
5 days after transfusion	−	+ + ±	−
6 days after transfusion	−	+ + ±	−
7 days after transfusion	−	+ + ±	−

The tests were made by mixing 2 drops of patient's serum with 1 drop of a 2 per cent blood suspension in a small tube, and allowing the mixtures to stand for two hours at a refrigerator temperature, after which time the reactions were read.

Q.N.S. = quantity not sufficient.

The most logical explanation for these findings was that although both donors were A_1M, for some reason the blood of the donor used for the first and last transfusions (donor 1) was incompatible, whereas the blood of the other donor (donor 2) was compatible. That this explanation is correct was established by the cross-matching tests. As is shown in table 2, the patient's serum before the fourth transfusion gave at best only a doubtful reaction with the blood of donor 1, and serum obtained shortly after the transfusion gave no reaction at all. However, on the fourth day following the transfusion and thereafter, it could be shown by the sensitive technic described that the patient's serum agglutinated the blood of donor 2 but not the blood of donor 1. No agglutination was observed in mixtures of the patient's cells with the serum of either donor.

A series of individuals was available whose bloods had been tested with the serum of the patient in case 1. Blood samples were drawn from these persons in order to ascertain whether or not the agglutinable property of the blood cells detected by the serum of the patient in case 2 corresponded with the agglutinogen Rh. As is shown in table 3, the reactions of the two sera are identical so that both sera contain the same antibody, anti-Rh.

* For the technic see: WIENER, A. S.: Blood groups and blood transfusion, pages 55–57.

2312 ALEXANDER S. WIENER AND H. RAYMOND PETERS

TABLE III

Comparison of Agglutination Reactions Obtained with the Sera of the Patients of Case 1 and Case 2

Tests Made With	Bloods (All Group O) of Type													
	M			N		MN								
	1	2	3	4	5	6	7	8	9	10	11	12	13	14
Serum From Patient in Case 1	−	+++	−	++	+++	+++	+++	−	+++	+++	−	+++	+++	−
Serum From Patient in Case 2	−	++	−	++	+++±	++	++±	−	++	++	−	++	+++±	−

Let us now summarize the second case in the light of the serological findings. A patient, group A (Rh—) was given a series of blood transfusions from two donors, one group A (Rh+) the other group A (Rh—). The first transfusion from the donor A (Rh+) gave rise only to a subclinical reaction. The following two transfusions from donor A (Rh—) were perfectly compatible, so that the donor's cells could be demonstrated in the circulation of the patient (with the aid of the M–N tests) for a long time afterwards. On the other hand, the blood from the first transfusion was gradually hemolysed and eliminated, this being accompanied by the appearance of Rh antibodies in the patient's plasma. Later, when a second transfusion of blood from the first donor, A (Rh+), was given, a hemolytic reaction followed. The long interval between the two transfusions from this donor probably allowed time for a fall in the titer of the anti-Rh agglutinins, so that these were not demonstrable either by the hanging drop or centrifuge technic before the last transfusion. The reason why the Rh agglutinins were not demonstrable immediately after the transfusion is that they had been completely absorbed by the Rh+ blood introduced into the recipient's circulation. By the fourth day, however, the antibodies had reformed in sufficient amount to be detectable.

That the property Rh is a true antigen is established by its capacity to stimulate the formation of immune antibodies in our two patients. The anti-Rh agglutinins in the patient's serum had the same properties as most other specific agglutinins, since its activity was not appreciably affected by heating at 56° C. for 30 minutes, and, as shown in table 4, it is absorbable

TABLE IV

Specific Absorption of the Agglutinin Anti-Rh

Tests Made With	Tested Against			
	Rh Positive Blood		Rh Negative Blood	
	1	2	3	4
Untreated Serum	+ + ±	+ + ±	—	—
Serum Absorbed with Rh+ Blood	—	—	—	—
Serum Absorbed with Rh− Blood	+ + ±	+ + ±	—	—

The absorptions were set up by mixing the patient's serum with one-third volume of packed washed cells in test tubes. After the mixtures had stood for an hour, the tubes were centrifuged in cups containing ice-water, and the supernatant serum pipetted off for the tests. Two drops of serum were mixed with one drop of cell suspensions (2 per cent) in small test-tubes and the readings made after these had stood for two hours in the refrigerator.

by Rh+ blood but not by Rh— blood. The serum from the patient in case 2 like that of the first patient reacted most strongly at low temperatures and not at body temperature. As is shown in table 5, even at ice-box temperature, the reactions were only of relatively low titer. Corresponding

2314   ALEXANDER S. WIENER AND H. RAYMOND PETERS

TABLE V

Titration of the Anti-Rh Agglutinins in the Serum of Patient 2

Tested Against	Dilution of Patient's Serum				
	Undil.	1 : 2	1 : 4	1 : 8	1 : 16
Rh Positive Blood	+ + ±	+ +	+ ±	±	—
Rh Negative Blood	—	—	—	—	—

Two drops of each serum dilution were mixed with one drop of cell suspension (2 per cent) and readings were made after the mixtures had stood for 2 to 3 hours in the refrigerator.

with the low titer of the anti-Rh antibody was its lability, for after only one month of storage in the refrigerator, the activity of the serum had diminished noticeably. On the other hand, serum obtained from the patient more than one month after the transfusion was almost as active as the sample originally tested. Three months later, however, the antibody could no longer be detected in the patient's serum.

Of interest is the relative incidence in the general population of Rh positive and Rh negative bloods. In addition to the bloods previously tested with the serum of patient 1, a series of group O and group A bloods was examined with the serum from patient 2. (Group A as well as group O bloods could be tested with the latter serum as it contained no α agglutinins.) Among a total of 101 individuals (not including the patients or donors of our two transfusion cases) 14 persons were encountered whose bloods did not agglutinate in the anti-Rh sera. This incidence of Rh— bloods (about 1 in 7) closely approximates that previously reported by Landsteiner and Wiener.

Our findings presented above confirm the occurrence of hemolytic reactions after transfusions of blood of the proper group, due to agglutinogens unrelated to the four blood groups. One may also consider that such incompatibilities might be detected before-hand by tests made at low temperatures. In this connection, a case seen by one of us several years ago is of interest.

Case 3. The patient was a female child, 4½ years of age, when first referred for blood transfusion by Dr. S. Katz in 1935. The patient first became ill during the winter of 1933 while in Florida, where she is said to have been handled and kissed by a nurse recuperating from acute rheumatic fever. The patient was taken home to Brooklyn where she ran an intermittent and remittent fever. During this illness, the patient also complained of pain and swelling of her thumb. She was treated at the Jewish Hospital for a time, where she was given a blood transfusion without any untoward reaction. Agglutination tests for typhoid, paratyphoid, etc. were negative. The patient recovered 16 weeks after the onset of the illness, following a tonsillectomy.

She again became ill at the end of November 1934, with remittent and intermittent fever ranging as high as 104° F. This was accompanied by migratory joint pains. In January 1935, because of a developing anemia, the patient, who belonged to group A, was given a transfusion of 180 c.c. of blood from a group A donor without any untoward reaction. (The bloods were also shown to be compatible by the usual open slide technic.) On February 14, 1935, the patient was given a second transfusion of 100 c.c. of blood from the same donor (after re-grouping and cross-matching the bloods). One hour after this transfusion, the patient had a severe chill and the temperature rose to 106° F. As reexamination of the bloods of patient and donor again corroborated the previous results, this was interpreted as a non-specific reaction, the clinical condition being blamed as a contributing factor. After the transfusion the patient's temperature remained normal for two days, then intermittent fever ranging up to 105° F. and 106° F. recurred and continued for two weeks. As the patient's hemoglobin was dropping and her clinical condition continued downhill, a third transfusion of 150 c.c. of blood was given from the same donor. This was followed by a sharp chill, rise in temperature to 107° F. and hemoglobinuria. The patient developed a hemorrhagic tendency, and blood oozed from all puncture wounds, including that of the transfusion, and from the mucous membranes. Another transfusion seemed urgently needed, but since retests again proved patient and donor to belong to group A, and the cross-matching tests were again negative, this idea was abandoned, there being no assurance that a different donor's blood would not also be incompatible. (Indeed additional tests even showed that the bloods of recipient and donor both belonged to subgroup A₁ and type MN, so that neither the subgroups nor the properties M and N could be implicated as the cause of the reaction.) The oozing of blood continued and the patient died two days later from exsanguination.

In the case just described, it seems certain that the hemolytic reaction must have been due to the appearance in the patient's plasma of immune iso-antibodies for the donor's blood cells. It is possible that agglutinins might have been demonstrable in the recipient's serum, if the sensitive technic outlined in the present paper had been used; namely, incubation of the mixtures of serum and cells in the refrigerator, with or without centrifugation. Possibly the cases reported by DeGowin and Baldridge,[9] Johnson and Conway,[18] and Goldring and Graef,[10] etc., could have been explained in a similar way. However, there is evidence that not all intra-group transfusion reactions can be traced to the formation of Rh antibodies in a Rh-individual. For example, in Zacho's case,[41, 42] the agglutination reactions given by the patient's serum were of highest titer at 37° C. and weakest at low temperatures. Aside from this peculiarity of the antibody, the difference in the frequency of bloods containing the agglutinable factor proves that the property Rh played no part in the reaction. The appearance following a transfusion of an immune isoagglutinin with properties similar to those of Zacho's case has been reported by Neter.[27] With regard to the transfusion reaction reported by Mandelbaum,[23] the blood of the patient was retested by us and found to be Rh positive. Accordingly the property Rh cannot be blamed for that reaction either. In the case reported by Levine and Stetson,[22] the incidence of bloods agglutinable by the patient's serum (based on 104 tests) was about 80 per cent, which is not significantly different from the frequency of Rh plus blood (about 85 per cent), but the antibodies gave just as intense reactions at 37° C. as at low temperatures. Whether or not the agglutinogen Rh was the responsible factor in the two cases reported by Culbertson and Ratcliffe[6] or in the cases reported by Bauer[2] cannot be decided from the data given in their papers. As to Mosonyi's report[26] of a hemolytic reaction following repeated transfusions of group B blood to a group B patient, the writer's conclusion that the reaction was due to the formation of immune iso-agglutinins specific for group B blood is not intelligible to the present authors.

In addition to those cases where hemolytic reactions followed repeated transfusions of blood of the homologous group, there are a number of reports of intra-group hemolytic reactions in patients who had never received a previous blood transfusion, or where the previous transfusion had been given so long ago (several years) that they could hardly be blamed for the reaction. Such instances have been reported by Zacho,[41] Parr and Krischner,[29] Culberston and Ratcliffe,[6] McCandless,[25] Johnson and Conway,[13] Smith and Haman,[34] Mandelbaum [28] and Levine and Stetson.[22] Remarkably enough in all of these cases except the one reported by McCandless * the patients were women who had recently given birth or had had a miscarriage.† Culbertson and Ratcliffe remarked concerning this coincidence in their two cases but did not attempt any explanation. In the case reported by Levine and Stetson, the patient, who had just had a stillbirth, was transfused with blood from her husband and a hemolytic reaction resulted. These authors suggest that the fetus inherited an antigenic substance from the father which was lacking in the mother, and the latter became immunized to the antigen after carrying the fetus for a long time after it had died in utero. In support of their interpretation that the agglutinin found in their patient's serum was an immune antibody rather than a natural one, Levine and Stetson cite the gradual drop in its titer and its eventual complete disappearance several months after the transfusion. In the other instances referred to above, a similar explanation may hold, though the individual antigenic differences responsible need not be the same in every case.

In support of this idea can be cited the report by Jonsson,[14] who found the average titer of the isohemolysins α and β to be higher than normal in women who had recently given birth, and who attributes this phenomenon to the specific stimulation provided in instances of heterospecific pregnancy. If the presence of a group A or group B fetus in a group O mother can cause a rise in titer of the isoantibodies α and β, respectively, it does not seem improbable, that, for example, a Rh— woman carrying a Rh+ fetus might

* With regard to the McCandless case, this is actually not an instance of an intragroup hemolytic reaction, since retests of the donor's blood by Hoxworth [12] have shown that the donor actually belongs to group A (subgroup A_2) not to group O as stated in the original case report. The case reported by Von Deesten and Cosgrove [36] of renal insufficiency following a blood transfusion is not a true hemolytic reaction since the hemoglobin rose from 70 per cent before the transfusion to 87 per cent after the transfusion. The rise in hemoglobin resulting from the transfusion corresponds closely with the predicted rise from a transfusion of 750 c.c. of blood, which was the amount given. If hemolysis had occurred there should have been no rise in hemoglobin. Moreover, the symptoms were not typical of a transfusion reaction and could be more logically attributed to the slight kink of the right ureter detected subsequently by pyelogram.

Incidentally, Thalhimer's case [35] frequently cited as an example of the danger of repeated blood transfusions from the same donor is not an example of an intragroup reaction, since the donor belongs to group B and the patient to group O.

† While this paper was in press, our attention was called to another instance of intragroup incompatibility reported by Pondman,[43] occurring in a postpartum case.

react by producing Rh antibodies.   However, the paucity of reports of intra-group hemolytic reactions even in postpartum cases indicates that this phenomenon must be rare.   Possibly in normal pregnancy the placenta offers a barrier to the passage of antigens from fetus to mother, and, in addition, as pointed out above, because of constitutional differences not all individuals will respond to the foreign antigens by producing specific antibodies.

An important question is what bearing other known individual differences of human blood, namely, those dependent on differences in the agglutinogen A (A_1 and A_2) and on the agglutinogens M, N and P, have on the occurrence of intra-group transfusion reactions.   With respect to the subgroups of groups A and AB, it has been shown by Landsteiner and Levine [18] that a small percentage of individuals belonging to these groups have in their plasma irregular agglutinins acting on blood of the opposite subgroup.   Some writers [3,7] assert that differences in the subgroups can cause hemolytic reactions and warn that only donors of the homologous subgroup be used for transfusions.   As a matter of fact no case has yet been reported where the subgroups were conclusively proved to be responsible for a serious reaction.   In our own experience with over 3,000 transfusions [39] the incidence of even minor reactions among patients of group A when donors are selected without regard to the subgroups is not significantly higher than among patients in groups O and B, the blood cells of the donor persisting in the patient's circulation whether donor and recipient belong to the same or different subgroups.   Similar has been the experience of Hoxworth [12] in a series of 2950 transfusions.   As is illustrated by case 2, in hemolytic transfusion reactions, even if it is found that patient and donor are not in the same subgroup this does not prove the difference in subgroups to be responsible. To the best knowledge of the writers, no report has appeared in the literature which proves that agglutinogen A_1 can be antigenic for A_2 persons, or vice versa, but recently two such cases have come to our personal attention.[39] One patient (of subgroup A_2) had received repeated transfusions of A_1 blood; the other (also of subgroup A_2) was a postpartum case.   Both had α agglutinins in their sera of titer 16 at room temperature.   Accordingly, the most practical procedure, and the one followed by us, is to disregard the subgroups when selecting donors for transfusion except in the infrequent cases where the patient's plasma contains the irregular isoagglutinins α_1 or α_2 and then to use donors of the homologous subgroup.   Such instances can be detected by the usual cross-matching tests.

With regard to the agglutinogens M and N, the situation is similar. Despite the performance of hundreds of thousands of transfusions every year, in which donors are selected without regard to their M–N types, not a single hemolytic reaction can be traced to this source.   The report by Martinet [24] that he observed the formation of specific hemolysins for M and N following transfusions is unconvincing, and in the present authors' experience repeated injections of type M blood into type N individuals or vice-versa has not stimulated the production of isoantibodies for M or N.   Evidently, therefore, these agglutinogens, unlike A and B, are not antigenic, or at most very feebly antigenic, for human beings. Accordingly, the prominence given them by certain writers [31] as a possible source of hemolytic reactions after repeated transfusion is not warranted, though the possibility that such cases may ultimately be found cannot be excluded. Only three cases (among hundreds of thousands of persons tested) are known of human beings with natural anti-M isoagglutinins, none having been encountered to date with anti-N agglutinins. In patients with such isoagglutinins, it would of course be wise to take the agglutinogens M and N into account when selecting the blood donor.

At least one case is known where the injection of blood containing agglutinogen P into an individual lacking the agglutinogen stimulated the formation of isoantibodies for P. In this case, seen by Dr. S. H. Polayes, there was difficulty in finding a compatible donor for a patient of group A, since her serum agglutinated most other bloods of group A. This patient had had a previous transfusion without untoward reaction from a group A donor whose cells were now also agglutinated by her serum. The patient's blood was referred to one of us [39] for study and it was found that the abnormal reactions of its serum corresponded with the agglutinogen P. For this patient, accordingly, only blood of group A(P—) would be suitable for transfusion.

With regard to the rôle played by irregular agglutinins in general in hemolytic reactions, it may be said that they show marked differences as to their significance in transfusions. In a number of instances [18, 19] where patients were transfused with blood acted on by atypical agglutinins in their sera, no untoward symptoms resulted, although the in vitro reactions were at times as strong as those described here. This indicates the existence of some as yet undescribed qualitative difference among the various irregular isoantibodies.

No evidence exists that pseudoagglutination (or pronounced rouleaux-formation) can cause untoward transfusion reactions. Also, in the authors' experience autoagglutinins have not caused hemolytic reactions. (In patients with autoagglutinins, however, we take care to keep the blood at body temperature during its infusion, while ordinarily we are content with blood at room temperature.) Indeed, injudicious attempts to warm up the blood as a routine are dangerous, and in at least one case the injection of blood damaged by overheating gave rise to a fatal hemolytic reaction.[1] Another non-specific cause of severe or even fatal hemolytic transfusion reactions that has come to the fore in recent years is the use of preserved blood stored for too long periods of time before injection. As is pointed out elsewhere,[33, 40] the safe time limit for the storage of blood for transfusion is between five and 10 days.

DISCUSSION

The danger of intra-group hemolytic reactions has been shown to be greatest in patients receiving repeated blood transfusions and in postpartum cases. With regard to the warning [15] not to use the same donor for patients receiving repeated transfusions, our findings show that this measure is not sufficient to exclude transfusion reactions, since the antigens responsible may occur in a considerable percentage of individuals. In fact, the patients in cases 1 and 2 would have been safer with repeated transfusions from a single Rh— donor. With regard to the postpartum patients who had hemolytic reactions following transfusions of blood of the proper group, though never transfused previously, these should belong to the same category as the patients immunized by repeated transfusions, if the theory suggested is correct; namely, that the patients became immunized while the fetus was in utero to antigens shared by fetus and blood donor (usually the husband) but absent from the patient's body. Incidentally, some writers consider leukemia and hemolytic icterus contraindications to blood transfusion, as hemolytic reactions have been observed following transfusions of apparently compatible blood in these diseases. The formation of immune isoantibodies seems the most plausible explanation for these observations, because such patients are usually given many blood transfusions.

With regard to the prophylaxis of intra-group hemolytic reactions, no single in vitro technic will cover every exigency, as while most of the irregular isoagglutinins act best at low temperatures, others have been found that react more strongly at body temperatures. However, the following technic of cross-matching is advised in addition to the usual grouping and cross-matching tests, as it will anticipate most reactions of this sort.

1. Two drops of patient's serum, preferably separated from the clot at refrigerator temperature, are mixed with one drop of donor's cell suspension in a small test tube.
2. In a second tube a similar mixture of patient's serum and patient's cells is set up.

The tubes are placed in ice-water for 5 minutes, then centrifuged while still cold and the mixtures are gently shaken. The reactions are read both macroscopically and microscopically. If neither tube shows a reaction, the donor is compatible. If both show a reaction, we are dealing with an autoagglutinin and the donor probably can be used without danger. If tube 1 shows agglutination and tube 2 does not, the donor is incompatible and others must be tested in order to find a suitable one.

In any event, in patients receiving repeated transfusions and in postpartum cases the serological test should be supplemented by a biological test,[28] if time permits. In citrate transfusions it is a simple matter to inject the first 50 or 100 c.c. of blood very slowly in order to determine whether a reaction will occur. If a chill * results, the infusion should be stopped and another donor tried. This procedure would probably prevent any serious consequences since 100 c.c. of incompatible blood are hardly enough to cause a fatal reaction. In a series of 15 hemolytic reactions with 10 fatalities analysed by Bordley, all patients receiving less than 350 c.c. of blood recovered.

Our findings are also of interest since they demonstrate by another method the large number of individual differences in human blood. With

* A chill caused by a blood transfusion usually begins within an hour.

2320   ALEXANDER S. WIENER AND H. RAYMOND PETERS

the agglutinogens A_1, A_2, B, M, N, P and Rh alone as many as 72 different types of human blood are readily distinguished. Also remarkable is the correspondence between the reactions of the sera of our two patients and the anti-rhesus immune sera prepared by Landsteiner and Wiener.

SUMMARY

Three cases are reported in which repeated transfusions of blood of the proper group gave rise to hemolytic reactions, two of the three reactions resulting in the death of the patient.

In two cases there was noted the appearance in the patient's serum of an isoagglutinin designated as anti-Rh. This is explained as the immune response to the injection of Rh+ blood into Rh— individuals, the blood group playing no rôle. Following the appearance of the anti-Rh agglutinins the transfusion of Rh+ blood gave rise to hemolytic reactions. Remarkably the reactions of the anti-Rh sera corresponded with those of immune rabbit sera prepared by Landsteiner and Wiener by the injection of rhesus blood. The frequency distribution of agglutinogen Rh in the general population is approximately 85 per cent Rh+ and 15 per cent Rh—.

Our cases were compared with others reported in the literature and various similarities and differences pointed out. A hypothesis is offered to explain the occurrence also of hemolytic intra-group reactions in certain individuals who had not received previous blood transfusions. The rôle played by the properties A_1, A_2, M, N and P in transfusion reactions is discussed. Methods are suggested for the prevention of occurrence of intra-group hemolytic reactions.

ADDENDUM

While this article was in press, an additional case of intragroup incompatibility, based on individual blood differences with respect to the property Rh, was observed. The history of this case is as follows:

Case Report. The patient was a woman, 58 years of age, admitted to the private service of Dr. Frank Teller at the Jewish Hospital of Brooklyn, with the diagnosis of diabetic gangrene of the toes of one foot. Amputation was performed, and following the operation, the patient's condition was poor. A transfusion of 500 c.c. of citrated, group A, compatible blood was given by the gravity method. Despite the transfusion, the hemoglobin dropped from 78 to 70 per cent; the red blood cell count from 3.95 million to 3.14 million per cu. mm. Following this transfusion, which was given on April 18, 1940, there was no detectable untoward reaction. On April 25, a second transfusion was performed; this time 300 c.c. of group O blood were given. One hour after the transfusion, the patient had a severe chill lasting 30 minutes, and there was an abrupt rise in temperature. Moreover, again there was no appreciable improvement in the hemoglobin or red count, and it was decided to investigate the cause of this transfusion reaction in greater detail.

The grouping tests revealed:

Blood of	Group	Subgroup	Type
Patient	A	A_2	M
1st donor (patient's son)	A	A_2	MN
2d donor (professional)	O	—	M

HEMOLYTIC REACTIONS FOLLOWING TRANSFUSIONS OF BLOOD 2321

It is clear that the fate of the blood received at the first transfusion could be determined by testing the patient's blood with anti-N serum; the fate of the blood received at the second transfusion by tests with anti-A serum. Tests made on a sample of blood drawn four days after the second transfusion showed that all the blood received at the two transfusions had been eliminated from the circulation, while transfused cells ordinarily survive for periods up to three and four months. This indicated the existence of some incompatibility between the blood of the patient and those of the two donors. Tests were then set up by the centrifuge method in the cold, and it was found that while no agglutination occurred in mixtures of the patient's serum with her own cells, strong clumping was evident in the tubes containing the bloods of the donors. This phenomenon was evidently connected in some way with the transfusion reaction, and supplied the key to the explanation for the rapid disappearance of the donors' cells from the patient's circulation. A series of blood specimens from individuals who had previously been tested for the property Rh was then tested with the patient's serum, and the results proved that we were dealing once more with an incompatibility reaction based on the property Rh.

REFERENCES

1. BAKER, S. L.: Urinary suppression following blood transfusion, with report of case probably due to overheating blood, Lancet, 1937, i, 1390.
2. BAUER, M.: Ein Bluttransfusion Zwischenfall bei wiederholter Verwendung des gleichen Spenders, Ärztl. Sachverst. Ztg., 1935, xli, 1.
3. BLINOV, N.: Die Isohamoagglutinationsuntergruppen A₁ und A₂ und ihre praktische Bedeutung für die Bluttransfusion, Deutsch. Ztschr. f. Chir., 1934, ccxliii, 400.
4. BORDLEY, J.: Reactions following transfusion of blood with urinary suppression, Arch. Int. Med., 1931, xlvii, 288.
5. COCA, A. F.: Selection of donors for blood transfusion, with special reference to preliminary blood tests and use of universal donor, Am. Jr. Med. Technol., 1938, iv, 28.
6. CULBERTSON, C. G., and RATCLIFFE, A. W.: Reaction following intragroup blood transfusion. Irregular agglutinin demonstrated by the sensitive centrifuge test method, Am. Jr. Med. Sci., 1936, cxcii, 471.
7. DAVIDSOHN, I.: A method for recognition of blood subgroups A₁ and A₂, as a means of avoiding transfusion reactions, Jr. Am. Med. Assoc., 1939, cxii, 713.
8. DEGOWIN, E. L.: Hemolytic transfusion reaction from use of a universal donor, Jr. Am. Med. Assoc., 1937, cviii, 296.
9. DEGOWIN, E. L., and BALDRIDGE, C. W.: Fatal anuria following blood transfusion. Inadequacy of present tests for incompatibility, Am. Jr. Med. Sci., 1934, clxxxviii, 555.
10. GOLDRING, W., and GRAEF, I.: Nephrosis with uremia following transfusion with incompatible blood, Arch. Int. Med., 1937, xcxii, 471.
11. HESSE, E. R., and FILATOV, A. N.: Complications following transfusions, Sovet. khir., 1936, no. ix, 408.
12. HOXWORTH, P. I.: Personal communication.
13. JOHNSON, R. A., and CONWAY, J. F.: Urinary suppression and uremia following transfusion of blood, Am. Jr. Obst. and Gynec., 1933, xxvi, 255.
14. JONSSON, B.: Zur Frage der heterospezifischen Schwangerschaft, Acta path. et microbiol. scand., 1936, xiii, 424.
15. KEYNES, G.: Blood transfusion, p. 96, Oxford, London (1922).
16. LANDSTEINER, K.: Zur Kenntnis der antifermentativen, lytischen und agglutinierenden Wirkungen des Blutserums, und der Lymphe, Zentralbl. f. Bakteriol., 1900, xxvii, 357.
17. LANDSTEINER, K.: Über Agglutinationserscheinungen normalen menschlichen Blutes, Wien. klin. Wchnschr., 1901, xiv, 1132.
18. LANDSTEINER, K., and LEVINE, P.: On isoagglutinin reactions of human blood other than those defining the blood groups, Jr. Immunol., 1929, xvii, 1.

2322   ALEXANDER S. WIENER AND H. RAYMOND PETERS

19. LANDSTEINER, K., LEVINE, P., and JANES, M. L.: On the development of isoagglutinins following transfusions, Proc. Soc. Exper. Biol. and Med., 1928, xxv, 572.

20. LANDSTEINER, K., and WIENER, A. S.: An agglutinable factor in human blood recognized by immune sera for rhesus blood, Proc. Soc. Exper. Biol. and Med., 1940, xliii, 223.

21. LEVINE, P., and MABEE, J.: Dangerous "universal donor" detected by direct matching of bloods, Jr. Immunol., 1923, viii, 425.

22. LEVINE, P., and STETSON, R. E.: An unusual case of intra-group agglutination, Jr. Am. Med. Assoc., 1939, cxiii, 126.

23. MANDELBAUM, H.: Hemolytic reaction following blood transfusion; report of a case of intra-group incompatibility, ANN. INT. MED., 1939, xii, 1699.

24. MARTINET, R.: Contribution a l'étude des caractères sanguins M et N, Thése No. 1601, Univ. de Genève, Liege, 1936.

25. McCANDLESS, H. G.: A hemolytic blood transfusion reaction with oliguria, Jr. Am. Med. Assoc., 1935, cv, 952.

26. MOSONYI, L.: Das Auftreten von Immun-Isoantikörpern nach mehrmahliger Transfusion, Klin. Wchnschr., 1936, xv, 1675.

27. NETER, E.: Observations on abnormal isoantibodies following transfusions, Jr. Immunol., 1936, xxx, 255.

28. OEHLECKER, F.: Direct vein-to-vein transfusion of blood, Arch. f. klin. Chir., 1921, cxvi, 705.

29. PARR, L. W., and KRISCHNER, H.: Hemolytic transfusion fatality with donor and recipient in the same blood group, Jr. Am. Med. Assoc., 1932, xcviii, 47.

30. PINCOFFS, M. C., and PETERS, H. R.: In preparation.

31. RIDDELL, V. H.: Blood transfusion, Oxford University Press, London 1939.

32. ROBINSON, D. R.: Surg., Gynec. and Obst. (in press).

33. SCHAEFER, G., and WIENER, A. S.: Limitations in the use of preserved blood for transfusions, Quart. Bull. Sea View Hosp., 1939, v, 17.

34. SMITH, C. E., and HAMAN, J. O.: Reaction following blood transfusion; report of unusual case, Calif. and West. Med., 1934, xli, 157.

35. THALHIMER, W.: Hemoglobinuria after a second transfusion with the same donor, Jr. Am. Med. Assoc., 1921, lxxvi, 1345.

36. VON DEESTEN, H. T., and COSGROVE, S. A.: Renal insufficiency following blood transfusion; recovery after venesection, ANN. INT. MED., 1933, vii, 105.

37. WIENER, A. S.: Blood groups and blood transfusion, 1939, 2d edition, C. C. Thomas, Springfield, Ill.

38. WIENER, A. S.: Technique of blood grouping tests preliminary to blood transfusions, Am. Jr. Clin. Path., 1939, ix, 145.

39. WIENER, A. S.: Unpublished observations.

40. WIENER, A. S., and SCHAEFER, G.: Limitations in the use of preserved blood for transfusions, Med. Clin. N. Am., 1940, xxiv, 705.

41. ZACHO, A.: "Incompatibility" between blood of same blood type due to presence of irregular agglutinin and of hitherto undescribed receptor, Hospitalstid., 1935, 225.

42. ZACHO, A.: "Unverträglichkeit" zwischen Blutproben von gleichen Blutypus, beruhend auf dem Vorhandsein eines irregulären Agglutinins gegenüber einen bisher unbekannten Rezeptor, Ztschr. f. Rassenphysiol., 1936, viii, 1.

43. PONDMAN, A.: Moeilijkheden bij. Bloedgroepbepaligen (Difficulties in blood group determination), Nederl. Tidjschr. von Geneesk., 1938, lxxxii, 6111.

44. WIENER, A. S., OREMLAND, B. H., HYMAN, M. A., and SAMWICK, A. A.: Transfusion reactions. Experiences with more than 3000 blood transfusions, Am. Jr. Clin. Path., in press.

Paper 5

5. Levine, P., Burnham, L., Katzin, E. M. and Vogel, P. (1941). The role of iso-immunization in the pathogenesis of erythroblastosis fetalis. *Amer. J. Obst. and Gynec.*, *42*, 925-937.

Commentary

It is in this paper that the knowledge previously discussed is brought to bear on the problem of haemolytic disease of the newborn (HDN), and it shows unequivocally that most cases are due to immunisation of Rh-negative mothers by their Rh-positive fetus, the Rh antigen being inherited from the father. Many of the immunological features of the disease are described here for the first time.

The first point to note is that the patient described in Paper 2 was shown, three years after the transfusion accident, to be Rh-negative and her husband Rh-positive, and the donors who were selected as compatible for the uneventful transfusion in 1937 were found to be Rh-negative in 1940.

The second point is the observation by the authors that intra-group (i.e. of the same ABO blood group) transfusion accidents *tend to be associated with pregnancy*, and this is because the mother may have been previously immunised by an Rh-positive fetus, antibodies not being demonstrable before the transfusion because the standard cross-matching procedure was done at ordinary room, rather than at body, temperature. (The different findings as regards temperature, in Papers 2 and 4, can be explained by the fact that agglutination of Rh-positive cells takes place better in a tube, even in the cold, than on a slide).

The third point is that it was noted that there was a high incidence of toxaemia, spontaneous abortions and stillbirths in the *past* obstetric histories of women who later had had transfusion reactions, and this indicated that these women particularly should be investigated for their Rh group.

The main part of the paper concerns the Rhesus status of 153 mothers who had borne children with HDN, but before the results on these were presented the authors carried out a preliminary study on 37 pregnancies from seven patients. Six of the seven were Rh-negative and Rh antibodies were present in their blood.

The main data on the 153 cases showed that about 90% of the women were Rh-negative, in contrast to 15% in the general population, and in Table IV is shown that the husbands and infants were always Rh-positive.

The authors also point out that the reason for only one of several pregnancies resulting in an affected infant in some families is because the father is heterozygous for the gene, and if he is, only approximately 50% of his offspring will be Rh-positive. Another characteristic of the disease, namely that the firstborn is frequently but not always spared, is explained by the supposition that more than one pregnancy with an Rh-positive fetus may be required before a sufficient degree of iso-immunisation is attained.

A very important serological finding in this paper concerns the proportion of Rh-positive individuals in the population depending on the source of the antibody used for testing. Table II shows the results using anti-Rh serum from three different patients: that from E.B. giving 87% Rh-positive and that from M.S. only 73%. The reason for this was not clear at the time but it was subsequently shown that there were several different Rh antigens (called later in the Fisher-Race nomenclature C,c,D,d, and E,e) usually with their corresponding antibodies (Papers 9 and 10). Later testing demonstrated that E.B. had anti-D+C, M.F. had anti-D and M.S. anti-C only.

Furthermore, the authors mention for the first time (page 69, penultimate paragraph) a serum (which later turned out to be anti-c) which gave strong reactions with blood which was Rh-negative with other sera.

In this paper Levine *et al.* take the first step in preventing HDN in advising that

5. Commentary cont.

when Rh-negative mothers need transfusions the donor should be Rh-negative. They also suggest that, where the affected infant needs transfusion, higher levels of haemoglobin are maintained if Rh-negative rather than Rh-positive blood is given.

From P. Levine et al. *(1941). Am. J. Obst. and Gynec.,* **42,** *925-937, Copyright (1941), by kind permission of the authors and The C. V. Mosby Company, St. Louis*

American Journal of Obstetrics and Gynecology

VOL. 42   DECEMBER, 1941   No. 6

Original Communications

THE ROLE OF ISO-IMMUNIZATION IN THE PATHOGENESIS OF ERYTHROBLASTOSIS FETALIS*

PHILIP LEVINE, M.D., NEWARK, N. J., LYMAN BURNHAM, M.D.,
ENGLEWOOD, N. J., E. M. KATZIN, M.D., NEWARK, N. J., AND
PETER VOGEL, M.D., NEW YORK, N. Y.

(From the Division of Laboratories of the Newark Beth Israel Hospital, and the Woman's Hospital of New York)

STUDIES on the cause of intra-group transfusion accidents associated with pregnancy have established the importance of the concept of iso-immunization of the mother by blood factors in the fetus transmitted from the father.[1-5] More recently it was found that the same theory of iso-immunization may serve as the basis for a theory on the pathogenesis of erythroblastosis fetalis, the well-described familial hemolytic disease of the newborn.[3, 4, 6]

The data to be presented indicate that erythroblastosis fetalis results from (1) iso-immunization of the mother by dominant hereditary blood factors in the fetus, as evidenced by the production of immune intra-group agglutinins and (2) the subsequent passage of these maternal agglutinins through the placenta and their continuous action on the susceptible fetal blood. In the great majority of the cases the blood factor involved has been shown to be either identical with or related to the Rh (Rhesus) agglutinogen first described by Landsteiner and Wiener with the aid of rabbit sera prepared by injection of Rhesus blood.[7] In other words, the rabbit anti-Rhesus immune sera and the sera of pregnant women suffering from intra-group transfusion accidents gave almost identical agglutination reactions on all human bloods tested. Accordingly, a pregnant woman whose blood does not contain the Rh factor (Rh–, occurring in about 15 per cent of the general population) if married to an Rh husband (85 per cent in the random population), may produce anti-Rh agglutinins as a result of immunization with the Rh fetal blood. Should these agglutinins penetrate the placenta in suitable concentration they may serve as the source of the intrauterine hemolysis of fetal blood, the characteristic feature of erythroblastosis fetalis.[4]

The term iso-immunization denotes immunization within the same species, i.e., the individual being immunized and source of the antigenic (immunizing) stimulus belong to the same species. It is obvious that

*Aided by a grant from the Blood Betterment Association of New York City.

patients receiving repeated blood transfusions may be subjected to iso-immunization. A prerequisite condition is an antigenic difference in the bloods of recipient and donor. In each instance, this difference is expressed by the presence of a particular blood factor in the donor and its absence in the recipient. Although this condition is frequently satisfied in many cases of repeated transfusions, immune agglutinins are rarely produced because many human blood factors which immunize animals are not antigenic in man. An exception to this rule is the Rh factor which has recently been shown to be responsible for transfusion accidents in Rh– recipients who in the course of several transfusions produced anti-Rh agglutinins.[5, 8, 9] In short, the Rh factor is a good antigen for Rh– mothers as well as for Rh– recipients.

Iso-immunization in pregnancy as the cause of the production of atypical agglutinins responsible for an intra-group transfusion accident was suggested by Levine and Stetson[1] in 1939. In this case the patient (Group O), who harbored a dead fetus for two months, was transfused with her husband's blood (Group O) after the delivery of a macerated fetus (October, 1937). This transfusion was followed by an immediate severe reaction resulting in jaundice, anuria, and ultimate recovery. It was later shown that this patient's blood contained an atypical agglutinin which agglutinated about 80 per cent of Group O bloods. As was to have been expected, this agglutinin gradually diminished in titer and entirely disappeared from the blood at the end of one year. In 1940, or three years after the transfusion accident, it could be shown that the patient was Rh– and her husband Rh+. There is still further evidence that the atypical agglutinin in this patient was anti-Rh in its specificity since the same donors selected as compatible* for subsequent uneventful transfusions in 1937 were later (1940) found to be Rh– in tests with a human anti-Rh serum.

Recent studies have shown that intra-group transfusion accidents previously reported in the literature[5] and additional cases recently observed by Levine, Katzin, and Burnham,[2, 3, 10] occurred frequently in conditions associated with pregnancy. It is characteristic of this group of cases that the accident occurs at the first transfusion. Accordingly, the immune agglutinin which must have been present prior to the transfusion but could not be demonstrated with the usual cross-matching procedure, was probably induced by the pregnancy.

The atypical agglutinins in some of these cases were shown to have the unusual property of greater activity at 37° C. than at 20° C. (low room temperature). For this reason, the term "warm agglutinins" was applied to these antibodies.[10] This observation offers a possible explanation for the frequent failure of the cross-matching tests to detect this form of intra-group incompatibility. It is therefore recommended that in performing the compatibility test, the patient's serum and donor's blood cell suspension be incubated at 37° C. for thirty minutes before the mixture is centrifuged (one minute at 500 r.p.m.) for sedimentation and subsequent resuspension.[4, 11, 12]

The relationship of iso-immunization and certain pathologic states in the pregnant woman or in the fetus was pointed out by Levine and Katzin.[2] In an analysis of 12 intra-group transfusion accidents associated with pregnancy in which atypical agglutinins were demonstrated, these authors observed a high incidence of toxemia, spontaneous abortions and miscarriages, and stillbirths in the past obstetric histories.

---

*These tests were carried out by Dr. E. M. Katzin.

Accordingly, it was assumed that "there does appear to be a correlation of the complications with the incidence of atypical agglutinins, and one can speculate as to their relationship."

This observation made it possible to enlarge the source of the material to be studied instead of limiting it to the comparatively rare transfusion accidents in pregnancy.

Shortly thereafter, one of us (L. B.) observed a patient who suffered from a severe transfusion accident following the delivery of an infant in whom a diagnosis of erythroblastosis fetalis was established. The obstetric history in this case (R. C.)* and in still another case (J. L.) not transfused, were so striking as to suggest a theoretical basis for the pathogenesis of erythroblastosis fetalis.[3, 4] One of these mothers (R. C.) had three pregnancies, the first and third of which resulted in infants with erythroblastosis fetalis and the second pregnancy terminated in a macerated fetus. In the other case (J. L.), there had been 10 pregnancies, the first of which resulted in a normal infant; there were 3 spontaneous abortions and the remaining 6 pregnancies resulted in infants who survived one to three days. In at least 3 of these neonatal deaths there was sufficient evidence to support a diagnosis of erythroblastosis fetalis. This woman's blood was tested in the eighth month of her eleventh pregnancy. Since atypical agglutinins were already present, it was anticipated that the baby to be born would be affected. Actually, the infant suffered from anemia of the newborn, one of the several manifestations of erythroblastosis fetalis.

The two cases mentioned were among the seven patients with 37 pregnancies which formed the basis for the preliminary observation that the pathogenesis of erythroblastosis fetalis depends on iso-immunization of the mother by the fetus. The findings in these 37 pregnancies are reproduced in Table I.

TABLE I. OUTCOME OF 37 PREGNANCIES IN 7 PATIENTS

(*Modified After Levine, Katzin and Burnham*[3])

Normal babies	10
Babies with erythroblastosis	7
Neonatal deaths	3
Stillbirths	5
Abortions or miscarriages (at least 6 spontaneous)	10
No data available	2

In 6 of these 7 women in whose blood atypical agglutinins were demonstrated, there were indications that the specificity of the antibodies corresponded to the anti-Rh. Obviously, the blood cells of these women did not contain the Rh factor and were therefore Rh–. These considerations suggested a statistical study of the bloods of women known to have given birth to infants in whom a diagnosis of erythroblastosis fetalis was established. If iso-immunization with the Rh factor plays a significant role in the pathogenesis of this disease, one should expect to find (1) a high incidence of Rh– reactions in this group of selected mothers and (2) a high incidence of anti-Rh agglutinins in their sera.

Whenever possible, the bloods of the fathers and the affected children were also tested, for, if the iso-immunization theory is correct, then 100 per cent of the fathers and the affected children in the series of Rh– mothers should be Rh+.

----

*Another patient of Dr. Burnham (G. B.) who died from a transfusion anuria following the delivery of an infant with fetal hydrops, was mentioned in previous papers.[2, 3, 10] These two cases were the first to show the relationship of intra-group transfusion accidents and erythroblastosis fetalis. A more detailed discussion is given in a paper by Burnham.[13]

In each case, suspensions of red blood cells were tested with potent human anti-Rh agglutinins to determine whether the blood was Rh– or Rh+. Since the Rh factor is a constant immutable hereditary property of the red blood cells, it is obvious that such tests could be made at any interval after the last delivery of an affected infant.

The presence or absence of atypical agglutinins was determined by testing each serum with blood suspensions of at least 10 individuals of Group O, of which at least 1 was Rh–. It is obvious that the possibility of demonstrating atypical agglutinins was better if the serum was studied soon after birth of the affected infant.

EXPERIMENTAL

Selection of the Cases.—This study is based chiefly on blood tests of 153 mothers who delivered one or more infants suffering from one of three clinical forms of erythroblastosis fetalis, i.e., fetal hydrops, icterus gravis, or anemia of the newborn. Of these, 115 were under observation either by one of the authors or by other collaborators.* Thirty-eight mothers were referred to us from several sources mainly outside of the metropolitan area of New York. The diagnosis in the affected infants in the latter group could be accepted on the basis of a history submitted by the physicians referring the case. In each case, some or all characteristic features were present, such as a significant obstetrical history of previous miscarriages or stillbirths, or infants with erythroblastosis fetalis—and the accepted diagnostic criteria such as severe icterus at or shortly after birth, enlarged liver and spleen, excess of normoblasts in the peripheral circulation, progressive anemia, and in fatal cases post-mortem findings of extramedullary hematopoiesis.

In addition to the 153 mothers of infants in whom a diagnosis of erythroblastosis fetalis was established, data will be presented below (p. 933) in a smaller number of women whose pregnancies terminated in habitual abortion, miscarriages, stillbirths, or macerated fetuses.

Technique of the Agglutination Tests.—*Diagnosis of Rh+ and Rh– blood:* One or more drops of anti-Rh serum are mixed in small test tubes (75 × 10 mm.) with 2 drops of a washed 1 per cent to 2 per cent cell suspension (this corresponds to a suspension made by adding one drop of whole blood to 4 c.c. saline). The cell suspension is preferably prepared from the clot.

The tubes are shaken and incubated in a water-bath at 37° C. for one hour, at the end of which period each tube is properly identified and all tubes are centrifuged at low speed (500 r.p.m.) for one minute. After replacing the tubes in the rack, the sedimented cells are resuspended by gentle shaking and readings are recorded. Those mixtures in which no gross agglutination is visible are examined microscopically (low magnification) by withdrawing with the aid of a glass rod some of the mixture onto a slide. Bloods showing no agglutination are Rh–.

Detection of Anti-Rh in Human Sera.—Two drops of the serum to be tested are added to each of 10 small test tubes and each tube receives two drops of washed cell suspension of ten different Group O bloods. As a rule, at least one Rh– blood is included. The tests are incubated at 37° C. for one hour, and readings are made after centrifuging the tests and resuspension of the sediments as indicated above.

All cases were tested with one or more of three potent anti-Rh sera. Since the first serum employed (December, 1940) was of Group A (patient M. F.) all bloods of Groups O and A could be tested directly.

*Drs. L. Goldman, C. Javert, S. Polayes, and H. Schwartz.

In order to test bloods of Groups B and AB, it was necessary to treat this serum with an Rh– blood of Group B, in order to remove the normal iso-agglutinin anti-B. In April, 1941, the second potent anti-Rh serum was found (Patient E. B.). Since this serum belonged to Group AB, it could be used directly on bloods of all groups. In May, 1941, the third anti-Rh serum (M. S.) of Group O became available.

In the latter part of these studies, bloods of all groups could be tested in parallel with three anti-Rh sera. This became possible because of the availability of Witebsky's group specific soluble Substances A and B,[15]* the addition of which in small quantities inhibited the action of agglutinin anti-A and anti-B without affecting the activity of anti-Rh.

In any event, each of the three sera gave distinct agglutination reactions so that there was never any doubt as to the diagnosis of Rh+ or Rh–, in any blood tested with a particular serum.

A brief obstetric history of these patients is given below:

1. *M. F. (Group A):* A patient of Dr. P. Vogel had 7 pregnancies of which 6 were full term and one terminated at six months. A diagnosis of erythroblastosis fetalis was made in the last two infants, the most recent one in December, 1940. Serum obtained several weeks post-partum contained potent anti-Rh agglutinins. The agglutinins remained very active though they were somewhat weaker in the blood specimen drawn in May, 1941.

2. *E. B. (Group AB):* A patient of Dr. Freed had two full-term pregnancies. The first infant was very pale at birth and survived but one and one-half hours. No other data were available. The second infant, born April, 1941, showed classical symptoms of congenital anemia.

3. *M. S. (Group O):* A patient of Dr. Paul delivered a normal infant in 1931; this pregnancy was followed by a long interval of sterility. The second pregnancy (April, 1941) resulted in an infant suffering from icterus gravis.

Specificities of the Anti-Rh sera, M. F., E. B., and M. S.—A complicating feature in the behavior of the human anti-Rh sera is their failure to give entirely parallel reactions when tested with numerous bloods.[14, 17] Thus these sera give varying incidences of Rh– reactions (Table II).

TABLE II. RESULTS OF PARALLEL TESTS ON 334 RANDOM BLOODS OF ALL GROUPS

ANTI-Rh SERUM FROM PATIENT	PER CENT	
	Rh+	Rh–
E. B.	87	13
M. F.	85	15
M. S.	73	27

The greater incidence of Rh– reactions with serum M. S. is manifested by the fact that some bloods diagnosed as Rh+ in their reactions with sera E. B. or M. F. are not agglutinated by serum M. S.● This fact is applicable to the bloods of only 3 of the 29 mothers which were tested with each of the three sera.

These serologic observations which are of more than academic interest, will be published in detail elsewhere, but reference will be made later (page 932) to the significance of these findings in connection with the iso-immunization by the fetus.

_____

*Supplied by courtesy of Eli Lilly & Co.

●Very rarely, the converse specific effect is obtained, i.e., blood Rh– with serum M. F. is Rh+ with serum E. B. or M. S.

Statistical Data on the Rh Blood Factor in 153 Mothers of Infants with Erythroblastosis Fetalis.—This study reveals an incidence of about 90 per cent Rh– reactions in contrast to 15 per cent Rh– reactions in the random population. The actual analysis is rendered somewhat complex because not all bloods were tested with each of the three anti-Rh sera (Table III).

TABLE III

ANTI-Rh SERUM	NUMBER OF MOTHERS' BLOODS TESTED	PER CENT	
		Rh+	Rh–
M. F.	142	10	90
E. B.	60	15	85
M. S.	28	7	93
Combined results	153	7	93

The higher incidence of Rh+ with serum E. B. is due to the fact that more mothers Rh+ with serum M. F. were tested with serum E. B. than with serum M. S. At least one of the bloods Rh+ with serum E. B. can be considered Rh–, because this blood contains very active anti-Rh agglutinins.

Three mothers whose blood was Rh+ with serum M. F. or E. B. were Rh– with serum M. S. These three cases listed as Rh– could be considered as instances in which iso-immunization could occur, because in two instances the husband's blood, and in the third the affected child's blood were Rh+ with each of the three sera.

The striking difference in the incidence of the Rh factor in the selected population of mothers with erythroblastic babies and in the random population strongly supports the concept of iso-immunization. Since the incidence of Rh– bloods is very high in these mothers, it could be anticipated on the basis of the iso-immunization theory that the affected infants and the fathers in the series of Rh– mothers are exclusively Rh+. As will be shown such results were obtained in tests on 89 fathers and on 76 infants in whom a diagnosis of erythroblastosis fetalis was made (Table IV).

TABLE IV. INCIDENCE OF Rh+ AND Rh– IN HUSBANDS AND AFFECTED INFANTS OF THE 141 Rh– MOTHERS

	NUMBER TESTED	Rh+	Rh–	EXPECTANCY OF Rh– IN RANDOM POPULATION
Husbands	89	89	0	13 (89 × 15%)
Affected infants	76	76	0	11 (76 × 15%)

The findings in this table are based on tests with serum M. F. which gives an incidence of 15% Rh– reactions.

The findings in Tables III and IV strongly indicate the iso-immunization of the Rh– mother by the Rh factor in fetal blood. The final proof for such iso-immunization can be supplied only by the demonstration of anti-Rh agglutinins in the mother's blood. Obviously, the likelihood of finding such agglutinins will be greater if the mother's blood is tested soon after the delivery of an infant suffering from erythroblastosis fetalis. This is borne out by the findings presented in Table V.

TABLE V. INCIDENCE OF ANTI-Rh AGGLUTININS IN 141 Rh– MOTHERS

INTERVAL AFTER LAST DELIVERY OF AN AFFECTED INFANT	AGGLUTININS PRESENT	AGGLUTININS NOT FOUND
2 months post partum	33	37
2 months to 1 year past partum	5	15
1 year or longer post partum	2	39
During next pregnancy	2	5
No data	0	3
Total	42	99

The failure to detect anti-Rh agglutinins in many cases tested shortly after the delivery of an affected infant does not exclude their presence at some previous period during the course of their pregnancy. Since the course of antibody production in general is characterized by a gradual rise, a period of maximum activity, and gradual disappearance, it is conceivable that in some cases anti-Rh agglutinins, after exerting their lytic effect on the fetus, rapidly disappeared from the blood so that none could be demonstrated at the time of delivery. It is therefore indicated that the bloods of mothers known to have delivered babies with erythroblastosis fetalis be studied at several intervals during course of future pregnancies. Furthermore, it is conceivable that antibodies capable of reacting in vivo cannot be demonstrated because of limitations in the sensitivity of the technique employed.

It is of great interest that the anti-Rh agglutinins may be demonstrable for such unusually long periods, as two years post partum. Probably the long duration indicates an intense degree of iso-immunization which may perhaps influence the outcome of the next pregnancy with an Rh+ fetus. More specifically, reference is made to the clinical observation on the high incidence of spontaneous abortions and miscarriages in mothers of infants with erythroblastosis fetalis (p. 933).[3, 18, 19]

The results shown in Tables III, IV, and V indicate that a combination of Rh− mother, Rh+ father, and affected infant can be used as a laboratory test to support a diagnosis of erythroblastosis fetalis. Such results which are present in about 90 per cent of the cases should be of value in the diagnosis of mild, atypical, or borderline cases of this condition.

The 11 Cases in Which Iso-immunization with Rh is Excluded.— When these exceptional cases were first observed, it was assumed that blood factors other than Rh may also induce iso-immunization. This explanation seemed plausible since Levine and Polayes[20] had already demonstrated a new blood factor by means of an atypical hemolysin found to be the cause of a post-partum transfusion reaction.* Indeed, this antibody seemed to differentiate the bloods of several of the Rh+ mothers from those of their husbands or affected children in a manner compatible with the concept of iso-immunization. However, the results were only suggestive and further study was hampered by the weak activity of the antibody.

More decisive results, however, were obtained with the reactions of an atypical agglutinin found in the serum of one of the 11 Rh+ mothers (patient K. F.).[21] This patient of Dr. Javert had one full-term, normal pregnancy; one infant with erythroblastosis fetalis (1937) and a missed abortion. When tested she was again several months pregnant. The antibody in this serum gives strong reactions almost exclusively on bloods which are Rh− with serum M. S. Accordingly, the blood factor identified by this atypical agglutinin must have some genetic relationship with Rh. Since this serum became available late in the course of this study, the bloods of the remaining mothers of this group must be retested with this new agglutinin.

Reference again is made (p. 931) to the bloods of 3 mothers of erythroblastic babies which were Rh+ with two anti-Rh sera but Rh− with the third serum M. S. These cases were included in the Rh− series because in one instance the husband and in the other the affected child were Rh+ with each of the three anti-Rh sera.

---

*This mother had 4 miscarriages and 8 full-term, presumably normal infants.

The Theory of Heterospecific Pregnancy.—The Distribution of Blood Factors A, B, and Rh in Red Blood Cells, Tissue Cells, and Body Fluids.—It is of interest that a difference in the blood groups of mother and infant was the basis of an older theory on the pathogenesis of familial icterus gravis.†[22, 23] In the literature, this concept has been referred to as "heterospecific pregnancy." The theory, since abandoned for lack of evidence, does not differ in principle from the iso-immunization theory in which the Rh factor plays such a prominent role. According to the concept of heterospecific pregnancy, given a mother of Group O and an infant of Group A (or Group B), the maternal anti-A (or anti-B) agglutinins are theoretically capable of acting on the Group A (or Group B) fetal blood. Actually, there is now evidence that in the example cited the mother's normal iso-agglutinin anti-A (or anti-B) is increased in titer as a result of iso-immunization with the A (or B) blood of the fetus.[24, 25] Nevertheless, the maternal agglutinins are specifically inhibited from acting on the fetal blood because of the wide distribution of the A and B factors in tissues and body fluids.

However, this applies to about 80 per cent of all individuals (secretors)[26] and if a fetus of Group A belongs to the class of non-secretors (20 per cent), it is conceivable that the maternal iso-agglutinin anti-A may serve as the source of the intrauterine hemolytic process. Accordingly, the older theory of heterospecific pregnancy may have to be invoked at least for selected cases of erythroblastosis fetalis in which the Rh or other blood factors fail to indicate iso-immunization by the fetus.

From these considerations on heterospecific pregnancy and in view of the established importance of the Rh factor in the pathogenesis of erythroblastosis fetalis, it can be assumed that the Rh factor is probably not present in tissue cells or body fluids, but rather is limited to red blood cells only. Otherwise, the maternal anti-Rh agglutinins would be specifically inactivated and therefore incapable of inducing the hemolytic action on the Rh+ fetal blood. Tests made by Levine and Katzin[27] with numerous specimens of saliva, a few specimens of sperm cells, and seminal fluid, indicate that the Rh factor is not present in the material tested.*

Iso-immunization in Habitual Abortion and Stillbirth.—Reports from the literature indicate that the obstetric history of mothers of infants with erythroblastosis fetalis reveals a high incidence of abortions, miscarriages, and stillbirths. Macklin[18] and Darrow[19] stated that the mechanism responsible for the pathogenesis of erythroblastosis fetalis applies also for these abortions and stillbirths. This view is supported by the results in the present study. That iso-immunization by the fetus and subsequent action of maternal agglutinins on fetal blood may be the mechanism of these abortions and stillbirths is indicated in the data presented in Table I.[3, 4]

Another group of women were investigated because of their history of habitual abortion and stillbirths, but these women had no infants with erythroblastosis fetalis. Many of these women were Rh− but a satisfactory statistical analysis similar to the study on erythroblastosis fetalis is more difficult because habitual abortions and stillbirths may be manifestations of many conditions. Nevertheless, there is sufficient evidence

†At that time (1923) the more comprehensive term, erythroblastosis fetalis, was not yet in use

*Similar observations on saliva were recently reported by Wiener and Forer.[28]

in at least five† cases of this group to include them with the mothers of erythroblastic infants, because iso-immunization by the Rh factor in the fetus could be demonstrated. In each of these cases, anti-Rh agglutinins were observed. Three of these patients suffered from intragroup transfusion accidents following an abortion or stillbirths.

Two of these 5 patients had just delivered presumably normal infants in spite of the presence of moderately active anti-Rh agglutinins. Unfortunately, hematologic and other clinical data were not obtained so that a mild form of erythroblastosis fetalis could not be entirely excluded. However, the obstetric histories reveal that one of these patients (H. H.) had three consecutive miscarriages and the other (L. L.) had two miscarriages and one premature infant who survived for ten days.

The association of intragroup transfusion accidents, in the presence of atypical agglutinins, in three patients following an abortion, a miscarriage, and a stillbirth, respectively, was observed by us in the analysis of reports by Parr and Krischner,[29] Johnson,[30] and Zacho.[31] Other instances of intragroup transfusion accidents following abortions, miscarriages, or stillbirths, in the absence of atypical agglutinins have been reported by several authors.[32, 33] Very probably the transfusion accidents reported in the five papers quoted are ultimately attributable to iso-immunization by the fetus.

In any event, it is the action of maternal immune agglutinins on the fetus which may cause its death at any stage of its development so that the same mechanism may be responsible for erythroblastosis fetalis in the surviving infant as well as some cases of habitual abortion.

DISCUSSION

The numerous theories on the pathogenesis of erythroblastosis fetalis were recently reviewed by Darrow[19] who, in a hypothetical discussion, anticipated the iso-immunization theory. This author suggested an antigen-antibody reaction based on differences in maternal and fetal hemoglobin or other constituents of red blood cells as the most plausible explanation. A similar view was previously mentioned by Ottenberg,[23] but neither author presented experimental data to support their theses.

The findings presented establish the significant role of iso-immunization of the mother by blood factors in the fetus in the pathogenesis of erythroblastosis fetalis. Of prime importance is the Rh factor in the fetal blood which is transmitted as a dominant mendelian gene from the father.[14] Statistical evidence was offered to prove that its presence in the blood of the father and affected infant is a prerequisite condition for the iso-immunization of the Rh– mother. But in the final analysis, the proof of iso-immunization by the Rh factor was the demonstration in many instances of anti-Rh agglutinins in the mother's blood. It is the continuous intrauterine action of anti-Rh agglutinins with the Rh positive fetal blood over a period varying from weeks to months which causes a progressive hemolysis of fetal blood.

The reaction of anti-Rh antibody and Rh blood takes the form of agglutination in the test tube but in the fetal circulation the end result is hemolysis. Attempts to demonstrate corresponding hemolytic reaction in the test tube by the addition of fresh human serum have so far failed.

One of the most striking features of erythroblastosis fetalis is the wide variety of clinical syndromes it embraces, such as, the extremely fatal form of fetal hydrops and the mild, frequently unrecognizable

---

†Four of these patients were discussed in our previous papers.[1-3]

anemias of the newborn.[34] These clinical forms are probably the result of varying degrees and duration of iso-immunization during the course of the pregnancy. Nothing is as yet known concerning the exact time and conditions during the course of the pregnancy when iso-immunization begins. If some cases of habitual abortions are a manifestation of iso-immunization, then the process may start shortly after conception occurs. At any rate, it is conceivable that the prolonged action of immune iso-agglutinins on the susceptible fetal blood may induce more severe damage than the action of agglutinins produced very late in the course of a pregnancy.

The clinical observation has been made that some infants may be born apparently free from the condition, but in the course of a few days, severe anemia and jaundice make their appearance. It is difficult to correlate this fact with the iso-immunization theory since the infant after birth should be free from any further action by the maternal agglutinins. The source of the delayed hemolysis has been suspected to be the colostrum, but in a number of these cases the infant was not breast fed. An alternative explanation is the storage of mother's agglutinins by the tissue of the fetus so that their subsequent release may then induce the hemolysis several days after birth.

A few practical applications based on these studies are of importance to the obstetrician. In the first place the data presented make it clear why caution must be exercised in selecting compatible donors for transfusing mothers of infants with erythroblastosis fetalis or those with a history of habitual abortions, a stillbirth, or a neonatal death. It is of interest that 8 of the 141 Rh– mothers suffered from severe intragroup transfusion reactions. Such accidents can be prevented if Rh– donors are available for Rh– mothers[3] and if the modified compatibility (cross-matching) test be employed for the detection of the "warm" anti-Rh agglutinins (p. 927).[4, 11, 12]

Furthermore, there are indications from a small number of cases that the affected infant maintains higher levels of hemoglobin and red blood cell counts if he is transfused with Rh– blood instead of Rh+ blood. The rationale for this suggestion is drawn from the fact that the infant's own Rh+ blood is undergoing destruction.[35]

The hereditary nature of erythroblastosis fetalis, hitherto unknown, can now be stated in terms of the iso-immunization theory. In some families, every pregnancy but perhaps the first, terminates in either an abortion, a stillbirth, or an infant with erythroblastosis fetalis; while in other families, only one of several pregnancies results in an affected infant. Since the Rh factor is inherited as a simple mendelian dominant,[14] it is obvious from a genetic standpoint, that this striking difference in familial incidence of the disease is determined by the homozygosity (RhRh) or heterozygosity (Rhrh) of the father's blood.[36] The genetic details and evidence supporting this concept will be given elsewhere. It is, however, appropriate to state at this point, that the first born is frequently but not always spared because more than one pregnancy with an Rh+ fetus may be required before a sufficient degree of iso-immunization is attained.

It has been recorded by Javert[37] that erythroblastosis fetalis in one of its several forms, occurs once in 400 deliveries, but it is probable that this condition has a still higher frequency, especially if some cases of habitual abortion and stillbirths are manifestations of iso-immunization. Actually, the incidence of matings in which iso-immunization with Rh may occur (Rh+ husband and Rh– wife) is 85 by 15 or 13 per cent of all matings. Consequently, one would expect a much higher incidence of erythroblastosis fetalis. There are, however, a number of factors tending to reduce this incidence, such as, for example, the current tendency to small families and the inability of many Rh– women to respond to iso-immunization.

The data on erythroblastosis fetalis and the recent studies on the iso-immunization with the blood factors A and B in the absence of any pathologic conditions in the mother or the infant indicates that immunizing substances derived from the fetus make their way through the placental barrier into the maternal circulation. Since the Rh factor, in contrast to the A and B substances, is probably limited to only red blood cells, it is assumed that fetal blood in one form or another penetrates the villus in sufficient quantity to induce immunization in the mother.

SUMMARY AND CONCLUSIONS

1. In 93 per cent of the cases investigated, erythroblastosis fetalis results from the iso-immunization of the Rh– mother by the Rh factor in the red blood cells of the fetus.

2. In the remaining cases, blood factors other than Rh are responsible for the iso-immunization.

3. Agglutination tests for the Rh factor are of value as a laboratory aid in the diagnosis of erythroblastosis fetalis.

4. The pathologic manifestations of this disease are produced by the intrauterine action of maternal immune agglutinins on the susceptible red blood cells of the fetus.

5. It is probable that iso-immunization is also the cause of a certain proportion of habitual abortions and stillbirths.

6. Intra-group transfusion accidents associated with pregnancy can now be prevented by the use of Rh– donors and by means of modified cross-matching test.

The authors wish to express their appreciation to Dr. William Antopol, Pathologist and Director of Laboratories, Newark Beth Israel Hospital, for examination of the histologic sections and valuable suggestions, and to Miss Estelle Richardson for her technical assistance.

REFERENCES

(1) Levine, Ph., and Stetson, R.: J. A. M. A. 113: 126, 1939. (2) Levine, Ph., and Katzin, E. M.: Proc. Soc. Exper. Biol. & Med. 45: 343, 1940. (3) Levine, Ph., Katzin, E. M., and Burnham, L.: J. A. M. A. 116: 825, 1941. (4) Levine, Ph.: AM. J. OBST. & GYNEC. 42: 165, 1941. (5) Wiener, A. S., and Peters, H. R.: Ann. Int. Med. 13: 2306, 1940. (6) Levine, Ph., Vogel, P., Katzin, E. M., and Burnham, L.: Science 94: 371, 1941. (7) Landsteiner, K., and Wiener, A. S.: Proc. Soc. Exper. Biol. & Med. 43: 223, 1940. (8) Levine, P., Katzin, E. M., Vogel, P., and Burnham, L.: Symposium of the American Human Serum Association, June 2, 1941, Cleveland. (9) Wiener, A. S.: Arch. Path. 32: 227, 1941. (10) Levine, P., Katzin, E. M., and Burnham, L.: Proc. Soc. Exper. Biol. & Med. 45: 346, 1940. (11) Levine, P., Katzin, E. M., and Vogel, P.: In preparation. (12) Levine, P.: Cited by Wiener.[9] (13) Burnham, L.: AM. J. OBST. & GYNEC. 42: 389, 1941. (14) Landsteiner, K., and Wiener, A. S.: J. Exper. Med. 74: 309, 1941. (15) Witebsky, E., Klendshoj, N. C., and Swanson, P.: J. A. M. A. 116: 2654, 1941. (16) Levine, Ph.: Unpublished observations. (17) Levine, Ph., and Katzin, E. M.: Unpublished observations. (18) Macklin, M. T.: Am. J. Dis. Child. 53: 1245, 1937. (19) Darrow, R. R.: Arch. Path. 25: 378, 1938. (20) Levine, Ph., and Polayes, S. H.: Ann. Int. Med. 14: 1903, 1941. (21) Levine, Ph., Javert, C., and Katzin, E. M.: In preparation. (22) Hirszfeld, L.: Konstitutionsserolgie und Blutgruppenforschung, 1928, Berlin, Julius Springer. (23) Ottenberg, R.: J. A. M. A. 81: 295, 1923. (24) Jonsson, B.: Acta path. et Microbiol. Scandinav. 13: 424, 1936. (25) Levine, Ph.: Unpublished data. (26) Schiff, F., and Sasaki, H.: Ztschr. f. Immunitätsforsch. u. exper. Therap. 77: 129, 1932. (27) Levine, Ph., and Katzin, E. M.: Proc. Soc. Exper. Biol. & Med. (In press.) (28) Wiener, A. S., and Forer, S.: Proc. Soc. Exper. Biol. & Med. 47: 215, 1941. (29) Parr, E. L., and Krischner, H.: J. A. M. A. 98: 47, 1932. (30) Johnson, R. A., and Conway, J. F.: AM. J. OBST. & GYNEC. 26: 255, 1936. (31) Zacho, A.: Ztschr. f. Rassenphysiol. 8: 1, 1936. (32) Goldring, W., and Graef, I.: Arch. Int. Med. 58: 825, 1936. (33) Bernstein, A.: AM. J. OBST. & GYNEC. 39: 1045, 1940. (34) Diamond, L. K., Blackfan, K. D., and Baty, J. M.: J. Pediat. 1: 269, 1932. (35) Katzin, E. M., Vogel, P., and Levine, P.: Unpublished data. (36) Levine, Ph.: In preparation. (37) Javert, C.: AM. J. OBST. & GYNEC. 34: 1042, 1937.

Papers 6 & 7

6.   Levine, P. (1943). Serological factors as possible causes in spontaneous abortions. *J. Hered., 34,* 71-80. (Extracts).

7.   Race, R. R. and Sanger, Ruth. (1950). *Blood Groups in Man.* (1st ed.). pp 234-6. Blackwell, Oxford. (Extract).

Commentary

One of the striking phenomena associated with Rh incompatibility between mother and fetus is how infrequently the baby is in fact affected, and there are numerous reasons for this. One important one is ABO incompatibility between mother and fetus. It was Levine (1943) who first drew attention to the fact that in the matings of Rh-negative mothers who had produced erythroblastotic infants the incidence of ABO incompatible matings was lower than normal, i.e. 25% compared with 35% in a random sample. Levine did not however draw the inference that this incompatibility was protective, though he is often quoted as doing so. His paper simply drew attention to the fact that blood factors other than Rh may be responsible for abortions and stillbirths.

The relevant section of Levine's paper follows (extract 1, page 76). It should be noted that it first deals with ABO compatibility or incompatibility in women who had produced abortions and stillbirths *not* attributable to Rh, and the details of the compatible matings, are given in Table V. In Table VI it will be seen that ABO incompatibility is associated with a higher abortion or stillbirth rate than would be expected. But where Levine's Rh-negative series is concerned the reverse is the case.

In the last category of Table VI Rh-positive mothers with erythroblastotic babies show a higher incidence of ABO incompatibility than the general population. Levine suggests later in the paper that this may be connected with the secretor status of the baby, meaning presumably that, if the baby is a non-secretor*, the blood group substances in its body fluids 'mop up' some of the mother's antibody, and therefore the baby is more likely to have ABO HDN. The second extract deals with women who abort and have a high titre of anti-A or anti-B and yet whose babies are not jaundiced.

The idea that ABO incompatibility might actually be protective against Rh immunisation was first put forward by Race and Sanger in 1950 (Paper 7), and it was their fundamental suggestion which raised the hope that prophylaxis might be possible (Paper 25). Race and Sanger give three possible explanations as to how this protection might be brought about. They are a model of clarity and require no comment, except that we think Fisher's view (last paragraph) is incorrect because of the experiments of Stern *et al.* on Rh-negative men (Paper 28).

*Some individuals not only have the ABO blood group antigens on their red cells but also in their body fluids, and when this is so they are termed 'secretors'.

From P. Levine (1943). J. Hered., 34, 71-80. Copyright (1943), by kind permission of the author and the Longman Group

SEROLOGICAL FACTORS AS POSSIBLE CAUSES IN SPONTANEOUS ABORTIONS*

PHILIP LEVINE[†]

Division of Laboratories, Newark Beth Israel Hospital

Extract 1

Shortly after the pathogenesis of erythroblastosis fetalis was established, the writer had an opportunity to study the bloods of women having histories of abortions and stillbirths not attributable to erythroblastosis fetalis. It soon became evident that the *Rh* blood factor played only a comparatively minor role in these cases.[22] However, a difference was observed in the blood group of the mother on the one hand and of the father and of the fetus on the other, which could be interpreted as isoimmunition by the blood factors *A* and *B*. In these instances the mother's blood was lacking the blood factors *A* and *B,* one of which was present in the father and in the affected fetus. This sort of mating is defined as incompatible in contrast to those compatible matings in which the blood factors of the father and of the mother either are identical or in which the mother carries the dominant blood factor.

The two sorts of matings are classified in Table V.

TABLE V. Blood Group Matings.

Compatible		Incompatible
	♂ × ♀	
♂ × ♀	B × AB	♂ × ♀
O × O	AB × AB	A × O
O × A		B × O
O × B		A × B
A × A		B × A
B × B		AB × O
O × AB		AB × A
A × AB		AB × B

If we assume random mating between individuals of the four blood groups in the proportions found among the white population of the United States ($O =$ 45 per cent, $A = 41$ per cent, $B = 10$ per cent and $AB = 4$ per cent), 65 per cent of all matings would be compatible and 35 per cent incompatible In a group of cases selected because of two or more instances of unexplained early or late fetal death it is significant that this ratio is altered so that there is a higher incidence of incompatible matings. This evidence along with other significant data is tabulated in Table VI.

It is noteworthy that in the matings of the *Rh—* mothers with erythroblastotic infants the incidence of incompatible blood group matings is even lower than normal. Furthermore, in the exceptional group, i.e., where the mother is *Rh+*, the incidence of incompatible matings is considerably higher than normal. Shortly after these observations were made on a smaller series, the author found Taussig's reference[35] to the significant findings of Paroli and Tranquilli-Leali which are also recorded in Table VI.

The values given by the Italian workers in terms of homospecific and heterospecific pregnancy do not correspond with the figures given in Table VI which were derived by the author from an analysis of their data in terms of the concept of isoimmunization.

Although the statistical data presented in Table VI are most suggestive and very likely significant, they are not as convincing as the studies in erythroblastosis fetalis. This is to be expected since the heterogenous group studied is not by any means as clearly defined a clinical

TABLE VI. Isoimmunization by Factors *A* and *B*.

Matings	Compatible	Incompatible
Random	65%	35%
115 with two or more miscarriages	46	54
43 with two miscarriages or stillbirths	44	56
41 with fetal death*	41.5	58.5
215 Rh— mothers[†]	75	25
28 Rh+ mothers[†]	50	50

*Paroli[32] and Tranquilli-Leali.[36]
[†]Mothers of erythroblastotic infants.

*Read June 19, 1942, at the Conference on Abortions Problems sponsored by the National Committee on Maternal Health.

[†]Aided by grants from the Blood Transfusion Association of New York and the National Committee on Maternal Health.

entity as is erythroblastosis fetalis. There are obviously several factors responsible for fetal death in this group, but these preliminary studies strongly suggest that at least one of them will be found to be isoimmunization of the mother by the incompatible *A* or *B* blood of the fetus.

Extract 2 The significant fact is that in contrast to the *Rh* factor, the *A* and *B* blood factors are present not only in the red blood cells, but also in the tissue cells and body fluids of the fetus. However, this applies to more than 80 per cent of the cases (secretors), and in the remaining cases, described as non-secretors, the *A* and *B* blood factors may perhaps be limited to red blood cells.[25] Nevertheless, proof is still to be provided that this is the explanation for the high incidence of incompatible blood group matings in the small group of *Rh+* mothers of erythroblastotic infants included in Table VI.

Literature Cited

22. LEVINE, P., L. BURNHAM, E. M. KATZIN, and P. VOGEL. *Am. J. Obst. and Gyn.* 42: '65 1941.

25. LEVINE, P., and E. M. KATZIN *Proc. Soc. Exp. Biol. and Med.* 48:126. 1941.

32. PAROLI, G. *Rivista Ital. di Ginecologia* 7:388. 1928.

35. TAUSSIG, F. J. Abortions, Spontaneous and Induced. P. 100. C. V. Mosby, 1936.

36. TRANQUILLI-LEALI, K. *Rivista Ital. di Ginecologia* 14:492. 1932.

BLOOD GROUPS IN MAN

The ABO groups: an index of one protective agency

Levine[9] in 1943 drew attention to the curious fact that mothers of children with haemolytic disease due to anti-*Rh* were more often compatibly mated on the *ABO* system than were unselected women. A compatible mating in this sense is one in which the husband could be a blood donor to his wife (as far as the *ABO* groups are concerned). There is no longer any doubt about the magnitude of this effect, as Table 77 shows.

Three conceivable explanations of this effect of the *ABO* groups on the production of anti-*Rh* suggest themselves. The first has received attention because of its possible bearing on the problem of

TABLE 77

THE *ABO* GROUP RELATIONSHIP BETWEEN HUSBAND AND WIFE IN
FAMILIES WITH HAEMOLYTIC DISEASE DUE TO ANTI-*Rh*

(From van Loghem and Spaander,[10] 1948)

Pourcentages prévus de combinaisons matrimoniales:		*Compatibilité du système* ABO	*Incompatibilité du système* ABO
Pourcentages trouvés par:	*Nombre de cas examinés*	(66%)	(34%)
		%	%
Bessis	48	89·5	10·5
Levine	215	75	25
Race	247	84	16
Wiener	96	71	29
Broman	33	81	19
Van Loghem et Spaander	240	87	13

prevention of *Rh* sensitization; if an *Rh*-negative mother of, say, group *O* has group *A* children, her antibody-making tissues may be too fully occupied in making more anti-*A* to make anti-*Rh*. It is our impression, however, that people who can make one antibody are perhaps unusually capable of making others, but we have too little evidence for this to be considered a serious objection to the hypothesis. There is, however, another explanation which seems more likely; if *Rh* sensitization is due to foetal red cells entering the maternal circulation, it seems possible that if they carry, for example, the *A* antigen, and the maternal serum contains anti-*A*, then these invading cells may be eliminated before they have time to act as an *Rh* antigen.

A third possibility has been suggested by Fisher.[11] Levine, in the paper referred to, gave figures collected from the literature that pointed towards an elimination of *ABO* incompatible children

BLOOD GROUPS IN MAN

irrespective of *Rh* groups, for there were relatively fewer *A* children counted when the mother was *O* and the father *A* than when the mother was *A* and the father *O*. Fisher suggested that the latter observation might explain the former; if *ABO* incompatible foetuses were being eliminated early in pregnancy they would not be so effective in stimulating the production of anti-*Rh* as would *ABO* compatible foetuses. Van Loghem and Spaander[10] independently came to the same conclusion as Fisher.

REFERENCES

[9] LEVINE, P. (1943). 'Serological factors as possible causes in spontaneous abortions.' *J. Hered.*, **34**, 71–80.

[10] VAN LOGHEM, J. J., and SPAANDER, J. (1948). 'L'influence de l'incompatibilité du système ABO sur l'antagonisme *Rh*.' *Rev. d'Hém.*, **3**, 276–286.

[11] FISHER, R. A. (1944). Personal communication.

Papers 8, 9 & 10

8.   Wiener, A. S. (1944). A new test (blocking test) for Rh sensitization. *Proc. Soc. Exp. Biol. Med.,* 56, 173–6.
9.   Race, R. R. (1944). An 'Incomplete' antibody in human serum. *Nature, (London) 153,* 771–2.
10.   Coombs, R. R. A., Mourant, A. E. and Race, R. R. (1945). Detection of weak and "incomplete" Rh agglutinins: a new test. *Lancet, ii,* 15–16.

Commentary

These three papers have great clinical relevance and are closely interrelated. After the discovery of the Rh blood group system it was found that although children with HDN usually had mothers who were Rh-negative, quite frequently anti-Rh could not be detected in the maternal serum. This was explained in 1944 by Wiener and by Race independently, when they discovered a hidden antibody which was called "blocking" by Wiener and "incomplete" by Race.

In Paper 8 Wiener states that in 1941 he tried the first blocking experiments when he retested some of the stored post-transfusion sera of patients described by him and Peters the year before (see Paper 4) and found them to be no longer active. It occurred to Wiener that antibodies might still be present and capable of combining with the Rh-positive test cells but not capable of agglutinating them. He showed that this was so when a mixture of Rh-positive test cells and an apparently inactive serum were first allowed to combine and then active anti-Rh serum (i.e. one capable of agglutinating Rh-positive cells in control experiments) was added, for in these circumstances it was found that the test cells were not agglutinated, apparently because the action of the active antibody had been blocked. However, the results obtained were irregular and Wiener temporarily abandoned the work. By 1944, however, more satisfactory anti-Rh testing sera had become available and the experiments were resumed.

It then became clear that when no agglutination occurred or if it was markedly weakened, blocking antibody was consistently present, and Wiener demonstrated that this had become fixed to the red cells (see Table 1 for the experiment which proves this).

Wiener's paper was published in June, 1944, and in same month of that year there appeared quite independently one by Race (Paper 9).

Before discussing the results, it is necessary to mention that here is put forward for the first time the Fisher hypothesis (see also Paper 15). This postulates three pairs of Rh alleles, Cc, Dd and Ee, and in the first table are set out the serological reactions observed up to that time, in terms of the CDE notation. Wiener, on the other hand, considers that multiple alleles at a single locus control the Rh antigens and is strongly critical of the British nomenclature (see Paper 14).

In Paper 9 Race showed, as Wiener did independently, that the hidden Rh antibody could be detected by its inhibitory effect on an agglutinating anti-Rh antibody, and also by its direct action on Rh-positive cells. Thus if the latter were suspended in serum containing blocking (or incomplete) anti-D, the mixture then centrifuged and the cells washed and re-suspended in saline, the treated cells were no longer agglutinable by agglutinating anti-D, though they still were by anti-c, anti-C and anti-E. Thus the blocking was shown to be specific, but whether the unblocked antigens would still evoke an antibody response *in vivo* is uncertain (see Paper 48 for evidence on this point—the anti-Kell experiment).

Race also found that mixtures of antisera which might have been expected to agglutinate red cells of certain genotypes did not always do so, e.g. anti-D mixed with anti-C did not agglutinate cDE cells. This was because the mixture contained a blocking anti-D and 'it seems as if the incomplete antibody wins the race for antigen'. It

8. 9. 10.   Commentary   cont.

was in fact the agglutinating anti-C in the mixture which contained the hidden blocking anti-D, since when Rh$_2$ (cDE) cells were suspended in it (the anti-C) and then washed and re-suspended in saline, the treated red cells could no longer be agglutinated by standard anti-D. It was a long time before a *pure* anti-C was obtained.

Paper 10 (Coombs, Mourant and Race, 1945) is most important. It describes a method of testing whether there is *any* antibody present, and in the case of Rh whether the D-antigen sites are coated. Rh-positive red cells in saline are added to the serum being investigated and if there is no agglutination the cells are washed to remove any serum. To these washed cells is added an equal volume of rabbit anti-human globulin (AHG) (made by immunising a rabbit with normal human serum). This will cause agglutination if the D sites are coated, and show that there was incomplete anti-D in the original serum (the indirect Coombs test). In the case of Rhesus immunisation, the first part of this test will have been performed *in utero,* since the baby's cells have been in contact with the mother's serum there, so it is only necessary for the cells to be washed and put up against the AHG to see if they agglutinate. This is known as the direct Coombs test.

As will generally be known, the Coombs test is of the greatest importance and practical value, and in these days of verbosity it is pleasant to find that it is described in about 700 words.

From A. S. Wiener (1944). Proc. Soc. Exp. Biol. Med., 56, 173-6. Copyright (1944), by kind permission of the author and the Society for Experimental Biology and Medicine

14640

A New Test (Blocking Test) for Rh Sensitization.*

Alexander S. Wiener.

From the Transfusion Division of the Jewish Hospital of Brooklyn, and the Serological Laboratory of the Office of the Chief Medical Examiner of New York City.

As was first shown by Wiener and Peters,[1] sensitization of Rh-negative individuals against the Rh factor can often be detected by *in vitro* tests for anti-Rh agglutinins in the individual's plasma. However, it was soon found[2,3] that there are many Rh-negative patients who are strongly sensitized to the Rh factor, as proved by the occurrence of an intragroup hemolytic transfusion reaction or a baby with erythroblastosis (hemolytic disease of the fetus and newborn), yet the plasma does not contain demonstrable anti-Rh agglutinins. The purpose of this paper is to describe a new *in vitro* test, the "blocking test," with the aid of which Rh sensitization can be detected in many of these problem cases.

The first blocking experiments were tried in 1941, when retests of some of the stored post-transfusion sera from the patients described by Wiener and Peters the year before showed these sera to be no longer active. It occurred to the writer that the antibodies might still be present and capable of combining with the test cells but incapable of

agglutinating the cells. When the mixture of test cells and apparently inactive serum was first allowed to combine and subsequently active (capable of agglutinating Rh+ cells in control experiments), anti-Rh serum was added, it was found that the test cells were not agglutinated, apparently because the action of the active agglutinin had been blocked. However, the results obtained were irregular, and therefore experiments on this "blocking test" for Rh antibodies, which is a counterpart of the inhibition test for haptens and group-specific substances, were temporarily abandoned. Recently, when more satisfactory anti-Rh testing sera became available, the experiments were resumed. Tests have been carried out on a number of patients with erythroblastotic babies where the usual tests for anti-Rh agglutinins were unsuccessful, and in most of the cases clean-cut blocking reactions have been obtained, proving the presence of a special sort of anti-Rh isoantibody.

Table I presents the results of some blocking tests on a series of Rh-negative patients who have had erythroblastotic babies, as well as a control series of Rh-positive individuals. The technic of the test is simple: First, one drop of a 2% suspension of Rh-positive cells and a drop of the patient's serum are mixed in a small test tube and allowed to react in a water-bath at 38°C for 30 to 60 minutes. Then a drop of a suitable dilution of an active

---

* Aided by a grant from the United Hospital Fund of N. Y. C.

[1] Wiener, A. S., and Peters, H. R., *Ann. Int. Med.*, 1940, **18**, 2306.

[2] Wiener, A. S., *Arch. Path.*, 1941, **32**, 227.

[3] Levine, P., Burnham, L., Katzin, E. M., and Vogel, P., *Am. J. Obst. and Gyn.*, 1941, **42**, 925.

TABLE I.
Tests on a Series of Human Sera for Anti-Rh Blocking Antibodies.

Experiment	Test cells* (Group O)	Tests with sera from Rh-positive individuals							Tests with sera from Rh negative mothers of erythroblastotic babies					
		1	2	3	4	5	6	7	8	9	10	11	12	13
1	Rh_1	++±	++	++	++±	++±	++	+±	−	++	++	−	+±	−
2	Rh_2	++±	++	++	++	++	++	++	−	++	++	−	++	−

One drop of the serum being tested was mixed with a drop of test cells (2% suspension) in a small, narrow test-tube and the mixture allowed to interact in a water-bath at 38°C until sedimentation was complete (30 to 60 minutes). In experiment 1, the supernatant fluid was then removed, and a drop of diluted (1:5) anti-Rh_0 serum (original titer 60) was added to each tube. In experiment 2, the anti-Rh_0 serum was added directly without removing the supernatant. The tubes were shaken and then reincubated until sedimentation was complete, and the reactions were read grossly by inspecting the sediment in each tube, and microscopically after gentle shaking. Sera 8, 11, and 13 contain blocking antibodies.

* For nomenclature of the Rh blood types and Rh antisera, see Wiener, A. S., *Science*, 1944, **99**, 532.

TABLE II.
Titration of Agglutinating and Blocking Anti-Rh Isoantibodies in the Serum of a Patient with an Erythroblastotic Infant.

Date of tests	Nature of tests	Test cells (Group O)	Dilution of patient's serum in test									
			Undil.	1:2	1:4	1:8	1:16	1:32	1:64	1:128	1:256	1:512
6 days after delivery	Direct Titration	Rh_1	—	—	tr.	+	+±	+±	tr.	—	—	
		Rh_2	±	+±	++	++	++	++	++	+±	tr.	—
1 month after delivery	Direct Titration	Rh_1	—	—	—	tr.	+	—	—	—		
		Rh_2	—	—	—	—	—	—	—	—		
	Blocking	Rh_1	—	—	tr.	+±	++	++±	++±	++±		
		Rh_2	—	—	—	++	++±	++±	++±	++±		

The direct titrations were carried out in the usual manner, the readings being taken after 45 minutes in the water-bath at 38°C.

The blocking tests were carried out as described in Table I; in the tests with Rh_2 cells the supernatants were removed before adding the anti-Rh_0 serum, while in the tests with Rh_1 cells, the supernatants were not removed.

anti-Rh serum is added, and after an additional incubation period of 30 to 60 minutes, the reactions are read. If blocking antibodies are present, no agglutination will occur, or the clumping will be markedly weakened. That the reaction is specific follows from the fact that it has thus far been obtained only with sera from Rh-negative individuals sensitive to the Rh factor, such as mothers of erythroblastotic babies, and not with sera from Rh-positive patients or normal Rh-negative individuals not sensitized to the Rh factor. That the reaction is due to an antibody that becomes fixed to the test cells follows from experiment 1, Table I, in which the supernatant fluid was removed before the anti-Rh test-serum was added.

A number of human anti-Rh sera have been obtained which exhibit a marked prozone[*] effect.[4,5] Taylor et al.[4] have attempted to explain the behavior of such sera on the basis of optimal proportions of antigen and antibody, but if this explanation were correct, it would be difficult to explain why the phenomenon does not occur more frequently. The present author's experiments described above suggest that such prozone phenomena may be due to the presence in such sera of a mixture of blocking and agglutinating antibodies, the

[4] Taylor, G. L., Race, R. R., Prior, A. M., and Ikin, E. W., Brit. Med. J., 1942, 2, 572.

[5] Levine, P., Arch. Path., 1944, 37, 83.

latter being of higher titer. In support of this idea may be cited some observations recently made on a patient after she had given birth to an erythroblastotic baby (cf. Table II). Tests 6 days after delivery showed her serum to contain strong anti-Rh agglutinins exhibiting a distinct prozone effect. Direct tests performed only 3 weeks later were almost entirely negative for anti-Rh agglutinins, but quantitative blocking tests showed the presence of blocking antibodies of a titer 2 to 4. The most reasonable explanation of these findings is that immediately after delivery, this patient's serum contained a mixture of blocking and agglutinating antibodies, and that the latter diminished in titer more rapidly than the former. To test this hypothesis, the serum obtained one month after delivery was treated with Rh-positive cells in order to attempt to remove the blocking antibodies in case these masked the presence of low-titered anti-Rh agglutinins. It was indeed found that the absorbed serum then gave distinct and specific clumping, even though the original unabsorbed serum gave no or only faint reactions. Similarly, the serum obtained 6 days after delivery was improved instead of weakened by absorption with Rh-positive cells. Repetition of these absorption experiments gave irregular results, probably on account of the competition between the blocking and agglutinating antibodies.

If, as there is some reason to believe, of

---

[*] Prozone: the phenomenon exhibited by some sera, which give effective agglutination reactions when diluted several hundred fold but do not visibly react with the antigen when undiluted or only slightly diluted. In relation to this paper, the explanation is that with mixtures of complete and incomplete antibody dilution may weaken the blocking component.

the two sorts of Rh antibodies, the blocking antibodies prove to be of greater clinical significance in the causation of erythroblastosis, this would serve to explain the puzzling lack of correlation between the titer of anti-Rh agglutinins in the maternal serum and the severity of the disease in the infant.

Recently, studies have been conducted on the titer and specificity of Rh blocking antibodies in various human sera. To date, the highest titer encountered was 64, and all the blocking antibodies had specificities corresponding to anti-Rh_0. Thus, type Rh_1 blood suspensions treated with such blocking sera gave reactions indistinguishable from type Rh' blood with the three sorts of Rh antisera, and in the same way type Rh_2 blood suspensions could be "converted" into type Rh", etc.

The observations on blocking antibodies are of interest in connection with the problem of the nature of agglutination and precipitation reactions in general. According to Marrack's "framework" hypothesis,[6] the second stage as well as the first stage of these reactions is assumed to be specific, in contrast to the classic theory which postulates that the second stage is non-specific. Some observations on mixed agglutination reactions were previously reported which were more readily explained under Marrack's hypothesis than the classic theory.[7] The present observations can also be more easily explained under the framework hypothesis, if one postulates that the blocking antibodies are monovalent antibodies, in contrast to the usual agglutinating and precipitating antibodies which are assumed to be bivalent.[8]

In conclusion, it seems highly improbable that blocking antibodies are peculiar to the Rh factor. Doubtless, study of other antigen-antibody systems will reveal the existence of analogous phenomena.[9]

---

[6] Marrack, J. R., Report No. 230, Medical Research Council, His Majesty's Stationery Office, London, 1934; second edition, 1938.

[7] Wiener, A. S., and Herman, M., *J. Immunol.*, 1939, **36**, 255.

[8] Pauling, L., Campbell, D. H., and Pressman, D., *Physiol. Rev.*, 1943, **23**, 203.

[9] *Cf.* Jones, F. S., and Orcutt, M., *J. Immunol.*, 1934, **27**, 215; Kleckowski, A., *Brit. J. Exp. Path.*, 1941, **22**, 192; Hooker, S. B., and Boyd, W. C., *Ann. N. Y. Acad. Sci.*, 1942, **43**, 107.

From R. R. Race (1944). Nature (London), 153, 771-2. Copyright (1944), by kind permission of the author and Macmillan and Co Ltd

LETTERS TO THE EDITORS

The Editors do not hold themselves responsible for opinions expressed by their correspondents. No notice is taken of anonymous communications.

An 'Incomplete' Antibody in Human Serum

A STUDY of the properties of mixtures of different types of human anti-*Rh* sera has led to the recognition of what appears to be an incomplete antibody. The research arose out of a suggestion by Prof. R. A. Fisher that this technique might throw some light on the problem of antibody absorption.

Human anti-*Rh* serum of the type called by Wiener "standard" agglutinates red cells of the gene Rh_1 and also those of Rh_2. 'Anti-Rh_1' serum agglutinates the former cells but not the latter[1,2]. If, however —and this was the observation that started the present work—cells of the genotype Rh_2Rh_2 or Rh_2rh are added to a mixture of these two sera, the expected agglutination due to the standard anti-*Rh* serum does not occur. It was then found that the sera need not be mixed, for if the Rh_2 cells are suspended in anti-Rh_1 serum—which causes no agglutination—and after a few minutes are separated from the serum, washed and re-suspended in saline, then these treated cells can no longer be agglutinated by standard anti-*Rh* serum.

In January of this year Fisher drew up the following formulation of the relationships found in the Rhesus factor, designed to distinguish the three categories, antigens, genes or allelomorphs and antibodies for which provision must be made in a satisfactory notation.

Name of serum:	Anti-Rh_1	St	Anti-*Rh* Standard	Anti-Rh_2	Not yet found	
Antibody present:	Γ	γ	Δ	H	δ	η
Genes						
Rh_z CDE	(+)	(−)	(+)	(+)		
Rh_1 CDe	+	−	+	−		
Rh_y CdE	(+)	−	(−)	+		
Rh' Cde	+	−	−	−		
Rh_2 cDE	−	+	+	+		
Rh_0 cDe	−	+	+	−		
Rh'' cdE	−	+	−	+		
rh cde	−	+	−	−		

Those reactions not yet determined serologically are given in brackets.

The three forms of allelomorphic antigens are arbitrarily denoted by *C, c, D, d, E, e,* chosen to avoid confusion with any symbols so far used. The antibodies with which these react are denoted by corresponding Greek letters. These single letters refer to antigens and their corresponding antibodies only. Every gene of the system seems to be associated with a selection of three antigens from these three pairs. The system thus predicts an eighth allelomorph, Rh_z, which could not be recognized in a single individual, but could be identified in a favourable pedigree. It also suggests the possibility of two more antibodies not yet known reacting with *d* and *e* respectively.

Wiener[1] has supposed that the presence of the Rh_1 gene results in there being two "partial antigens" on the red cell (*C* and *D* of the table), and our recent work with *St* and other sera seems to make three

parts necessary to the total antigen resulting from the Rh_2 gene, namely, *c, D* and *E*.

It is only one of these three antigens in the Rh_2 cells, called *D* in the table, which is being blocked by the anti-Rh_1 serum. *E* and *c* are left uncoated and ready for agglutination.

	Rh_2 cells untreated				Rh_2 cells coated with anti-Rh_1 serum			
Serum dilutions	1/1	1/2	1/4	1/8	1/1	1/2	1/4	1/8
Anti-Rh_1 serum (Γ)	−				−			
Standard anti-*Rh* serum (Δ)	+	+	+	+	−	−	−	−
St serum (γ)	+	+	+	+	+	+	+	+
Anti-Rh_2 serum (H)	+	+	+	+	+	+	+	+

The coating of this same *D* antigen in Rh_1 cells can be demonstrated, but first it is necessary to remove the agglutinin (Γ) in the anti-Rh_1 serum for Rh_1 cells. This was done by absorption of the serum by $Rh'rh$ cells which remove the agglutinin but not the coating factor, since these cells contain *C* but not the coatable antigen *D*. With the resulting absorbed serum, cells of the genotype Rh_1Rh_1 can be coated without agglutination confusing the result. There is no blocking of the antigen *C* in Rh_1 cells.

Absorption with untreated Rh_2 cells diminishes the agglutinin titre of standard anti-*Rh*, (Δ), anti-Rh_2 (H) and *St* (γ) sera. Absorption with coated Rh_2 cells diminishes the titre of anti-Rh_2 and *St* sera but not that of standard anti-*Rh* serum. Thus, absorption experiments confirm that in Rh_2 cells it is only the antigen *D* which is being blocked, *E* and *c* being left free.

The coating factor may be looked on as the standard anti-*Rh* serum antibody (Δ), which can combine with its appropriate antigen, but is defective in that it is not a suitable partner for the second stage of the antigen-antibody reaction which results in agglutination of the cells. It may be called an incomplete antibody (Δ′). Varying salt concentrations failed to produce agglutination of the coated cell suspensions, so did variations in the *p*H.

The incomplete standard anti-*Rh* antibody (Δ′) has been found in good strength in four anti-Rh_1 sera (from *Rh* negative mothers) and in a weak amount in our remaining anti-Rh_1 serum (from an *Rh* negative mother). With the removal of the incomplete antibody, these five sera gained no fresh agglutinating range; they did not, for example, then behave as anti-*Rh'* sera. In other words, there is no complete standard anti-*Rh* serum antibody present which is being masked by the presence of the incomplete form of this antibody.

One standard anti-*Rh* serum in our collection contains the incomplete antibody (Δ′) as well as the complete agglutinin (Δ). Titration results with this serum and Rh_1 or Rh_2 cells had previously given what was a puzzling and unique appearance—weak reactions, with intervening negatives, continuing up to a high dilution (1/1,000). Preliminary absorption with, say, Rh_2 cells removes the incomplete antibody leaving the normal antibody, which now gives strong reactions up to the same titre with more of the same Rh_2 cells. It seems as if the incomplete antibody wins the race for antigen.

Incomplete antibodies have been looked for but not found in three *St* sera, four anti-Rh_2 sera, one standard anti-*Rh* serum, two sera from normal *Rh*

NATURE

JUNE 24, 1944, VOL. 153

negative donors, and eleven sera from normal *Rh* positive donors. The appropriate antigen *D* in all cells so far tried has been coatable; the cells were Rh_1Rh_2 (1), Rh_1Rh_1 (3), Rh_1rh (3), Rh_2rh or Rh_2Rh_2 (6) and Rh_0rh (1). The incomplete antibody can be removed from serum by appropriate but not by inappropriate (for example, *rhrh*) cells, nor by saliva from an Rh_1Rh_1 A_1B secretor. Heating to 56° C. all the sera involved made no difference to the reactions.

I do not know of any similar phenomenon in hæmagglutination or hæmolysis. The inhibition by normal serum of the tissue hæmolysis of red cells recently reported by Magraeth, Findlay and Martin[3] is evidently of a very different nature. The inhibitor described by these workers was not species specific, whereas the incomplete antibody now being described is specific down to one antigen.

In bacterial agglutination a more striking resemblance is found in the agglutinoid phenomenon studied by Shibley[4]. The most obvious differences are that agglutinoid was made by partial heat denaturation of the serum and showed itself only as a zone of inhibition followed in higher dilutions by normal agglutination; whereas in the anti-Rh_1 sera, which had not been heated but stored at − 20° C., all the standard anti-*Rh* antibody was in the incomplete form while all the anti-Rh_1 antibody was in the complete form. The behaviour of anti-*Rh* sera, heated to 65–70° C., is now being investigated.

Very recently a sixth anti-Rh_1 serum has been found, locally. The incomplete antibody was present in good strength immediately after taking the blood.

R. R. RACE.

Medical Research Council,
Emergency Blood Transfusion Service.
May 17.

[1] Wiener, *Proc. Soc. Exp. Biol. and Med.*, **54**, 316 (1943).
[2] Race, Taylor, Cappell and McFarlane, NATURE, **153**, 52 (1944).
[3] Magraeth, Findlay and Martin, NATURE, **151**, 252 (1943).
[4] Shibley, *J. Exp. Med.*, **50**, 825 (1929).

From R. R. A. Coombs, A. E. Mourant and R. R. Race (1945). The Lancet, ii, 15-16. Copyright (1945), by kind permission of the authors and The Lancet Ltd

Preliminary Communications

DETECTION OF WEAK AND "INCOMPLETE" Rh AGGLUTININS : A NEW TEST

IN most cases of hæmolytic disease of the newborn, and of transfusion reactions due to Rh incompatibility, agglutinins can be detected by direct microscopic agglutination tests. The "incomplete" Rh antibody (see Race [1] and Wiener [2]) differs from the true Rh agglutinin in that it fails to agglutinate the red blood-cells which it sensitises ; nevertheless, it is probably just as important in the causation of the disease (Wiener [2]). Until recently, its presence has only been detected by an inhibition test, in which appropriate cells treated with this antibody do not agglutinate when subsequently exposed to the action of homologous agglutinating serum. Also in a number of cases of hæmolytic disease and transfusion reaction, when the history and Rh groups strongly suggest immunisation, antibodies either cannot be detected or are present in such small amount as to leave their existence in doubt.

A technique has been evolved by which cells sensitised by weak agglutinins or "incomplete" antibody are made to agglutinate strongly. The method developed from the idea that such sensitised cells presumably have adsorbed antibody globulin at some points on their surface ; and that an anti-human-globulin serum might be expected to react with this in some observable way.

The method in brief is as follows. Two drops of a 2% suspension of washed blood-cells of an appropriate Rh genotype are added to an equal volume of the serum under investigation. This is incubated at 37° C for half an hour. A small sample of the deposited cells is then carefully withdrawn with a fine Pasteur pipette, placed on a glass slide, and examined microscopically. The results at this stage should be the same as those found in the routine test for agglutinins. The demonstration of agglutination indicates the presence of anti-Rh agglutinin. However, the absence of agglutination may mean either that the serum is compatible with the cells or, on the other hand, that the agglutinin is too weak to be detected or is of the "incomplete" variety. To exclude these latter two possibilities the cells are now thoroughly washed with saline to remove any human serum, and to a suspension of these washed cells is added an equal volume of an appropriate dilution of rabbit anti-human-globulin serum which has had all agglutinins to human red cells absorbed from it. After a further incubation of half to one hour the tubes are re-examined macroscopically and microscopically for agglutination ; though in practice the macroscopic reading has in every case proved sufficient. In our hands the test has proved most specific and reliable, showing up weak Rh sensitisation and sensitisation with "incomplete" antibody. A detailed description of the immunological procedure and technique involved, with a full survey of the results, will be published shortly.

This test may have useful applications in detecting fine degrees of sensitisation in other antigen-antibody systems where for some reason the second stage of agglutination is not manifested. The opportunity is also afforded to determine whether the red cells of an infant suffering from hæmolytic disease are in fact sensitised in vivo even when no free agglutinin is demonstrable in its serum. All that is necessary is to expose the washed blood-cells of the infant to a rabbit anti-human-globulin serum.

Wiener [3] has recently reported on a "conglutination" test by which he also claims to have succeeded in producing agglutination of cells sensitised with "incomplete" antibody, by a completely different method.

R. R. A. COOMBS,* B SC EDIN., M R C V S
Department of Pathology, University of Cambridge
A. E. MOURANT, D PHIL OXFD   R. R. RACE, M R C S
Medical Research Council Emergency Blood Transfusion Service

1. Race, R. R. Nature, Lond. 1944, 153, 771.
2. Wiener, A. S. Proc. Soc. exp. Biol., NY, 1944, 56, 173.

Paper 11

11. Morton, J. A., and Pickles, M. M. (1947). Use of trypsin in the detection of incomplete anti-Rh antibodies. *Nature, London, 159,* 779—780.

Commentary

It has been seen from Paper 10 that Rh-positive cells coated with an incomplete anti-D antibody can be made to agglutinate by exposing them to an anti-human globulin after they have been washed (the Coombs test).

Pickles (1946)* showed that red cells similarly coated and washed were agglutinated by a filtrate of a broth culture of vibrio cholera. From its reactions, the filtrate appeared to have the properties of an enzyme. At the time of this discovery, it was not suggested that the procedure had any advantages over the Coombs test for the routine detection of incomplete anti-Rh antibodies.

Subsequently, Morton and Pickles (Paper 11) showed that trypsin had the same effect as the cholera filtrate, but also, and this is very important, it enhanced the specific agglutination of other haemagglutinins in the absence of any detectable incomplete antibody by the Coombs test. In other words, this enzyme technique is more sensitive than the Coombs test.

Paper 11 also discusses the method of action of trypsin. It appears to act on the surface of the red cell but it does not affect the character of the blood group antigen loci, nor does it ever change the type of reaction of the sera from the incomplete to the agglutinating form.

Even though enzyme tests are most valuable and are routine in most laboratories, yet they can be difficult to assess and are not such a reliable or certain indication of immunisation (see Paper 46) as that given by the Coombs test.

*(Pickles, M. M. (1946). Effect of cholera filtrate on red cells as demonstrated by incomplete anti-Rh antibodies. *Nature, (London), 158,* 880.

From J. A. Morton and M. M. Pickles (1947). Nature (London), 159, 779-780, Copyright (1947), by kind permission of the authors and Macmillan and Co Ltd

Use of Trypsin in the Detection of Incomplete Anti-*Rh* Antibodies

IN an attempt to define the properties of the enzyme present in the filtrate of a culture of vibrio cholera, which causes cells sensitized with an 'incomplete' anti-*Rh* antibody to agglutinate[1], cultures of other organisms and pure enzyme preparations have been tested. During this investigation trypsin has been found to cause agglutination of cells sensitized with an 'incomplete' antibody, and also to enhance the specific agglutination of other hæmagglutinins in the absence of any detectable antibody of the 'incomplete' type.

If trypsin is added to the serum or to the cell antigen antibody mixture, its action may be inhibited by the natural trypsin inhibitor present in all sera[2]. This can be overcome by the addition of an excess of the enzyme or removal of the serum inhibitor, or by washing cells already sensitized before exposing them to the trypsin; if this latter method is used, a single washing is sufficient to remove the inhibitor. Test cells may also be incubated with trypsin and, on incubation with sera, show enhancement of agglutination with *iso*agglutinins and immune agglutinins, and agglutination with sera of the 'incomplete' type; and after such treatment are not susceptible to the normal serum inhibitor or to soya bean trypsin inhibitor. With fresh undiluted sera, however, there is also enhancement of rouleau formation, which can be abolished by the addition of saline.

In this investigation the trypsin preparations used have been crystalline trypsin (Plaut Research Laboratory, New Jersey) and *liquor trypsini co.* (Allen and Hanbury). The stock solution of crystalline trypsin has been a 1 per cent solution in $N/20$ hydrochloric acid, and has remained stable for three months. Before use the stock solution is diluted with phosphate buffer (pH 7·2) to a concentration of 1 : 400 to 1 : 10,000; and the *liquor trypsini co.* is diluted with buffer to give a final concentration of ·1 : 5 of the original solution. With a 1 : 400 solution of crystalline trypsin, complete agglutination of fully

sensitized cells occurs within 20 min. With increasing dilution of the enzyme the time of agglutination is lengthened.

As with the enzyme present in the filtrate of vibrio cholera, trypsin appears to act on the surface of the red cell but does not affect any of the known hæmagglutinogen loci. Neither removal of the normal trypsin inhibitor from an 'incomplete' serum nor the incubation of inhibitor-free serum with trypsin for up to 30 hr. has changed the type of reaction of the sera from the 'incomplete' to the agglutinating form. After incubation the sera still show the blocking reaction[3], though the 'Coombs'' test[4] is markedly weakened.

In the detection of incomplete anti-*Rh* antibodies some of the reagents are difficult to obtain or the methods are laborious for routine use. The trypsin method is very simple in execution and only requires a standard pharmaceutical preparation as a reagent. The crystalline trypsin solutions have given positive results in parallel with the Coombs' test with twenty incomplete anti-*D* sera and also with cells sensitized *in vivo* in infants suffering from hæmolytic disease of the newborn.

The full results of these findings, together with considerations of the part they play in agglutination and in the elucidation of the nature of the incomplete antibody, will be published later. We are indebted to Dr. Kunitz for the soya bean trypsin inhibitor and to Dr. A. H. T. Robb-Smith and Dr. R. G. Macfarlane for much help and advice.

J. A. MORTON
M. M. PICKLES

Division of Laboratories,
Radcliffe Infirmary,
Oxford.
Feb. 26.

[1] Pickles, M. M., *Nature*, 158, 880 (1946).
[2] Delezene, C., and Pozerski, E., *C.R. Soc. Biol. Paris*, 55, 327 (1903).
[3] Weiner, A. S., *Proc. Soc. Biol. Exp. and Med.*, 56, 173 (1944).
[4] Coombs, R. R. A., Mourant, A. E., and Race, R. R., *Brit. J. Exp. Path.*, 26, 255 (1945).

Papers 12, 13, 14 & 15

12.   Annotation. (1948). Anti-Rh serum nomenclature. *Brit. Med. J., i,* 400.

13.   Wiener, A. S. (1948). Anti-Rh serum nomenclature. *Brit. Med. J., i.,* 805.

14.   Wiener, A. S. (1949). Heredity of the Rh blood types, VII, Proc. 8th Int. Cong. Genetics (Stockholm; July 1948). Supplementary volume of *Hereditas.* (Extract).

15.   Race, R. R. (1964). (Extract). Some notes on Fisher's contributions to human blood groups. *Biometrics, 20,* 361–7.

Commentary

It is debatable how much space should be devoted in a book of this type to the controversy over nomenclature, but the arguments have been very much part of the Rh scene since the early days, and moreover there is nothing like a disagreement for stimulating interest and in this case for learning basic principles.

In the four papers selected we have tried to be fair, choosing two short and two long ones from opposing camps. The *British Medical Journal* annotation and the reply to it by Wiener give the essentials of the problem, but in the annotation it must be pointed out that though it is true that the anti-e serum was later found, anti-d never has been (lines 33 and 34).

Wiener's reply needs no comment except to point out that in the Rh/Hr nomenclature he is referring to reciprocal alleles in the Rh system, all at the same locus. He only uses the capital Rh when what Fisher and Race call D is present (which he calls Rh_0). Hr_0 is chosen for the hypothetical d, Hr' is c and hr'' is e.

Wiener's longer and later paper is reproduced because it states his genetic hypothesis, compares the two notations and also gives his criticisms of "CDE" in considerable detail.

Race's paper on the other hand is a commemorative tribute to a brilliant geneticist whose main contribution to Rh genetic theory and nomenclature was made many years earlier (see Fisher 1947*, and Paper 9).

After reading both points of view the reader must make up his mind on which side to cast his vote.

*Fisher, R. A. (1947). The Rhesus factor, a study in scientific method. *American Scientist, 35,* 95–103.

400   FEB. 28, 1948   BRITISH
                                                       MEDICAL JOURNAL

ANTI-Rh SERUM NOMENCLATURE

It is natural and common that when a new phenomenon has been discovered and as yet is only partly understood a system of nomenclature should be introduced which is proved by later work to be either inconsistent with the facts or inconvenient in practical use. It had been hoped by some that such a position would now be recognized in the case of the anti-Rh sera, and that the Review Board appointed by the Surgeon General of the United States Public Health Service to advise on nomenclature might have adopted without reservation the Fisher-Race system. as opposed to the earlier Wiener system, in favour of which priority is the chief argument. Reading only a little between the lines of the Review Board's report,[1] it can be assumed that its members would have liked to follow the above suggestion, but it seems they felt unable to go further for the present than to recommend the use of both systems in parallel, the Wiener nomenclature being given first on any label. and the Fisher-Race designation following in brackets. There is certainly no lack of candour in the Board's comments. In favour of the Wiener theory it is stated that it has priority and " is used by nearly all workers on the subject in the western hemisphere." Against it are " incomplete specifications, changed rapidly from year to year " : " complications, both typographical and genetic, of subscripts, superscripts, numbers, primes and other symbols " ; and " the doubtful assumption of multiple antigens produced by a single gene." It is recalled also that following publication of the Fisher-Race theory and proposals for nomenclature[2] Wiener not only denied the linkage postulate on which the theory is based but stated that his own views would preclude the existence of the two additional (d and e) factors propounded by Fisher, whereas in the event anti-e serum was found by Mourant and anti-d by Diamond, " thus bearing out Fisher's predictions." In favour of the Fisher-Race nomenclature the Board recognized that " it is in wide usage in England, is gaining in usage in the western hemisphere, and hence may become the international standard." Against it only two objections are raised—its lack of priority, already mentioned, and that it " is based on a genetic hypothesis which is unproved." In the strictest sense of the words that is a correct statement of the position, though a theory which makes a correct prediction is normally regarded as having been " confirmed " to that extent. " Proof " in these matters is a relative term, and the real question confronting the Board was what degree of proof was necessary to justify the abandonment of the prior, and in the United States the most widely used, system of nomenclature. While the immediate effect of the report in the United States will be to ensure the temporary confinement within brackets of the Fisher-Race descriptions, the Board's comments must none the less have gone a long way to encouraging its wider use by United States and other workers and thus rendering the present compromise transitional.

---

[1] *Science*, 1948, **107**, 27.
[2] *Nature*, 1945 **155**, 542.

From A. S. Wiener (1948). Brit. Med. J., i, 805. Copyright (1948), by kind permission of the author and the British Medical Association

APRIL 24, 1948   CORRESPONDENCE   BRITISH MEDICAL JOURNAL

Correspondence

Anti-Rh Serum Nomenclature

SIR,—In the annotation on " Anti-Rh Serum Nomenclature " (Feb. 28, p. 400) you discuss the recent edict of the National Institute of Health in the United States regarding the labelling of anti-Rh sera, namely to use the earlier Wiener Rh–Hr system as standard, with the corresponding Fisher–Race C-D-E notations in parentheses. You regard this decision as a " transitional compromise," implying that eventually the original notations will be abandoned in favour of the Fisher–Race system. However, this conclusion as well as the Board's own analysis fails to take into account all the available facts.[1][2][3][4] I have therefore prepared my own analysis of the situation, and after it is printed in your journal perhaps one of the C-D-E protagonists will attempt a reply. Only by publishing all the facts and both sides of every scientific problem can we ever hope to arrive at the correct solution.

Advantages of the Rh–Hr Nomenclature

1. They have priority, having been proposed by one of the discoverers.

2. They form a coherent and unified system, which readily lends itself to extension to include newly discovered blood factors belonging to the rhesus system.

3. The genetic theory on which the notations are based is amply supported by heredity studies on a large series of families, and statistical studies on the distribution of the types in the population. On the other hand, there is no evidence against the theory.

4. The notations are simple to use in writing and orally.

5. The notations clearly separate the designations for phenotypes and genotypes, and for agglutinogens and genes, leaving no room for ambiguity.

6. The phenotypes' names clearly indicate what tests have actually been made and what reactions were obtained, without including symbols for hypothetical blood factors which have not been tested for, and for which there is no clear experimental evidence.

7. The notations clearly indicate the relationship to the original rhesus factor, and separate the Rh–Hr types from other independent systems such as the A-B-O groups and M-N types.

8. For individuals who already know and understand the four blood groups and the three M-N types, the Rh–Hr notations are easy to learn almost instantaneously.

9. The notations lend themselves readily to clinical use, since the capital R's and small r's clearly indicate which types are Rh₀-positive and which are Rh₀-negative.

10. They take advantage not only of the reciprocal relationship between the Rh and Hr factors, but also of the special clinical, serologic, and genetic position of factor Rh₀.

11. They do not involve any incorrect assumption of one-to-one correspondence between genes and partial antigens.

12. They are self-sufficient.

13. None of the symbols used in the Rh–Hr notations have previously been applied to other agglutinogens.

14. The notations as used by workers throughout the world are uniform.

15. Simple tables are available for the Rh–Hr types and their genetics.

16. They are the *only* notations used in most standard textbooks, encyclopaedias, dictionaries, and articles.

Supposed Disadvantages of the Rh–Hr Notations

1. That they take longer to teach. Where this seems to be so, it is merely because one must *understand* the Rh–Hr types in order to use the Rh–Hr notations intelligently, and to teach them.

2. That they have been changed several times. This is true, but none of the changes are basic or really upsetting. Moreover, one need only learn the present nomenclature to understand the subject. The changes have served to improve and streamline the nomenclature, and are no more objectionable than the changes made from year to year in order to improve the performance and appearance of automobiles. One does not have to study the entire evolution of the automobile from 1905 to date in order to learn how to drive one's 1948 model.

Supposed Advantages of the C-D-E and Rh₁-Rh₂-Rh₃ Notations

1. Many workers have the false impression that they are easier to " learn " and teach. The reason for this is that one can speak about C-D-E and Rh₁Rh₂Rh₃ at once, without having any real understanding of the subject. These notations therefore serve as a convenient cloak for lack of knowledge and understanding, and actually discourage any desire to acquire such an understanding.

2. They make use of a one-to-one correspondence between genes and blood factors. This supposed advantage is based on the wrong concept that such a one-to-one correspondence must exist, which is not true.

3. They are gaining more adherents. This is true only because the protagonists of this system are teaching it, and because the new regulation passed by the National Institute of Health has forcibly called these notations to the attention of workers. The C-D-E and Rh₁-Rh₂-Rh₃ notations will naturally attract some adherents, just as the Moss and Jansky systems each gained their adherents. The resulting unnecessary confusion may take many years to clear.

Disadvantages of the C-D-E, Rh₁-Rh₂-Rh₃, and other Systems

1. They lack priority.

2. The genetic theory on which they are based is purely theoretical; there is no experimental evidence to support it, nor does it lend itself readily to experimental attack. On the other hand there is some statistical evidence based on the analysis of the distribution of the Rh–Hr types in the population that tends to refute the linkage idea.

3. The notations are cumbersome to use. For example type rh becomes small-c, small-d, small-e over small-c, small-d small-e. An error in printing in which a capital letter is substituted for a small letter or *vice versa* could prove fatal. Thus if anti-d is written instead of anti-D this would be very serious, but if anti-rh₀ is written instead of anti-Rh₀ the intention of the writer would still be obvious.

4. There is no clear separation of phenotypes and genotypes. The use of designations for " the most likely " genotype without indicating clearly all the time what is intended conveys to the reader the false impression that the actual genotype has been determined. The writings of users of these notations continually confuse genotypes with phenotypes, and it is impossible to tell from the designation used what tests have actually been made.

5. The letters C-D-E give no indication of any relationship to the rhesus system and convey instead the erroneous impression of a relationship to the A-B system of blood groups.

6. To learn the other notations suggested one must start from scratch, and all one's knowledge and understanding of the A-B-O and M N systems is wasted.

7. The notations are too awkward for clinical use. There is no clear indication in the notations which bloods are Rh₀-positive and which are Rh₀-negative.

8. While some of the proposed systems of notations take advantage of the reciprocal relationship between the Rh and Hr factors, none takes into account the special clinical, serologic, and genetic position of the factor Rh₀.

9. The notations are not self-sufficient or self-explanatory. Thus users of the C-D-E notations are compelled also to use the Rh–Hr notations, as can be seen by consulting the papers of Fisher and Race who originated the C-D-E notations.

10. The symbols C and E have already been applied to other agglutinogens in human blood. The introduction of the use of these letters for agglutinogens of the rhesus type would therefore result in ambiguity.

11. There is no uniform understanding among users of the C-D-E notations as to terminology for the phenotypes. Thus blood reacting with " anti-C," " anti-D," and " anti-c," but not with " anti-E " is variously designated as CDe, or CcDe, or CDe/cde, etc. Under the Rh–Hr notations, the blood would be designated simply as Rh₁rh, a name which clearly indicates positive reactions with sera anti-rh', anti-Rh₀, and anti-hr', and negative reactions with anti-rh".

12. No simple unified tables regarding the types and their heredity involving the other proposed systems of notations are available for use.

13. The C-D-E and other proposed notations are not mentioned in most standard laboratory texts, and are therefore unintelligible to the average reader.

—I am, etc.,

New York.   A. S. WIENER.

REFERENCES

[1] Wiener, A. S., " Theory and Nomenclature of the Rh Types, Subtypes, and Genotypes," *British Medical Journal*, 1946, 1, 982.
[2] —— " Rh System in the Chimpanzee," *Science*, 1946, 104, 578.
[3] —— " Nomenclature of the Rh Factors," *Lancet*, 1948, 1, 343.
[4] —— *Blood Groups and Transfusion*, 3rd edition, 1943. C. C. Thomas, Springfield, Ill.

From A. S. Wiener (1949), Hereditas, Supplementary Volume, July 1948. Copyright (1949), by kind permission of the author and Hereditas

HEREDITY OF THE Rh BLOOD TYPES

VII. ADDITIONAL FAMILY STUDIES, WITH SPECIAL REFERENCE TO THE GENES R^z AND r^y

BY *ALEXANDER S. WIENER*

SEROLOGICAL LABORATORY OF THE OFFICE OF THE CHIEF MEDICAL EXAMINER
OF NEW YORK CITY

IN previous papers of this series,[1,2,3,4,5,6] studies were described on the heredity of the Rh—Hr blood types in a series of 525 families with 925 children. The results of these family studies, as well as the statistical analysis of the distributions of the Rh—Hr type in various populations throughout the world have confirmed the accuracy of the theory of heredity of the Rh—Hr blood types by multiple allelic genes.

In fact, based on these findings, the Rh—Hr blood types are now used routinely alongside of the A—B—0 groups and M—N types in medicolegal cases of disputed parentage in the U. S. A.[7,8,9]. The genetic studies on the Rh—Hr types have been continued, and the purpose of this paper is to present some of our more recent results, and especially to discuss the rare genes R^z and r^y.

NOMENCLATURE OF THE Rh BLOOD TYPES.

Any worker who is familiar with the history of the four LANDSTEINER blood groups and the confusion caused by the MOSS and JANSKY numberings should be anxious to avoid a repetition of these mistakes in the case of the nomenclature of the Rh blood types. As soon as the existence of the three factors was established by the writer, designations were selected which took into account the serologic and genetic facts, especially the unique position of factor Rh_0. When the experimental findings justified it, the notations were later extended to include the reciprocally related Hr blood factors.[10] From the onset, an infinite number of possible notations were available to the writer, such as the numerical notations Rh_1, Rh_2, Rh_3, etc. and the literal notations U, V, W, etc., but these were discarded in favor of the present notations Rh_0, rh′ and rh″ because the latter summarize the facts most simply and at the same time are the most rational. However, later workers, undeterred by the history of the MOSS—JANSKY mix-up have attempted to introduce other notations for the Rh types, none of which incorporate any novel concept. In fact, these later workers mostly made no actual genetic studies of their own, but suggested their notations purely on philosophical rather than on experimental grounds. Luckily for persons obliged to learn the Rh blood types, all but one of these suggestions have fallen by the wayside. There still remains a duplicate system of notations involving the letters CDE, but these do not differ in principle from the UVW notations previously considered by the writer, but only to be discarded.

In previous papers, the disadvantages of the CDE, XYZ, UVW and other similar notations were clearly pointed out, and it is significant that the objections which were raised have not been answered satisfactorily to date. However, due to the prestige of the proposers,[11] the CDE notations have gained some followers, so that it is necessary to point out additional fallacies in these notations * before serious confusion results. In Table 1, therefore, are compared the WIENER and the

TABLE 1. *Comparison of* WIENER *and* FISHER—RACE *notations for the eight Rh blood types.*

| WIENER notations for phenotypes * | Reactions with sera | | | FISHER—RACE notations for phenotypes in use | | | |
	Anti-Rh_0 (Anti-D)	Anti-rh' (Anti-C)	Anti-rh" (Anti-E)	a	b	c	d
rh	—	—	—	?	cde/cde	cde	cde
rh'	—	+	—	C	Cde/cde	Cde	Cde
rh"	—	—	+	E	cdE/cde	cdE	cdE
rh'rh"	—	+	+	CE	Cde/cdE	CdE	Cde/cdE
Rh_0	+	—	—	D	cDe/cde	cDe	cDe
Rh_1	+	+	—	CD	CDe/cde	CDe	CDe
Rh_2	+	—	+	DE	cDE/cde	cDE	cDE
Rh_1Rh_2	+	+	+	CDE	CDe/cDE	CDE	CDe/cDE

* Rh_1 is short for Rh_0'; Rh_2 is short for Rh_0''.

FISHER—RACE notations for the eight Rh blood types. It will be seen that in the original notations for the Rh—Hr types, the phenotypes clearly indicate which of the Rh factors tested for are actually present. Two abbreviations are used in order to streamline the notations, namely, Rh_1 for Rh_0', and Rh_2 for Rh_0''. Moreover, blood reacting with anti-Rh_0 and anti-rh' but not anti-rh" is written as Rh_1 (or Rh_0') instead of Rh_0rh' in order to indicate the genetic fact that the agglutinogen in this type blood ordinarily represents the effect of a single gene R^1, rather than the combined action of the two genes R^0 and r'. On the other hand, type Rh_1Rh_2 is so designated because it ordinarily results from the combined action of the two genes R^1 and R^2.

Since there is disagreement among the CDE protagonists as to the proper phenotype notations under their system, four methods that have been used by those workers are given in the table. As CASTLE, WINTROBE and SNYDER [16] point out, the phenotype name should only include the agglutinogens actually *proved to be present* by the tests, as shown in column (a), but this system lacks a suitable name for type rh. Moreover, while the genetic possibilities are practically self evident when the matings are written as rh × Rh_1, rh × Rh_1Rh_2, etc., it would be impossible to forecast the types of the children correctly if the matings were written as Neg. × CD, Neg. × CDE, etc. Other CDE workers [17] use as the phenotype designation the "most likely genotype", as shown in column (b). These notations, however, are misleading in

* To avoid repetition, the reader is referred to previous papers,[12],[13],[14],[15] listing numerous fallacies of the FISHER—RACE notations. In this paper, only points not previously mentioned will be discussed.

that they imply that tests for the three Hr factors have been performed. Moreover, in particular cases these workers become hopelessly confused when the actually genotype of the individual proves to be different from the "most likely" genotype. A third group of CDE workers [18, 19] have adopted the notations shown under column (c). Like notations (b), these notations are misleading since they imply that tests have actually been made for the Hr factors, and frequently the notations are contrary to the facts. For example, the designation CDE for type Rh_1Rh_2 implies that this type blood contains no Hr factors, while as a matter of fact such blood usually has the two Hr factors hr' and hr", namely, in individuals of genotype R^1R^2. Moreover, type Rh_1Rh_2 blood may also have only a single Hr factor (genotypes R^1R^z, R^2R^z, r^yR^z, etc.), or as many as three Hr factors (genotypes $r'R^2$, R^1r'', R^zr, R^0r^y, etc.) and only rarely does it completely lack Hr factors (genotype R^zR^z). Still a fourth group [20] of CDE workers use the phenotype designations listed in column (d). This "system" can be dismissed immediately as a complete fraud, since it merely plagiarizes the Rh—Hr notations of the first column with the aid of the substitutions rh = cde, rh' = Cde, rh" = = cdE, etc.

TABLE 2. *Reactions determined by the Rh genes, including genes* r^y *and* R^z.

Gene	Reactions with Anti-Rh sera			Reactions with Anti-Hr sera		
	Anti-rh'	Anti-rh"	Anti-Rh$_0$	Anti-hr'	Anti-hr"	Anti-Hr$_0$
r	—	—	—	+	+	(+)
r'	+	—	—	—	+	(+)
r''	—	+	—	+	—	(+)
r^y	+	+	—	—	—	(+)
R^0	—	—	+	+	+	(—)
R^1	+	—	+	—	+	(—)
R^2	—	+	+	+	—	(—)
R^z	+	+	+	—	—	(—)

The WIENER notations have been criticized by the CDE protagonists on the ground that they do not include the Hr factors in the phenotype and genotype symbols. To answer this objection, it is necessary only to refer to Table 2 giving the reactions determined by the various allelic genes. It will be seen that each gene can be identified completely by the reactions it determines with the three Rh antisera, since the reactions with the Hr sera are always opposite to those obtained with the corresponding Rh sera. For example, since gene R^1 by definition determines positive reactions with sera anti-Rh$_0$ and anti-rh' and negative reactions with anti-rh", it necessarily determines negative reactions with anti-Hr$_0$ and anti-hr' and positive reactions with anti-hr". Similarly, genotype R^1r' for example, is obviously positive for Rh$_0$, rh', hr" and Hr$_0$, and negative for rh" and hr'. The situation is entirely analogous to the reciprocal relationship between agglutinogens and agglutinins in the case of the four blood groups. Yet no one but the neophyte feels the need for designations such as group O, anti-A, anti-B; group A, anti-B; etc., when naming these blood groups.

In conclusion, it should be mentioned that the recent rediscovery by British workers of the intermediate genes described by the writer[21] in 1944 has caused still further confusion among the CDE workers. They have now adopted designations such as C^uDE and CD^ue, which besides being cumbersome also incorrectly imply that the so-called C^u and D^u agglutinogens share a factor "u" in common. This predicament has latterly forced RACE[22] to consider still other less desirable notations, using sets of symbols such as a^1, a^2, a^3 ..., b^1, b^2, b^3 ..., c^1, c^2, c^3 ... or C^1, C^2, C^3 ..., D^1, D^2, D^3 ..., etc. These systems of notations like the others that have been proposed all fail to take into account the special position of factor Rh_0 which is the key to the Rh—Hr system. All this unnecessary confusion, which is retarding the progress of the work of the British investigators, could have been avoided by adhering to the original, simplest and most rational nomenclature.

REFERENCES.

1. WIENER, A. S., SONN, E. B., and BELKIN, R. B. 1944. Heredity of the Rh blood types. — J. Exp. Med., 79: 235—253.
2. WIENER, A. S., DAVIDSOHN, L., and POTTER, E. L. 1945. Heredity of the Rh blood types. II. Observations on the relation of factor Hr to the Rh blood types. — J. Exp. Med., 81: 63—72.
3. SONN, E. B., and WIENER, A. S. 1945. Heredity of the Rh blood types. III. Observations on the rare genes *Rh'* and *Rh''*. — J. Heredity, 36: 301—304.
4. WIENER, A. S., and SONN, E. B. 1945. Heredity of the Rh blood types. IV. Medicolegal applications in cases of disputed parentage. — J. Lab. and Clin. Med., 30: 395—405.
5. WIENER, A. S., SONN, E. B., and POLIVKA, H. 1946. Heredity of the Rh blood types. V. Improved nomenclature; additional family studies with special reference to Hr. — Proc. Soc. Exp. Biol. and Med., 61: 382—390.
6. WIENER, A. S., and SONN-GORDON, E. B. 1947. Heredity of the Rh blood types. VI. Additional family studies, with special reference to the theory of multiple allelic genes. — J. Immunol., 57: 203—214.
7. WIENER, A. S. 1946. Application of the Rh blood types and Hr factor in disputed parentage. — J. Lab. and Clin. Med., 31: 575—583.
8. — 1946. Recent developments in the knowledge of the Rh—Hr blood types; tests for Rh sensitization. — Amer. J. Clin. Path., 16: 477—497.
9. SCHATKIN, S. B. 1948. Disputed paternity proceedings, 2nd ed., 614 pp. — Matthew Bender and Co., New York, N. Y.
10. WIENER, A. S. 1945. Theory and nomenclature of the Hr blood factors. — Science, 102: 479—482.
11. FISHER, R. A. 1944. Cited by RACE, R. R.: An "incomplete" antibody in human serum. — Nature (London), 153: 771.
12. WIENER, A. S. 1946. Theory and nomenclature of the Rh types, subtypes, and genotypes. — Brit. Med. J., 1: 982—984.
13. — 1946. The Rh system in the chimpanzee. — Science, 104: 578—579.
14. — 1948. Nomenclature of the Rh factors. — Lancet, 1: 343.
15. — 1948. Anti-Rh serum nomenclature. — Brit. Med. J., 1: 805—806.
16. CASTLE, W. B., WINTROBE, M. W., and SNYDER, L. H. 1948. On the nomenclature of the anti-Rh typing serums; report of the advisory review board. — Science, 107: 27—31.

17. RACE, R. R. 1946. A summary of present knowledge of the human blood groups, with special reference to serological incompatibility as a cause of congenital disease. — Brit. Med. Bull., 4: 188—193.
18. MATSON, G. A., and PIPER, C. L. 1948. Distribution of the blood groups, M—N, Rh types and secretors among the Indians of Utah. — Amer. J. Phys. Anthrop., 5 N. S.: 357—368.
19. ZOUTENDYK, A. 1947. Rhesus factor blood types in South African Bantu. — South Afr. J. Med., Sci., 12: 167—169.
20. DONAHUE, W. L., and FREME, I. A. 1948. Maternal isoimmunization without evidence of clinical erythroblastosis fetalis in the newborn. — J. Lab. and Clin. Med., 33: 526—531.
21. WIENER, A. S. 1944. The Rh series of allelic genes. — Science, 100: 595—597.
22. RACE, R. R. 1948. Sur la nomenclature des groupes Rh. — Rev. d'Hématol., 3: 112—115.
23. RACE, R. R., and TAYLOR, G. L. 1944. The rare gene Rh_y in mother and son. — Nature, 153: 560.
24. MURRAY, J., RACE, R. R., and TAYLOR, G. L. 1945. Serological reactions caused by the rare human gene Rh_z. — Nature, 155: 112.
25. STANCU, A. G., CLARK, P. C., and SNYDER, L. H. 1947. Studies in human inheritance. XXIX. A statistical analysis of Rh—Hr incompatibility, with illustrative data from cases of dementia precox. — Ohio State Med. J., 43: 628—631.
26. WIENER, A. S. 1943. Blood groups and transfusion, 3rd ed., p. 254. — C. C. Thomas, Springfield, Ill.
27. WIENER, A. S., and LANDSTEINER, K. 1943. Heredity of variants of the Rh type. — Proc. Soc. Exp. Biol. and Med., 53: 167—170.
28. WIENER, A. S. 1943. Genetic theory of the Rh blood types. — Proc. Soc. Exp. Biol. and Med., 54: 316—319.
29. RACE, R. R., TAYLOR, G. L., IKIN, E. W., and PRIOR, A. W. 1944. The inheritance of allelomorphs of the Rh gene in fifty-six families. — Ann. Eug., 12: 206—210.
30. RACE, R. R., TAYLOR, G. L., IKIN, E. W., and DOBSON, A. M. 1945. The inheritance of allelomorphs of the Rh gene; a second series of families. — Ann. Eug., 12: 261—265.
31. STRATTON, F. 1945. The inheritance of the allelomorphs of the Rh gene, with special reference to the Rh' and Rh" genes. — Ann. Eug., 12: 250—260.
32. McFARLANE, M. 1946. The inheritance of allelomorphs of the Rh gene in fifty families. — Ann. Eug., 13: 15—17.
33. RACE, R. R., MOURANT, A. E., and MACFARLANE, M. N. 1946. Travaux récents sur les antigènes et anticorp Rh avec une étude particulière de la méthode de FISHER. — Rev. d'Hématol., 1: 9—12.

From R. R. Race (1964). Biometrics, 20, 361-7. Copyright (1964), by kind permission of the author and the William Byrd Press, Inc

SOME NOTES ON FISHER'S CONTRIBUTIONS TO HUMAN BLOOD GROUPS

R. R. RACE

*Medical Research Council Blood Group Research Unit,
The Lister Institute, London, S.W.1, England.*

The Rh system

By 1941 it was realized that the Rh groups were not as simple as they had first appeared, and in the two following years a system of what then seemed bewildering complexity unfolded itself. By the end of 1943 the stage illustrated in Table 1 had been reached by British workers who were one antibody ahead of the Americans. The four antibodies defined seven alleles. The + and − signs represent how the antibodies would react with the antigens produced by one allele. Apart from the present names of the antibodies, which are given in brackets, this was the table studied by Fisher.

The first observation was that serum 1 and serum 4 gave antithetical reactions, and Fisher assumed that the antigens and genes they detected were allelic and called them C and c.

TABLE 1

THE RH GENES, ANTIGENS AND ANTIBODIES AT THE END OF 1943

genes and 'haploid' antigens

antisera	R_1	R_2	r	R_0	R''	R'	R_z
1 (anti-C)	+	−	−	−	−	+	?
2 (anti-D)	+	+	−	+	−	−	?
3 (anti-E)	−	+	−	−	+	−	+
4 (anti-c)	−	+	+	+	+	−	−

The reactions of serums 2 and 3 were not antithetical to each other, nor did they bear any relation to those of serums 1 and 4, so they were called anti-D and anti-E, and their corresponding antigens and genes D and E. Fisher supposed that the antigens D and E would also have 'allelic' forms d and e which would be capable, in favourable circumstances, of stimulating their own antibodies anti-d and anti-e.

It was assumed that the three genes, if separable, must be very closely linked, for no recombination had been observed at that time (nor has it been since). Furthermore, if crossing-over could occur at all freely the frequencies of the various gene complexes would differ very greatly from those observed.

The synthesis (cited by Race [1944]) immediately brought order into the confusion and was welcomed almost universally. Unfortunately it aroused the bitter and enduring antagonism of Dr A. S. Wiener, a leading American expert.

The synthesis had certain obvious consequences which are indicated in Table 2. Two more antibodies, anti-d and anti-e, were anticipated, as well as an eighth allele. Anti-e was found two years later and the missing allele, CdE, five years later. In spite of various reports it is practically certain that anti-d has never been found: its absence remains unexplained unless some impediment is provided by the original rhesus antigen of Landsteiner and Wiener, which is now known to be present in both $D+$ and $D-$ red cells yet to be genetically independent of the CDE antigens (Levine *et al.* [1963]).

TABLE 2
CONSEQUENCES OF FISHER'S THEORY

genes and 'haploid' antigens

antisera	CDe	cDE	cde	cDe	cdE	Cde	CDE	CdE
	R_1	R_2	r	R_0	R''	R'	R_z	R_y
anti-C	+	–	–	–	–	+	+	+
anti-D	+	+	–	+	–	–	+	–
anti-E	–	+	–	–	+	–	+	+
anti-c	–	+	+	+	+	–	–	–
anti-d	–	–	+	–	+	+	–	+
anti-e	+	–	+	+	–	+	–	–

The reactions within the enclosure are those known before Fisher formulated his theory. The predictions made by the theory are shown outside the enclosure: save that no anti-d has been identified all the reactions have been confirmed serologically.

The crossing-over idea.

This, perhaps the most brilliant idea that has been contributed to the rather factual subject of blood groups, has given a great deal of pleasure though it has not yet been either confirmed or disproved. The following account is taken with slight modification from Race and Sanger [1962].

Noticing that in the English population there were three orders of frequency of the gene complexes, CDe, cde and cDE 12 per cent or over, then cDe, cdE, Cde and CDE less than 3 per cent and finally CdE with a frequency so low that it had not at that time been found, Fisher [1946b, 1947, 1953b] suggested that the rarer combinations might be maintained by occasional crossing-over from the common heterozygotes. For example, a cross-over happening between C and D in CDe/cde would produce cDe and Cde. All four second order complexes could be produced in this way, but not the third order CdE. The production of CdE would require a cross-over from a heterozygote, e.g. cDE/Cde, involving a second order complex Cde, itself according to the theory a cross-over. This would doubtless be a very rare event. The theory thus offered a very satisfactory explanation of the then puzzling absence of CdE.

Fisher carried this brilliant idea a step further in suggesting that the order of genes within the complex is such that C lies between D and E. The reason is that the frequency ratio of cdE to the heterozygote cDE/cde, which represents a cross-over between D and E, is considerably larger than the ratios of Cde to CDe/cde (cross-over between C and D) and of CDE to CDe/cDE (cross-over between C and E).

The crossing-over hypothesis does not pretend to offer an explanation of the frequent gene complexes in any population, but, given the frequent combinations, it may explain the less frequent.

It was hoped that the testing of populations which differ sharply from the English might, by the infrequent gene complexes revealed, provide a clear confirmation or refutation of the crossing-over idea, but this has not happened: some series have been strikingly for and some against.

Subsequent work, such as that on the gene complex $-D-$, on the combined antigens ce, Ce, etc., and on G, persists in associating C with E and D with C, but nothing has turned up so far to connect D with E: that is, the order DCE still seems to hold.

An almost complete story of Rh can still be told in terms of CDE, but the question is now being raised whether the scheme has anything more to offer, or whether it represents only a part of a larger pattern, so that thought about some of the latest observations is handicapped if attempts are made to fit them to the original pattern. Be that as it may, Fisher's synthesis has been of enormous use in describing observed relationships and in anticipating others; indeed, such successful prediction must be rare in biology.

After the elucidation of Rh, Fisher, who was R_1r (CDe/cde), had many injections of blood containing the antigen E, but to his disappointment he failed to make anti-E, which was much needed at the time.

In 1946 and 1947 Fisher applied his maximum likelihood method to the estimation of Rh gene frequencies from the results of tests on unrelated people.

It may be of interest to record that some time before the war, when only the A_1A_2BO, MN and P groups were known, Fisher suggested cross-injections of a few cubic centimetres of blood between the members of the Galton Laboratory, or at least those members who might prove as enthusiastic about the idea as he was. The medical men, Taylor and Race, remembering their Hippocratic oaths, were against it, and so the discovery of Rh was probably postponed for two years, and left to the Americans. Had Fisher's plan been carried out anti-Rh and perhaps anti-Kell would very likely have been produced by someone (Fisher himself was later found to be Kell $+$). Had the injections been confined to males they would probably have had no ill effects: later knowledge showed that the experiment could well have been disastrous to the offspring of some of the females who might have been involved.

In the world of blood transfusion Fisher is gratefully remembered by thousands of workers for making Rh understandable; but his main contribution was to the science of blood groups which has become a small branch of biology on its own. Furthermore, he brought together a team capable of doing the tests and induced in them habits of genetical and statistical thought which were amongst their most useful tools, and he provided unlimited enthusiasm and encouragement.

PAPERS BY R. A. FISHER WHOLLY OR IN PART DEVOTED TO BLOOD GROUPS

[1936] Heterogeneity of linkage data for Freidreich's ataxia and the spontaneous antigens. *Ann. Eugen., Lond.* 7, 17–21.

[1939] (with Janet Vaughan). Surnames and blood groups. *Nature, Lond. 144,* 1047–8.

[1939] (with G. L. Taylor). Blood groups in Great Britain. *Brit. med. J. ii, 826.*

[1940] (with G. L. Taylor). Scandinavian influence in Scottish ethnology. *Nature, Lond. 145,* 590.

[1943] (with J. A. F. Roberts). A sex difference in blood-group frequencies. *Nature, Lond. 151*, 640.

[1944] (with R. R. Race and G. L. Taylor). Mutation and the rhesus reaction. *Nature, Lond. 153*, 106.

[1945] G. L. Taylor, M. D., Ph.D., F.R.C.P. (Obituary). *Brit. med. J. i*, 463.

[1946a] The fitting of gene frequencies to data on *rhesus* reactions. *Ann. Eugen., Lond. 13*, 150–55.

[1946b] (with R. R. Race). Rh gene frequencies in Britain. *Nature, Lond. 157*, 48.

[1947] The Rhesus factor. A study in scientific method. *Amer. Scientist 35*, 95–103.

[1947] Note on the calculation of the frequencies of *rhesus* allelomorphs. *Ann. Eugen., Lond. 13*, 223–24.

[1949] (with P. H. Andresen, S. T. Callender, R. Grubb, W. T. J. Morgan, A. E. Mourant, M. M. Pickles and R. R. Race). A notation for the Lewis and Lutheran blood-group systems. *Nature, Lond. 163*, 580–81.

[1951] Standard calculations for evaluating a blood-group system. *Heredity 5*, 95–102.

[1952] Statistical methods in genetics. *Heredity 6*, 1–12.

[1953a] The variation in strength of the human blood group *P*. *Heredity 7*, 81–9.

[1953b] Population genetics. *Proc. Roy. Soc. B. 141*, 510–23.

[1954] Blood groups in anthropology (a review of *The Distribution of the Human Blood Groups*, by A. E. Mourant) *Brit. med. J. ii*, 1034.

[1956] Blood groups and population genetics. *Acta genet. 6*, 507–09.

[1957] Methods in human genetics. *Acta genet. 7*, 7–10.

OTHER REFERENCES

Dobson, A. M. and Ikin, E. W. [1946]. The *ABO* blood groups in the United Kingdom; frequencies based on a very large sample. *J. Path. Bact. 48*, 221–27.

Levine, P., Celano, M. J., Wallace, J. and Sanger, R. [1963]. A human 'D-like' antibody. *Nature, Lond. 198*, 596–97.

Race, R. R. [1944]. An 'incomplete' antibody in human serum. *Nature, Lond. 153*, 771–72.

Race, R. R. Ikin, E. W., Taylor, G. L. and Prior, A. M. [1942]. A second series of families examined in England for the A_1A_2BO and *MN* blood group factors. *Ann. Eugen., Lond. 11*, 385–94.

Race, R. R. and Sanger, R. [1952]. The inheritance of the Duffy blood groups: analysis of 110 English families. *Heredity 6*, 111–19.

Race, R. R. and Sanger, R. [1954, 1958 and 1962]. *Blood Groups in Man.* 2nd, 3rd and 4th Ed. Blackwell Scientific Publications.

Roberts, J. A. F. [1948]. The frequencies of the *ABO* blood groups in South-Western England. *Ann. Eugen., Lond., 14*, 109–16.

Taylor, G. L. and Prior, A. M. [1939]. Blood groups in England. III. Discussion of the family material. *Ann. Eugen., Lond. 9*, 18–44.

Section II

Methods of treating the established disease

Paper 16

16.   Diamond, L. K. (1947). Erythroblastosis foetalis or haemolytic disease of the newborn. *Proc. Roy. Soc Med.*, *40* 546-550. (Abstract).

Commentary

Though this paper was given 28 years ago at a meeting of the Section of Paediatrics at the Royal Society of Medicine in London, it reads in a remarkably modern way and the basic information about iso-immunisation by Rh remains correct, though some of the ways in which women become immunised (e.g. by intramuscular injections of blood for skin diseases) have fortunately disappeared.

The particular interest in Dr Diamond's paper is the tracing of the practice of transfusion in newborn infants suffering from jaundice and anaemia. This started in Dr Diamond's unit as far back as 1927, and at this time the babies were simply given ABO compatible blood from the father. 'Many transfusions were often necessary since the red cells did not seem to survive long, but eventually the majority of such children recovered'—though the author points out that there was a mortality of about 40%, so this majority was not large.

With the discovery of the Rh system, repeated transfusions of Rh-negative blood were given, and the mortality dropped to about 30%. When more became known about rising titres of Rh antibody, it seemed reasonable to deliver the sensitised woman 2—3 weeks before term, and when this was done and the baby then given frequent transfusions of Rh-negative blood the mortality was lowered still further to around 20%.

Finally came a major advance. Because sometimes free maternal Rh antibody was found in the baby's blood it seemed likely that this continued to act for several days after birth and was responsible for the occasional sudden worsening of the clinical condition. Exsanguination (i.e. 'exchange') transfusion was therefore initiated and the criteria for using this are given in the paper. The result was that 'infants very sick and anaemic at birth . . . survived' and in the 50 infants reported the mortality was near 10%; but the author concludes 'there is no justification for complacency or surety'.

*From L. K. Diamond (1947). Proc. Roy. Soc. Med., **40, 546-550**. Copyright (1947), by kind permission of the author and Longmans, Green and Co Ltd*

546   *Proceedings of the Royal Society of Medicine*

Erythroblastosis Fœtalis or Hæmolytic Disease of the Newborn
(*Abstract of Illustrated Talk*)

By Louis K. Diamond, M.D.

(*The Children's and Infants' Hospitals, and Harvard Medical School, Boston, Mass.*)

Recent and more widespread interest in erythroblastosis fœtalis or hæmolytic disease of the newborn has led to the erroneous impression that this is a new condition of recent origin. Actually it was well described, in the English literature, before 1900, being then recognized in the form of fœtal hydrops. Between 1900 and 1910, there were numerous articles, published in this country, dealing with familial icterus gravis, another manifestation of the same disease, and even the severe anæmia and erythroblastæmia were recorded as important features. Next, interest shifted to the pathology, studied and fully described by German investigators, between 1910 and 1920. Finally, the anæmia developing unexplainably in newborn infants was considered a new entity, shortly after 1920.

Our own interest in and experience with erythroblastosis fœtalis dates back twenty years, and in 1932 we collected and published records of 20 infants, suffering from œdema at birth, or jaundice and anæmia shortly after birth, splenomegaly and erythroblastæmia—all being manifestations of a single underlying morbid process.

The discovery of the Rhesus blood factor in humans in 1940 and in 1941, its important relation to erythroblastosis fœtalis, once more focused attention on this disease. In the succeeding five years, so much has been written on the Rh factor, and the disturbances which result from it, that it is worth while reviewing the subject and considering what is established fact and what is hypothesis.

The Rh blood factor is present in the red cells of 85% of the white population and absent in 15%. Since it is foreign to the system of the latter group, the Rh factor can act antigenically to start isoimmunization, when introduced into the body, either by transfusion or, in women—and even then only in a small percentage of them—by pregnancy. The antibodies produced by the Rh-negative individual, after sensitization, are agglutinins, capable of clumping and eventually destroying Rh-positive red cells. It usually requires one or more transfusions of Rh-positive blood into an Rh-negative patient, and an interval of two weeks or more, before a hæmolytic reaction is produced.

In women, subject to sensitization via pregnancy, even a first transfusion of Rh-positive blood may cause a serious untoward reaction. The factors which govern this are, first, the combination of an Rh-negative mother and an Rh-positive father, to whom are born Rh-positive children. These may serve to sensitize the woman when fœtal erythrocytes or tissues enter her circulation during gestation. Thereafter, the transfusion of this Rh-negative woman with Rh-positive blood will lead to a hæmolytic crisis.

Actually the danger of isoimmunization of the Rh-negative woman by pregnancies involving an Rh-positive fœtus is relatively small, since about 13% of all marriages are between an Rh-negative woman and an Rh-positive man, but only 1 in 150 deliveries produces an infant with erythroblastosis fœtalis, and even so the first Rh-positive infant almost always escapes. This means that less than one such woman in twenty need be concerned about becoming sensitized through pregnancy alone. However, a single transfusion of Rh-positive blood, followed by pregnancies, will increase the chances of trouble from 5% to over 50%.

Another hazard of isoimmunization following transfusion affects the fœtus. If an Rh-negative woman is given Rh-positive blood, the antibodies which develop may produce hæmolytic disease in any subsequent Rh-positive fœtus, even if it is a firstborn.

The modes of Rh sensitization of the Rh-negative woman then are, first, through transfusion of Rh-positive blood, second, through repeated pregnancies with Rh-positive babies, and third—a little appreciated menace—through the injection intramuscularly of even small amounts of Rh-positive blood, a mode of therapy fortunately now discarded for the treatment of hæmorrhagic diseases, pernicious vomiting of pregnancy and stubborn dermatitis. Although such intramuscular blood probably does little or no harm alone, if followed by Rh-positive pregnancies, even years later, it may be important in initiating isoimmunization.

The woman who, through any of the above mechanisms, has become sensitized against the Rh factor, may face several serious problems in subsequent child-bearing. If she is fortunate enough to marry an Rh-negative man—about one chance in seven—she need have no fears, since Rh-negative children will not be affected. If the sensitized woman has an Rh-positive husband who is homozygous, i.e. carries two Rh-positive genes, every infant will be Rh-positive and will be affected, usually with increase in severity of the disease. If the husband is heterozygous, Rh-negative children are possible and only the Rh-positive infants may have erythroblastosis fœtalis.

It is important, therefore, not only to determine the Rh type of every recipient of blood and every woman during child-bearing, but if Rh sensitization is detected in the woman, to test the husband's blood for homozygosity or heterozygosity and so be able to prognosticate the chances of successful pregnancy. For such special tests, the ordinary simple Rh-typing serum must be supplemented with special specific anti-Rh serums which can only be found in certain diagnostic laboratories.

Prior to 1944, tests for sensitization of Rh-negative individuals were often quite unsatisfactory since, even in instances of proven hæmolytic transfusion reaction or definite erythroblastosis fœtalis, the serum of the affected individual often failed to disclose Rh agglutinins. In 1944, new tests were developed which detected antibodies coating Rh-positive red cells or blocking their further agglutination in saline suspension, or clumping them only in protein media. These new and more complex antibodies were named "incomplete antibodies", "blocking antibodies" or "hyperimmune antibodies". The latter name arose from the finding that if human experimental subjects were injected repeatedly with Rh-positive blood cells, their serum first contained ordinary agglutinins acting against Rh-positive red cells suspended in saline. These were named "early antibodies". With continued injections, such Rh-negative persons gradually lost their simple Rh agglutinins, but developed the "incomplete" or "blocking" form which no longer agglutinated Rh-positive cells in saline but did become attached to such cells and could clump them in plasma, serum, or albuminous suspension media, and, of course, did produce agglutination within the body. These were named "hyperimmune antibodies". They are more complex, much more stable and long-lasting and probably can produce more damage, especially to Rh-positive infants developing erythroblastosis fœtalis.

Just as in these experimental subjects stimulated by blood injections, Rh-negative women bearing Rh-positive infants, tend first to develop early saline-acting agglutinins but with succeeding pregnancies, form more of the hyperimmune antibodies and, later, only this form. However, the form of Rh antibody and its concentration or titre bear no direct relation to the severity or the type of erythroblastosis fœtalis which develops in the child of the sensitized woman.

Certainly only the roughest parallelism is to be found between the type of Rh antibody and its amount during and after pregnancy, and the form of the disease or its severity in any given infant. In general, the hyperimmune and high titred Rh antibodies are found in association with the more serious or more often fatal types of hæmolytic disease in the newborn. But a prognosis based on antibody tests and titres, in any given case, must be offered with reservations.

With regard to the clinical problems faced by the pædiatrician or practitioner, our own experience began about twenty years ago, when we first treated newborn infants with jaundice and anæmia, using compatible blood from the father (therefore Rh-positive) for transfusion. Many transfusions were often necessary since the red cells did not seem to survive long, but eventually a majority of such children recovered, especially if they had no complications such as severe jaundice, œdema, diffuse hæmorrhage or cardiac failure with secondary pneumonia. Over a period of fifteen years, including the infants who were born dead and diagnosed by the pathologist, we found a gross mortality of about 40%. Several features were intriguing then, just as they are now. Often, newborn infants displayed very little anæmia, but developed early and severe jaundice. Transfusion did not materially benefit these and sometimes they developed signs of brain damage, about the fourth or fifth day of life, and fortunately did not recover. If they did improve, marked developmental retardation and muscle unbalance might result. Pathologically, kernicterus was usually found in such patients. This is a diffuse and symmetrical staining of nerve cells. It is unrelated to simple mechanisms such as intravascular thrombi or agglutination of red cells.

The tendency for the recurrence of infants with erythroblastosis fœtalis was always disturbing, especially since the disease became progressively more severe in succeeding siblings. Often, this resulted in the birth of hydropic stillborns, with severe anæmia, tremendous splenomegaly, hepatomegaly, and dilated hearts. Then again, a single child might escape serious damage and exhibit only moderate and easily repaired anæmia.

Not all of these clinical observations have been explained by the discovery of the Rh factor and the knowledge of the action of anti-Rh agglutinin on the Rh-positive infant's red cells. The serologists have tended to oversimplify the pathogenesis of the disease and draw too many analogies between what happens in the baby and what can be demonstrated in the test-tube.

With the disclosure of the role of maternal Rh antibodies in damaging the infant's Rh-positive red cells, it seemed logical to use only compatible Rh-negative blood for transfusion of the anæmic infant with erythroblastosis fœtalis. Such transfusions were given as frequently as needed, always into an easily accessible superficial vein, in amounts of about 10 c.c. per pound of body-weight, using a pressure system. More may be given, but if the infant has cardiac dilatation or a tendency to develop petechial hæmorrhage, sudden collapse may occur during large transfusions from cardiac decompensation or diffuse hæmorrhage.

During a period of about three years when our treatment consisted only of repeated small transfusions of Rh-negative blood, the gross mortality from erythroblastosis fœtalis seen in our clinic was about 30%. This improvement may have been due to earlier recognition and treatment of such infants as well as the use of Rh-negative blood transfusion.

By 1944, most of the obstetricians were well aware of the dangers of Rh antibodies in Rh-negative women, and were testing such patients more regularly. We had organized several prenatal clinics for the care of these problems and were following the titres in sensitized women throughout pregnancy. It was always distressing to detect a rising or a high titre, to wait for the delivery of the infant at term, and to have the infant succumb *in utero* only a few weeks from term, or even shortly after birth. In such cases, it seemed reasonable therefore to try to deliver the sensitized woman two or three weeks before term. During the years that this has been practised in conjunction with frequent transfusions of Rh-negative blood, as needed, the gross mortality has been lowered to 20%.

Finally, another improvement in therapy was attempted. We had shown for some time that the erythroblastotic infants who were most seriously ill or suddenly collapsed after being quite normal in appearance at birth, usually showed free maternal antibody in their cord blood. It seemed likely that this continued acting in the child's system and caused the sudden change for the worse in succeeding days. In addition, many of the babies' red cells were proved to be coated with maternal antibody. The removal of as much as possible of the affected infant's circulating blood, shortly after birth, in proper cases, seemed desirable.

The first attempts to do an early exsanguination-transfusion were complicated by mechanical difficulties. The longitudinal sinus is a dangerous vessel to puncture blindly, particularly in a newborn infant, whose head is moulded out of shape with normal anatomic relations distorted. Peripheral veins are small and fragile. Even arteries may be too small for ready cannulization and the exposure of a sick newborn infant for an hour or two while vessels are exposed and used may be a cooling and shock-producing procedure. Needles and tubing tend to clog as the blood thickens or the flow slows. The injection of heparin to prevent clotting is a decided risk in an infant who usually has hypoprothrombinæmia and a well-marked bleeding tendency.

Only through the development of special plastic catheters and their use in the umbilical vein were all these difficulties resolved and the techniques of exsanguination-transfusion made easier.

The indications for this operation have been fixed as follows until such time as sufficient data have been accumulated to evaluate the results. If the mother has been known, or is quickly demonstrated, to have Rh antibodies in her serum, and the infant shows definite clinical signs of erythroblastosis fœtalis, at or shortly after birth, treatment is begun at once. If the infant born to a sensitized mother exhibits no symptoms at birth, but is found, by immediate testing of the cord blood, to be Rh-positive and to have detectable Rh antibody still present in its serum, treatment is also indicated. If the infant not only looks well, but though Rh-positive has no free maternal antibody by suitable tests, no treatment is given at present. To date, about ten such infants have had no serious anæmia later, although a few of them have required single transfusion.

The results of exsanguination-transfusion have been quite satisfactory in many cases. Infants, very sick and anæmic at birth, have survived. Most of them have been ready for discharge with the mother in seven or eight days. Only a few have developed moderate anæmia by the third week and required another small transfusion.

Statistically, our mortality in about fifty sick infants has been near 10%. Several babies who succumbed had atelectasis, intracranial hæmorrhage and other signs of immaturity, rather than erythroblastosis fœtalis.

Much more study and data are needed before the problems of the management of blood incompatibility—antibody action between mother and child—and the best care of the newborn infant with hæmolytic disease are all solved. Notable advances have been made. But there is no justification for complacency or surety. Neither is there reason for undue anxiety when faced with the problems of Rh incompatibility.

[*June* 14, 1947]

MEETING HELD AT ROYAL VICTORIA INFIRMARY, NEWCASTLE-UPON-TYNE

The following papers were read:

Problems in the Organization of a Professorial Unit.—Professor J. C. SPENCE, M.C., M.D.

A Method of Recording Neonatal Infections in a Maternity Hospital.—MARY TAYLOR, M.D.

Prematurity in an Industrial Town.—F. J. W. MILLER, M.D.

Treatment and Prognosis of Bronchiectasis.—ALAN OGILVIE, M.D., F.R.C.P.

A Consideration of Acute Intussusception in relation to Medical Teaching.— DONALD COURT, M.R.C.P.

Paper 17

17. Mollison, P. L. and Walker, W. (1952). Controlled trials of the treatment of haemolytic disease of the newborn. *Lancet, i,* 429-433.

Commentary

Trials testing the efficacy of Diamond's therapy are given in this paper. It needed people of the calibre of Mollison and Walker to do this, because centres had to be persuaded either to use premature induction or to allow the pregnancy to go to term, or alternatively to give either exchange or simple transfusion. The point of inducing early is that the Rh-positive baby is exposed for a shorter period to the maternal antibodies, but on the other hand immaturity *per se* carries its own problems and the balance is a fine one. In the paper it will be seen that there were numerous complicating factors such as the level of the haemoglobin at which transfusion should be given, but all the cases referred to were of more than average severity.

In the induced versus spontaneous deliveries, 28 out of 77 (36·4%) of the former were either stillborn or died neonatally, as against 26 out of 108 of the latter (24·1%). This difference does not quite reach the conventional level of significance, but emphasises the importance of longer gestation.

In the exchange versus simple transfusion comparison (both procedures carried out within nine hours of birth) 8 babies died out of 62 in the former group and 21 out of 57 in the latter ($p = 0·002$). A considerable proportion of the infants in both groups were immature (though none were induced) and all were severely affected—that is to say, the figures do not indicate the mortality that would be expected in an ordinary consecutive series.

The results of the trials show (a) that the practice of premature induction alone was associated with a reduced incidence of stillbirths, but that this was outweighed by the increased incidence of neonatal deaths, and (b) that infants treated by exchange had a greater chance of survival and a very low incidence of kernicterus compared with those treated by simple transfusion. This can only be clearly demonstrated in two groups of cases; (1) mature infants who were severely affected (cord haemoglobin concentration 11 g/100 ml or less) and (2) immature infants who were only moderately affected (cord haemoglobin concentration above 11 g/100 ml). The benefits of exchange transfusion were most striking in the latter group. In mature infants who were only moderately affected the mortality following simple transfusion was about as low as after exchange transfusions. Immature infants severely affected had a low recovery rate even when treated with exchange transfusion.

From P. L. Mollison and W. Walker (1952). Lancet, i, 429–433. Copyright (1952), by kind permission of the author and The Lancet Ltd

THE LANCET]   **ORIGINAL ARTICLES**   [MARCH 1, 1952

CONTROLLED TRIALS OF THE TREATMENT OF HÆMOLYTIC DISEASE OF THE NEWBORN *

P. L. MOLLISON   W. WALKER †
M.D. Camb., M.R.C.P.   M.D. Durh.

From the Medical Research Council's Blood Transfusion Research Unit, Postgraduate Medical School of London, and the Children's Department, Royal Victoria Infirmary, Newcastle upon Tyne

THERE is at present no general agreement about the relative value of different methods of treatment for hæmolytic disease of the newborn. This confusion is due to a failure to make valid comparisons between different forms of treatment. Where comparisons have been attempted, they have been between groups of cases treated not only by different methods but at different periods of time. Inevitably there is doubt whether the cases that are compared are of equal severity and whether factors other than the type of transfusion have operated to the same extent during the period of observation.

The present paper records the results of controlled trials of treatment : that is to say, trials in which one type of treatment was given to approximately half the infants in a series and another type to the remaining half, the treatment to be given being determined beforehand by a system of chance. It is believed that, by this method, closely comparable series have been obtained, and that the data provide the best available evidence of the relative merits of the various forms of treatment of hæmolytic disease of the newborn which are now being practised ; in particular, they indicate unequivocally the value of exchange transfusion.

Exchange transfusion began to be practised in Britain in 1947, doubtless mainly because of the description of a simple and practical technique of performing the operation by the umbilical vein (Diamond 1947). At about the same time, many obstetricians began to practise premature induction of labour, a procedure which had also been recommended by Diamond (1947).

In 1948 a feeling arose that, owing to wide variations in the severity of cases, the merits of these new forms of treatment would be very difficult for any one person to assess. In order that sufficient material should be available for statistical analysis, it seemed desirable that several centres should pool their cases. It was realised at the outset that it would be essential to compare cases of equivalent severity and that, to ensure this, treatment would probably have to be decided by random selection.

At a preliminary meeting held in November, 1948, at which 17 centres from the British Isles were represented, it was discovered that approximately half were carrying out premature induction of labour as a routine measure, and that just over half were using exchange transfusion rather than simple transfusion. The criteria

---

* The trials whose conclusions are briefly summarised here were conducted by a group of people, representing several different centres—namely : Prof. J. C. McC. BROWNE and Dr. P. L. MOLLISON (Hammersmith), Dr. W. A. B. CAMPBELL (Belfast), Dr. W. R. F. COLLIS and Dr. P. C. D. MACCLANCY (Rotunda), Miss DOREEN DALEY (St. Helier), Dr. R. J. DRUMMOND (Cardiff), Dr. D. M. T. GAIRDNER (Cambridge), Prof. W. F. GAISFORD (Manchester), Dr. JOHN MURRAY (Queen Charlotte's), Mr. S. D. PERCHARD and Dr. V. W. PUGH (Mile End), Dr. MARGARET M. PICKLES (Oxford), Dr. G. H. TOVEY (Bristol), and Dr. W. WALKER (Newcastle). The scheme was organised by the Blood Transfusion Research Unit of the Medical Research Council, with assistance from the Council's Statistical Research Unit at the London School of Hygiene and Tropical Medicine. A full report of the trials is at present being prepared. Meanwhile we are very grateful to our colleagues for empowering us to publish this preliminary report.

† During the tenure of a Luccock Research Fellowship.

---

for the selection of cases for exchange transfusion varied from centre to centre, and up to that time relatively few infants had been treated in this way.

Infants not treated by exchange transfusion were usually treated by simple transfusion for the relief of anæmia developing during the course of the illness, but in some centres it was the practice to give simple transfusions to most affected infants without waiting for the development of severe anæmia.

The Plan of the Trials

In the early part of 1949 a subcommittee put forward a definite scheme for trials, the essentials of which were as follows :

(1) It was to be a condition of taking part in the trials that each centre should either compare premature induction of labour with spontaneous delivery, or should compare exchange transfusion with simple transfusion, or should compare both.

(2) Treatment was to be decided not later than the 35th week of pregnancy, by opening an envelope which would contain instructions either regarding premature induction of labour or the type of transfusion to be given to the infant, or both. The instructions to be included in each envelope of the series were to be decided by a system of random numbers.

(3) Various tests were laid down for the detection of Rh antibody in the mother and for the detection of disease in the infant at birth. Special steps were taken to obtain comparable hæmoglobin estimations on cord-blood : the most important of these steps was the insistence that each centre should use the " M.R.C. Photometer " (King et al. 1948).

(4) Methods of carrying out treatment were carefully defined. For example, it was stipulated that, when labour was to be induced prematurely, induction should be performed between 35 and 21 days before the expected date of delivery ; all transfusions were to be given within 9 hours of birth ; when exchange transfusion was called for by the instructions, the amount of blood exchanged was not to be less than 60 ml. per lb. body-weight and a concentrated suspension of Rh-negative red cells was to be used. It was agreed that if the cord-blood hæmoglobin concentration exceeded 15·5 g. per 100 ml. no treatment need be given.

(Hb concentrations are abbreviated to " g. " in this paper. Note that on the Haldane scale 15·5 g. = 105% ; 14·8 g. = 100% ; 11 g. = 75%.)

In putting forward these " rules " it was emphasised that any centre which had a firm impression that one of these treatments was better than another could not take part in the scheme. As a result some withdrew, and it was interesting to note that these withdrawals were based on mutually contradictory impressions. Thus some centres felt that they could not abandon routine premature induction of labour, whereas others regarded premature induction as a purely experimental procedure which they were not willing to adopt. A few centres were unwilling to abandon exchange transfusion but many more felt unable to depart from simple transfusion, regarding exchange transfusion as hazardous and of doubtful benefit. However, a sufficient number of centres were left who were willing to try either premature induction of labour against spontaneous delivery, or to try exchange transfusion against simple transfusion, or both. The results that follow are all derived from centres where treatment was varied. Thus, for example, if a centre practised routine premature induction of labour but varied between simple and exchange transfusion, its results are used only in the " simple versus exchange transfusion " comparison and are not contrasted with those of another centre practising routine spontaneous delivery, to assess the relative methods of premature induction of labour and spontaneous delivery.

THE LANCET]   ORIGINAL ARTICLES   [MARCH 1, 1952

Before finally deciding upon the rules there was some discussion about the type of treatment with which exchange transfusion should be compared. Two alternative treatments were considered :

(1) " Early simple " transfusion—i.e., the giving of a simple transfusion within a few hours of birth to any infant with a cord hæmoglobin of less than 15·5 g. per 100 ml.

(2) " Late simple " transfusion, that is, transfusion for the relief of anæmia, as and when it occurred.

The subcommittee finally decided to recommend " early simple " transfusion rather than " late simple " transfusion, feeling that if " late simple " transfusion was used and proved inferior to exchange transfusion, then it might still be said that exchange transfusion owed its superiority to the supply of some protective factors and that accordingly " early simple " transfusion might, if tried, be found as effective as exchange transfusion. Alternatively it might be held that " early simple " transfusion, by indirectly reducing the proportion of circulating Rh-positive red cells, might achieve much the same ends as exchange transfusion. It was therefore considered that a trial of exchange transfusion versus early simple transfusion would, in effect, solve two problems. Firstly, it would show whether exchange transfusion was better than simple transfusion, and secondly, if exchange transfusion proved better, it would indicate clearly that this was due to the removal of the bulk of the infant's red cells rather than to some other effect.

One centre (N) felt strongly that it was more important to compare exchange transfusion with transfusion given solely to relieve anæmia rather than with routine " early simple " transfusion. It also considered that the cord-hæmoglobin level of 15·5 g. that was to decide the giving or withholding of transfusion was rather too high. The following modified plan was therefore adopted by this centre :

Envelopes were opened only after birth and only if the cord-hæmoglobin concentration was less than 14·8 g. per 100 ml. (100% Haldane). When the instructions called for simple transfusion this was given only if the cord-hæmoglobin concentration was 11 g. or less, or if the hæmoglobin content subsequently fell below 11 g. At this centre there was no trial of premature induction and all women were allowed to go into labour spontaneously.

In the following analysis cases from centre N with cord-hæmoglobin concentrations of 11 g. or less are included in the comparison of exchange transfusion and " early simple " transfusion, since the treatment of these cases differed in no way from that used at other centres ; the cases with cord-hæmoglobin concentrations exceeding 11 g. are considered separately, since in these simple transfusion was given only for the relief of anæmia. Although at this centre no envelopes were opened for infants whose cord hæmoglobin exceeded 14·8 g., since these infants received no early treatment, records were kept of all such infants born during the period of the trials and these cases are considered as part of the series from centre N.

Results

The following results are based on observation upon 477 infants with hæmolytic disease of the newborn, all of whom were born either at term or within 35 days of the expected day of delivery. (Cases born earlier have been excluded.) However, for the various comparisons made below only certain infants were suitable. For example, in comparing exchange transfusion with simple transfusion, infants with cord-hæmoglobin concentrations exceeding 15·5 g. per 100 ml. could not be used since such infants were not treated. However, if the same cases occurred in the " premature induction of labour versus spontaneous delivery " comparison, they could be used.

In this preliminary account the results of treatment have been expressed simply in terms of death or survival, and all infants living for one month or more have been considered as " living " ; infants dying from causes other than hæmolytic disease have been included in the

" dying." In the fuller account of the trials which is now being prepared, the question of cerebral damage in surviving infants will be considered.

COMPARISON OF PREMATURE INDUCTION AND SPONTANEOUS DELIVERY

Cases for this comparison were drawn only from centres which were carrying out both premature induction and spontaneous delivery according to instructions in sealed envelopes. Some of the centres were using only one form of transfusion treatment while others were varying exchange with early simple transfusion according to random numbers.

Table I refers only to cases in which the rules of the trial were strictly complied with : however, although the rules stated that premature induction of labour should be carried out between 35 and 21 days before the expected day of delivery, infants born 18 days or more before the expected day were included. Note that all infants born more than 35 days before the expected date of delivery, whether born alive or dead, were excluded from the investigation. In addition any case in which the infant was known to have died in utero more than 35 days before term was excluded, even if the mother was delivered within 35 days of term.

Table I shows that the practice of premature induction was associated with a reduced incidence of stillbirths but that this was outweighed by the increased incidence

TABLE I—COMPARISON OF THE EFFECTS OF PREMATURE INDUCTION OF LABOUR AND SPONTANEOUS DELIVERY

Treatment	No. of cases	Living	Dying			
			Neonatal death	Still-birth	Total	Mortality
Induced ..	77	49	22	6	28	36·4 %
Spontaneous..	108	82	12	14	26	24·1 %

of neonatal deaths : hence the total death-rate in the " induced " group is higher than in the group allowed to go to spontaneous delivery. The probability of obtaining a chance difference of this magnitude is 1 in 14, which, although not reaching the usually accepted significance level of 1 in 20, is none the less very suggestive. It can also be calculated from the findings that the odds are 39 to 1 against premature induction improving the survival-rate by more than 1%.

It will be noted that the number of cases in the " induced " group is considerably smaller than the number in the " spontaneous " group. The difference is accounted for by the exclusion of cases from the induced group due to failure to carry out premature induction of labour within the time-limits specified by the rules. Further analysis of the data suggests that the effect of these omissions is not serious.

COMPARISON OF EXCHANGE AND EARLY SIMPLE TRANSFUSION

Before giving the figures it must be emphasised that the results refer to cases of more than average severity. A large number of infants who had cord-hæmoglobin concentrations exceeding 15·5 g. (14·8 g. at centre N) received no treatment and are thus excluded from the present analysis ; the great majority of these pursued a mild course, and they are considered separately below. The average severity of the cases was also substantially increased by including only those cases from centre N in which the cord hæmoglobin was 11 g. or less (see above). A few infants who were moribund at birth, and thus did not receive the intended treatment, were excluded. The figures in table II refer only to cases in which the rules for the trial were strictly complied with —e.g., exchange transfusion was carried out within 9

THE LANCET]   ORIGINAL ARTICLES   [MARCH 1, 1952

TABLE II—OVER-ALL COMPARISON OF EXCHANGE AND EARLY SIMPLE TRANSFUSION

—	Total	Living	Died
Exchange	62	54	8
Simple (early)	57	36	21

(p = 0·002.)

hours of birth. (Although the rules called for the exchange of 60 ml. of blood per lb. body-weight, only cases in which less than 50 ml. per lb. was used were in fact excluded.)

As table II shows, mortality was considerably lower in the group treated by exchange transfusion (13%) than in the group treated by simple transfusion (37%). As already emphasised, these figures do not indicate the mortality that would be expected in an ordinary consecutive series, for the cases treated are ones of more than average severity. It must also be remembered that a considerable proportion of the infants were immature.

A most informative comparison is obtained by dividing the cases, firstly according to maturity, and secondly according to whether the cord-hæmoglobin concentration did or did not exceed 11 g. This shows that the significance of the over-all difference between exchange transfusion and simple transfusion is due entirely to two of the four groups—namely, immature infants with cord-hæmoglobin concentrations exceeding 11 g., and full-term infants with cord-hæmoglobin concentrations equal to, or less than, 11 g. In full-term infants with hæmoglobin concentrations exceeding 11 g. the survival-rate is high with both simple and exchange transfusion, and in premature infants with cord-hæmoglobin concentrations of 11 g. or less the survival-rate is rather low with both treatments.

It seemed possible that cases excluded owing to non-compliance with the rules might be ones with a worse-than-average prognosis. Accordingly, a second analysis was made, including cases under their intended treatments, whether or not they actually received them. This analysis did not modify to any important extent the conclusions which have already been stated.

COMPARISON OF EXCHANGE AND "LATE SIMPLE" TRANSFUSION

The cases upon which this comparison is based are all drawn from a single centre (N) and consist only of infants whose cord hæmoglobin was between 11·1 and 14·8 g. per 100 ml. When the instructions were for exchange transfusion, this was carried out within 9 hours of birth, as usual. However, when the instructions were for simple transfusion, treatment was withheld unless the hæmoglobin concentration of a skin-prick sample subsequently fell below 11 g. Thus, 7 cases selected for simple transfusion never received any treatment; of these, 4 survived, while 3 died with kernicterus.

3 infants with cord-hæmoglobin values of over 11 g. were treated by simple transfusion on the first day of life, 1 because of bleeding from the cord and 2 because of a misunderstanding about the cord-hæmoglobin value: 2 of these infants survived while the other died with kernicterus. All 3 are excluded from the present comparison.

Table III shows a suggestive but not significant difference in favour of exchange transfusion as compared with simple relief of anæmia. The death-rates are not significantly different from those for similar groups included

TABLE III—COMPARISON OF EXCHANGE TRANSFUSION AND "LATE SIMPLE" TRANSFUSION IN INFANTS WITH CORD-HÆMOGLOBIN CONCENTRATIONS BETWEEN 11·1 AND 14·8 G.

—	Total	Lived	Died
Exchange	24	24	0
Late simple	23	20	3

in the comparison of exchange transfusion and early simple transfusion—namely, mature infants with cord hæmoglobin concentrations between 11·1 and 15·5 g.

RESULTS FROM CENTRE N CONSIDERED ALONE

The results from centre N are of special interest because they form by far the largest group treated at a single centre. In the above analysis, as explained, they have been split up, because those due for simple transfusion received the transfusion "early" or "late," depending upon the cord-hæmoglobin concentration. However, they may be considered together and then form two parallel series : (a) treated by exchange transfusion ; (b) treated by simple transfusion only if and when they were anæmic.

Of 44 infants treated by exchange transfusion 43 survived, whereas in 40 infants treated by simple transfusion only 29 survived. (p = 0·001.)

All the infants in this series were born spontaneously and only 4 were premature (birth weight 5½ lb. or less). By chance all 4 of these infants were treated by simple transfusion and 3 died, all with kernicterus. Even if these 4 infants are excluded from the analysis, the figures for exchange transfusion remain significantly better than those for simple transfusion. (p = 0·009.)

INFANTS WITH CORD-HÆMOGLOBIN CONCENTRATION EXCEEDING 15·5 G. (14·8 G. AT CENTRE N)

Of the 191 infants in this group none received transfusion during the first few days of life, though 24 of the 177 survivors did in fact become sufficiently anæmic during the first month of life to need transfusion.

The 191 cases have been divided into two groups : those born less than 18 days before the expected day of

TABLE IV—ANALYSIS OF DEATHS IN INFANTS WITH CORD-HÆMOGLOBIN CONCENTRATIONS OVER 14·8 G.

—	Cord-Hb concentration 14·9–17·5 g.		Cord-Hb concentration 17·6–21·5 g.	
—	Total	No. of deaths	Total	No. of deaths
Full-term	101	6 (5 kernicterus ; 1 other cause)	40	1 (other cause*)
Immature	38	6 (4 kernicterus ; 2 other cause)	12	1 (other cause)

* "Other cause" means death from a cause apparently unrelated to hæmolytic disease of the newborn, such as asphyxia.

delivery ("full-term") ; and those born between 18 and 35 days before the expected day of delivery ("immature"). The outcome in these cases is shown in table IV. Note that the mortality was about 1 in 7 in immature infants but only 1 in 20 in full-term infants.

If the cases are divided by birth weight rather than by length of gestation, a still more striking contrast results. Thus, taking only infants with cord-hæmoglobin concentrations between 14·9 and 17·5 g., amongst 11 infants weighing 5½ lb. or less there were 3 deaths (all from kernicterus) whereas amongst 128 infants weighing more than 5½ lb. there were 9 deaths (6 from kernicterus). In these selected groups mortality was thus about four times as high in premature infants as in mature infants.

CAUSES OF DEATH

Out of a total of 477 Rh-positive infants born at term, or within 35 days of term, 24 were stillborn. Among the remaining 453 infants born alive there were 79 deaths within the first week of life.

Amongst the 79 infants dying during the first week of life the cord-hæmoglobin concentration was estimated in all but 5 cases ; in these 5 cases death occurred within half an hour of birth in one instance, and at 3–7 days in

Paper 17

the remaining 4 : in at least 1 of these 4 latter cases death was due to kernicterus.

14 deaths occurred in infants whose cord-hæmoglobin concentration exceeded 15·5 g., and these have already been described : 9 were thought to be due to kernicterus and occurred between the 2nd and 6th days of life ; 5 were thought to be due to other causes and 4 of these deaths occurred on the 1st day of life.

There remain 60 deaths to describe, all of which occurred in infants whose cord-hæmoglobin concentration was less than 15·5 g. Of these, 9 infants were moribund at birth ; all had hæmoglobin concentrations below 7·4 g. (50% Haldane). A further 8 died within 18 hours of birth. These 8 deaths occurred amongst a total of 188 infants who received transfusion (either exchange or simple) within 9¹/₂ hours of birth. All these 8 infants were severely anæmic at birth (cord-hæmoglobin concentration below 8·8 g.) and 4 had definite signs of cardiac failure at necropsy. It was noteworthy that in the 2 cases in which death occurred within 18 hours of an exchange transfusion, the infant had been injected with 40 ml. more of blood than was withdrawn. It has been emphasised elsewhere that in infants with hæmolytic disease of the newborn severe anæmia at birth is usually accompanied by a raised venous pressure and that in performing exchange transfusion in these cases it is advisable to withdraw more blood than is injected (Mollison and Cutbush 1949, Mollison 1951).

Of the remaining 43 deaths, all of which occurred between 1 and 6 days after birth, 36 were considered to be due to kernicterus. In some cases the diagnosis of kernicterus was made from clinical signs although in the majority a post-mortem examination was made and the diagnosis based on the finding of yellow staining of the basal ganglia. The remaining 7 deaths were ascribed to such causes as intracerebral hæmorrhage and asphyxia, although in some instances kernicterus was not definitely excluded as a contributory cause.

It is noteworthy that the high death-rate in infants treated by simple transfusion was due entirely to a far higher incidence of fatal kernicterus. Thus, taking the groups set out in table II, among 57 infants treated by early simple transfusion, there were 21 deaths, 18 of which were due to kernicterus ; among 62 infants treated by exchange transfusion there were 8 deaths, 4 of which were due to kernicterus. Thus the incidence of fatal kernicterus was about five times higher in infants treated by simple transfusion than in infants treated by exchange transfusion. It must also be emphasised that in 4 infants who developed fatal kernicterus despite exchange transfusion, 3 were premature (birth weight 5¹/₂ lb. or less) ; thus the present experience does not conflict with the claim that the incidence of fatal kernicterus in mature infants treated by exchange transfusion is negligible (Allen et al. 1950b).

SUBSEQUENT PROGRESS OF INFANTS

Out of 374 surviving Rh-positive infants, 368 were examined at the age of 1 month and assessed as normal or abnormal. The intention was to detect infants with signs of damage to the central nervous system and the presence of anæmia or jaundice at this age was not regarded as abnormal for the present purpose. Out of 368 infants only 13 (3·6%) appeared to have signs of damage to the central nervous system.

The full report to be published later will deal with examinations at the age of 6 months and, if possible, at 1 year. Results analysed so far suggest that not more than 5% of the surviving infants will be recognisably abnormal.

Discussion

The practice of inducing labour 3–5 weeks before the expected day of delivery, as a routine, in women whose serum contained Rh antibody, was associated with a lower incidence of surviving infants than was the practice of allowing labour to occur spontaneously. Although this reduction in the survival-rate, following premature induction of labour, was small (about 10%) and could have been due to chance, it can be calculated that further trials would be very unlikely to show that the practice of premature induction actually increases the survival-rate.

Since it appears certain that any advantage that the affected (Rh-positive) infant derives from premature induction of labour is at the most small, the disadvantage to the mother cannot be ignored. Moreover, the unnecessary hazard to which occasional Rh-negative infants are exposed by premature induction of labour must be considered. These factors will be discussed in the full report of the trials.

The present investigation shows beyond reasonable doubt that infants treated by exchange transfusion have a greater chance of survival than infants treated by simple transfusion. Further analysis of the results shows that the improvement produced by exchange transfusion can be clearly demonstrated only in two main groups of cases—namely, mature infants who are severely affected (cord-hæmoglobin concentrations 11 g. or less) and immature infants who are only moderately affected (cord-hæmoglobin concentrations above 11 g.). In mature infants who were only moderately affected the mortality following " early simple " transfusion was about as low as it was after exchange transfusion. It is apparent that if a series consisting mainly of such infants were treated by simple transfusion, mortality would be low and it would be concluded that simple transfusion was a very satisfactory treatment (see, for example, Pennell 1950).

Immature infants who are severely affected (cord-hæmoglobin concentration 11 g. or less) have a low recovery-rate even when treated by exchange transfusion. Since many hospitals began the practice of premature induction of labour at the same time that they began to practise exchange transfusion, it is easy to see why mortality has sometimes remained disappointingly high.

The superiority of exchange transfusion over " early simple " transfusion is most striking in immature infants who are only moderately affected. It is possible that the results of exchange transfusion seemed particularly favourable to Diamond (1947) because he had been practising premature induction of labour for some time before he began to use exchange transfusion. It should be added that his group was the first to realise that premature infants are far more likely than mature infants to develop kernicterus (Allen et al. 1950a) and that the infant's best chance of survival lies in not being born prematurely and being treated by exchange transfusion (Allen et al. 1950b).

The present results provide very useful data for examining the relationship between the cord-hæmoglobin concentration and the chance of survival with various treatments ; this question will be considered in the full report of the trials. The only point to be emphasised here is that the curve published previously relating cord-hæmoglobin concentration to the chance of survival in infants treated by exchange transfusion (Mollison and Cutbush 1951) referred to a group of infants many of whom were immature. It has now become clear that the chance of survival following exchange transfusion is higher in mature infants than in immature infants. Indeed, mortality in mature infants treated by exchange transfusion is so low that it may prove difficult to construct a curve relating hæmoglobin concentration to survival in this group.

INDICATIONS FOR EXCHANGE TRANSFUSIONS

The present results indicate clearly that an immature infant affected with hæmolytic disease of the newborn whose cord-hæmoglobin concentration is below about

15 g. will be more likely to survive if it is treated by exchange transfusion. Although in the present series immature infants with cord-hæmoglobin concentrations above about 15 g. were not treated, the incidence of fatal kernicterus was as high as 1 in 12, and it seems extremely likely that this incidence could have been reduced to a low level by exchange transfusion. There was no case of kernicterus among the 12 affected immature infants with cord-hæmoglobin concentrations exceeding 17·5 g. (118% Haldane).

In severely affected mature infants exchange trans-fusion is again clearly the best treatment. In mature infants with cord-hæmoglobin concentrations between 11 and 15 g., " early simple " transfusion appeared to be as successful as exchange transfusion—although there was some suggestion that " late simple " transfusion gave worse results. Despite the failure to demonstrate any clear superiority of exchange transfusion in these cases, there seems little doubt that it is in fact superior. In mature affected infants with cord-hæmoglobin concentrations between 15 and 17·5 g. no treatment was given and the incidence of fatal kernicterus was about 1 in 21. In this group there are considerable differences between one infant and another and the problem is to detect those few infants who are going to become deeply jaundiced and be at risk from kernicterus. It is suggested that if a woman has previously lost an infant from hæmolytic disease of the newborn, it is always wise to treat the succeeding infant, however mildly it appears to be affected. Other indications will be discussed in the full report of the trials. Mature affected infants with cord-hæmoglobin concentrations over 17·5 appear to have so small a chance of developing kernicterus that treatment is not justified.

Since exchange transfusion will probably be practised increasingly in the future, it seems necessary to emphasise that the present trials have shown that, though highly experienced centres have no difficulty in performing successfully a series of exchange transfusions, centres with only small experience shared between frequently changing clinicians may sometimes fail to complete an exchange transfusion. Moreover in very ill infants the chance of survival following exchange transfusion is undoubtedly related to the way in which the procedure is carried out. It is of the first importance that a woman expected to give birth to an infant with hæmolytic disease of the newborn should be delivered in one of a limited number of institutions capable, by virtue of their experience, of maintaining a high degree of technical efficiency in the conduct of exchange transfusion.

Summary

1. Controlled trials of treatment of hæmolytic disease of the newborn were carried out in Britain from 1949 to 1951, the treatment to be given in any individual case being determined by a system of random numbers.

2. The practice of inducing labour 3–5 weeks before the expected day of delivery was associated with a lower proportion of surviving infants than was the practice of allowing delivery to occur spontaneously, though the difference did not quite reach the conventional level of significance.

3. Exchange transfusion was followed by a significantly higher survival-rate than was simple transfusion, both treatments being carried out equally early after birth. The incidence of kernicterus after exchange transfusion was very low.

4. Indications for exchange transfusion are discussed briefly, in the light of experience gained in these trials.

We should like to acknowledge our debt to Miss Marie Cutbush of the Blood Transfusion Research Unit for carrying out the laborious task of abstracting relevant information from all the record cards and tabulating it ; to Dr. J. A. Fraser Roberts for advice in planning these trials ; and to Dr. P. Armitage of the M.R.C. Statistical Research Unit for performing all the statistical tests and giving most valuable advice on the analysis of the data.

REFERENCES

Allen, F. H. jun., Diamond, L. K., Vaughan, V. C. (1950a) *Pediat.* **6**, 441.
— — — (1950b) *Amer. J. Dis. Child.* **80**, 779.
Diamond, L. K. (1947) *Proc. R. Soc. Med.*, **40**, 546.
King. E. J., Wootton, I. D. P., Donaldson, R., Sisson, R. B., Macfarlane, R. G. (1948) *Lancet*, ii, 971.
Mollison, P. L. (1951) Blood Transfusion in Clinical Medicine. Oxford.
— Cutbush, M. (1949) *Brit. med. J.* i, 123.
— — (1951) *Blood*, **6**, 777.
Pennell, S. (1950) *Ibid*, **5**, 107.

Papers 18 & 19

18. Bevis, D. C. A. (1950). Composition of liquor amnii in haemolytic disease of the newborn. *Lancet, ii*, 443.

19. Bevis, D. C. A. (1952). The antenatal prediction of haemolytic disease of the newborn. *Lancet, i*, 395-8. (Extract).

Commentary

The discovery of the Rh blood groups brought its own problems, and one of these was not knowing, in an immunised woman, how severely the next Rh-positive baby was likely to be affected. Statistically, though anti-D antibody titres tended to rise in successive pregnancies, and babies to be worse affected, yet there were many exceptions and the important information needed was an accurate prognosis in a particular case.

In this short but very informative preliminary communication on 30 patients (Paper 18), Bevis showed that the liquor amnii (a mixture of fetal urine and secretion of the amnion) obtained by rupturing the membranes in order to induce labour, contained increasing amounts of iron corresponding to the degree of severity of haemolytic disease in the fetus. Bevis comments, however, that since the haemolytic processes are often advanced by the time labour is induced, better information would be obtained if the liquor could be examined in the ante-natal period.

Two years later Bevis achieved this objective and in a paper published in the *Lancet* he summarises the findings (Paper 19). The extract needs no explanation.

From D. C. A. Bevis (1950). Lancet, ii, 443. Copyright (1950), by kind permission of the author and The Lancet Ltd

Preliminary Communication

COMPOSITION OF LIQUOR AMNII IN HÆMOLYTIC DISEASE OF NEWBORN

THE antenatal prediction of hæmolytic disease in the children of immunised Rh-negative mothers being notoriously unreliable, attempts have been made to obtain assistance from examination of the liquor amnii.

If the liquor amnii in late pregnancy is a mixture of fœtal urine and the secretion of the amnion, in hæmolytic disease bile pigments, amino-acids, or iron might possibly be found in the liquor. Liquor amnii has been obtained from cases of pre-eclampsia and postmaturity as well as from suspected cases of hæmolytic disease, high rupture of the membranes being used in St. Mary's Hospitals, Manchester, as a method of inducing labour. Care has been taken to avoid contamination of the liquor with maternal blood, and investigations have been made within twenty-four hours of obtaining the samples. All tests have been made on centrifuged liquor.

METHODS AND RESULTS

Bile-pigments.—Attempts to demonstrate the presence of bile-pigments with Fouchet's reagent and the van den Bergh reaction proved negative in all cases, including two in which the liquor had the characteristic golden colour seen in severe hæmolytic disease.

Urobilinogen.—Tests for urobilinogen (Watson 1937) have also been negative. This does not exclude the presence of urobilinogen, since protein is thought to inhibit Erhlich's reagent (Wilson and Davidson 1949).

Urobilin.—Schlesinger's test for urobilin has also been negative in all cases.

Amino-acids.—Tests for amino-acids by paper chromatography have proved disappointing, because the liquor seems to contain very little amino-acid. No difference has been discovered between affected and unaffected babies.

Iron.—The presence of iron was first sought with the prussian-blue reaction. Macroscopically this has always been negative, but the Gomori technique on dried "smears" of liquor shows that iron is always present. In cases of rhesus incompatibility the amount of iron is always increased, and the relative increase is a fairly reliable guide to prognosis. The method is, however, somewhat troublesome, and the results are not always easy to interpret. Simpler methods have therefore been sought, and the "spot reagents" produced and described by the British Drug Houses (1949) have been studied.

Tests with 'Ferron' (7-iodo-8-hydroxyquinoline-5-sulphonic acid) have been uniformly negative, indicating that the iron is present in the ferrous state.

$\alpha\alpha'$-Dipyridyl has been tried but has not proved so satisfactory as thioglycollic acid (mercaptoacetic acid). To 5·0 ml. of liquor amnii containing 1 drop of thioglycollic acid (B.D.H.) is added 0·5 ml. of ammonia (0·880); a change to purple indicates the presence of iron.

The following conclusions have been drawn from the results of 30 determinations : (1) if there is no purple, the child will be unaffected at birth but may become anæmic after the end of the first week of life ; (2) if there is a faint purple, the child will be unaffected at birth but may soon become jaundiced and is almost always anæmic by the end of the first week ; and (3) if there is a well-marked purple, the child will be affected at birth, and the prognosis is not good.

The colour seems to be due to ionised iron in the liquor amnii, because the amount of iron obtained after incineration of the liquor is appreciably greater. No purple is given by meconium in solution, although this too has been shown to contain iron on incineration. No false negative reactions have been obtained, but one false positive was found in an abortion at 16 weeks and the cause of the error is unknown.

SUMMARY

The precise origin of liquor amnii is doubtful, but it certainly seems to contain some fœtal urine.

A test for iron in liquor amnii is described which seems to have some prognostic value, but often the hæmolytic processes are found to be too far advanced when labour is induced. Possibly, if the test were applied to liquor obtained by paracentesis in the antenatal period, the induction of labour could be timed more accurately.

Thanks are due to Prof. W. I. C. Morris for suggesting that the presence of iron should be sought and for much help in the preparation of the paper.

REFERENCES

British Drug Houses (1949) The B.D.H. Book of Organic Reagents for Analytical Use. 9th ed., Poole.
Watson, C. J. (1937) *Arch. intern. Med.* **59**, 196.
Wilson, T. M., Davidson, L. S. P. (1949) *Brit. med. J.* i, 884.

D. C. A. BEVIS
M.B. Manc., M.R.C.O.G.
Senior Registrar, St. Mary's Hospitals,
Manchester.

From D. C. A. Bevis (1952). Lancet, i, 395-8. Copyright (1952), by kind permission of the author and The Lancet Ltd

THE LANCET]   ORIGINAL ARTICLES   [FEB. 23, 1952

THE ANTENATAL PREDICTION OF HÆMOLYTIC DISEASE OF THE NEWBORN

D. C. A. BEVIS

M.B. Manc., M.R.C.O.G.

SENIOR REGISTRAR, SAINT MARY'S HOSPITALS, MANCHESTER

SUMMARY

The results of analysis of the liquor amnii taken at various times in pregnancy indicate that the concentrations of non-hæmatin iron and urobilinogen offer a reliable guide to the outcome for the fœtus.

Methods of analysis and for obtaining specimens are described, and it is shown that the iron concentration tends to follow a sigmoid curve. The implications of this are briefly discussed.

REFERENCES

Bevis, D. C. A. (1950) *Lancet*, ii, 443.
Cantarow, A., Stuckert, H., Davis, R. C. (1933) *Surg. Gynec. Obstet.* **57**, 63.
Diamond, L. K., Vaughan, V. C., Allen, F. H. jun. (1950) *Pediatrics*, **6**, 630.
Flexner, L. B., Gellhorn, A. (1942) *Amer. J. Physiol.* **136**, 757.
King, E. J. (1951) Microanalysis in Medical Biochemistry. 2nd ed., London.
Kitzes, G., Elvehjem, C. A., Schuette, H. A. (1944) *J. biol. Chem.* **155**, 653.
Kropp, B. (1940) *Anat. Rec.* **77**, 407.
London, I. M., West, R., Shemin, D., Rittenberg, D. (1950) *J. biol. Chem.* **184**, 351.
Makepeace, A. W., Fremont-Smith, F., Dailey, M. E., Carroll, M. P. (1931) *Surg. Gynec. Obstet.* **53**, 635.
Mollison, P. L., Cutbush, M. (1951) *Blood*, **6**, 777.
Pommerenke, W. T., Hahn, P. F., Bale, W. F., Balfour, W. M. (1942) *Amer. J. Physiol.* **137**, 164.
Sandell, E. B. (1950) Colorimetric Determination of Traces of Metals. 2nd ed., New York.
Shrewsbury, J. F. D. (1933) *Lancet*, i, 415.
Tankard, A. R., Bagnall, D. J. T., Morris, F. (1934) *Analyst*, **59**, 806.
Uranga Imaz, F. A., Gascon, A. (1950) *Obstet. Ginec. lat.-amer.* **8**, 237.
Vanotti, A., Delachaux, A. (1949) Iron Metabolism and Its Clinical Significance. London.
Winternitz, M. (1926) *Klin. Wschr.* **5**, 988.

Paper 20

20. Liley, A. W. (1963). Intrauterine transfusion of foetus in haemolytic disease. *Brit. Med. J., ii,* 1107–9.

Commentary

Professor Liley begins this historic preliminary communication by pointing out that there is an irreducible minimum of perinatal deaths from HDN even with the best exchange transfusion technique. This is because occasionally babies become very severely affected early in the third trimester and such cases could not possibly be saved by standard treatment given *after* delivery. Here, as he points out, intraperitoneal transfusion seemed logical, and the rationale was to try to arrest the deterioration of the fetus and to gain a few weeks of gestation.

The management of an actual patient is described. The placenta was localised by a contrast medium (urografin) injected into the amniotic cavity. The fetus swallowed some of this, which enabled solid viscera to be avoided when the blood was being given. The method of introducing the needle and catheter into the fetal peritoneum was then described. On two separate occasions 100 ml and 110 ml respectively of group O Rh-negative cells were injected over 20 minutes. The baby survived after Caesarean section had been performed at 34 weeks and 4 days, but needed exchange transfusions postoperatively.

Liley points out that amniotic fluid analysis, particularly the spectral absorption curve, is the best criterion for deciding when to perform intrauterine transfusion. Liley's Chart (reproduced on page 124) relates the optical density of the liquor to the maturity of the fetus and the likely effect of the antibody on the baby.

* Holland, E. and Brews, A. (1969). *Manual of Obstetrics* (13th ed.) pp 195–6. (Ed: Robert Percival). London: J. and A. Churchill, Ltd.

*From A. W. Liley (1963). Brit. Med. J., ii, 1107-9. Copyright (1963), by kind permission of the author
and the British Medical Association*

Preliminary Communications

Intrauterine Transfusion of Foetus in Haemolytic Disease

In the management of the pregnancy complicated by rhesus sensitization the guidance given by amniotic-fluid pigmentation (Bevis, 1956; Walker, 1957; Mackay, 1961; Liley, 1961, 1963) has greatly reduced the perinatal mortality from haemolytic disease. In the National Women's Hospital, Auckland, with a policy of selective induction based on amniocentesis findings, this perinatal mortality has fallen steadily from 22% in 1957–8 to 9% in 1962. It was obvious that no further reduction could be expected from conventional treatment when of 7 perinatal deaths in 80 consecutive rhesus-sensitized pregnancies one baby had multiple congenital abnormalities and the other six were all hydropic before 34 weeks' gestation. Transfusion *in utero* appeared the logical procedure for these very severely affected babies early in the third trimester, and intraperitoneal transfusion seemed the simplest technique.

CASE REPORT

The mother, aged 32, was pregnant for the fourth time. Her first pregnancy was normal, with a surviving 4,090-g. male infant. In her second pregnancy intrauterine death occurred a few days before delivery at term. Antibodies were present at 10 weeks in her third pregnancy and reached a titre of 1:64 by indirect Coombs test at 29 weeks. Mild hypertension had developed and stillborn macerated twins were delivered at 30 weeks. In her fourth pregnancy at 30 weeks by menstrual dates a specimen of bright yellow amniotic fluid was sent by post to this hospital. The spectral absorption curve (Bevis, 1956; Walker, 1957) of this fluid showed a very large peak at 450 mμ, the optical density of the deviation from linearity at this wavelength being 0.536. In view of the hopeless prognosis indicated by this peak (Liley, 1961, 1963) the patient's practitioner transferred her to the care of the professorial unit.

On admission at 30 weeks 3 days by dates she was found to be obese at 91.6 kg. and mildly hypertensive; B.P. 145–155/85–90. The uterus was large for her dates, although there was no reason to challenge the maturity on menstrual history, quickening, or subsequent x-ray examination. The patient was group A, ccddee, D^u-negative with Hb 11.8 g./100 ml. An antibody screen confirmed anti-D to a titre of 1:128 with ficin-treated cells and by indirect Coombs test. This antibody level did not alter during the remainder of the pregnancy.

The patient and her husband were an intelligent couple, and the prognosis for the foetus, the possibility and uncertainty of intrauterine transfusion, and the potential hazards to the mother were fully explained to and discussed with them. However, any attempt on the foetus was deferred for 10 days while some weeping abdominal skin ulceration, a reaction to adhesive plaster, was vigorously treated. A glucose-tolerance test and isotopic renogram were normal and the blood-pressure settled to 110–140/70–80 without sedation or strict bed-rest.

At 32 weeks 1 day, under local anaesthesia, 20 ml. of 76% "urografin" was injected into the amniotic cavity and antero-posterior and supine lateral films were taken. These showed a left antero-lateral placenta and the foetus as a vertex R.O.L. with no evidence of hydrops or obvious ascites. Five hours later, with a premedication of 100 mg. of pethidine, 25 mg. of promethazine hydrochloride, and 0.6 mg. of atropine, the patient was returned to the x-ray department and a further antero-posterior film taken with paperclips attached with "sellotape" as skin markers. The swallowed contrast medium in the foetal gut defined the target in two dimensions and the previous lateral film indicated the depth. Under local anaesthesia an 8-cm. gauge 16 Tuohy needle was inserted into the amniotic cavity and the stylet withdrawn. A syringe of sterile saline was attached and the needle advanced until resistance to slow steady injection showed that the tip lay in the foetal abdominal wall. With a slight advance free injection was again possible into the foetal peritoneum. No ascitic fluid

could be aspirated. A "portex" epidural catheter shortened to 30 cm. was now fed up to the hub of the Tuohy needle and the needle withdrawn on to the mother's skin. The position of the catheter was checked by x-ray examination and 100 ml. of packed warmed group O, Rh-negative cells fully compatible with mother's serum was injected over 20 minutes. Antibiotic cover was provided by 1 g. of streptomycin and 1,000,000 units of penicillin injected into the amniotic cavity at amniography, half this dose injected slowly as the catheter was withdrawn through the foetal and maternal tissues, and a four-day course of penicillin and streptomycin given to the mother.

Eight days later an attempt to repeat the transfusion failed, since with uterine enlargement and a slight change in foetal position the 8-cm. needle could just reach but not penetrate the abdominal wall. However, two days later—that is, at 33 weeks 4 days by dates—a successful puncture was made easily with an 18-cm. gauge 16 Tuohy needle. An epidural catheter shortened to 45 cm. was fed through this needle. On withdrawal of the needle and injection of 3 ml. of urografin the characteristic biconcave shadows of dye between loops of bowel and crescents of dye under the domes of the diaphragm confirmed the correct placement of the catheter (see Fig.). Over 20 minutes 110 ml. of packed warmed cells was injected. Antibiotic cover was provided as on the previous occasion. The foetal heart gave no concern during either injection, and the mother had no discomfort during or after the procedure.

At 34 weeks 3 days surgical induction by Drew Smythe catheter was performed and a polythene catheter inserted. The cervix was firm and undilated and the foetus was lying obliquely as a breech. Twenty-eight hours later, with no progress and the foetal lie uncorrected after eight hours of oxytocin nasal spray and eight hours of oxytocin drip, caesarean section was performed. At laparotomy the sites of uterine puncture were well healed with no adhesions. A male infant weighing 2,560 g. was delivered. He was pale and slightly jaundiced. The abdomen was moderately distended, with a liver edge palpable 5 cm. below the right costal margin and an easily felt enlarged spleen. Two small pigmented scars in the left lower quadrant of the abdomen showed the puncture sites of the successful transfusions and four smaller scars the pricks of the unsuccessful attempts. The placenta weighed 700 g. and had the pale hyperplastic appearance of severe haemolytic disease. Cord blood showed Hb 8.4 g./100 ml., a strong positive direct Coombs reaction, bilirubin 6.8 mg./100 ml., and 350 nucleated R.B.C./100 W.B.C. Central venous blood at the start of

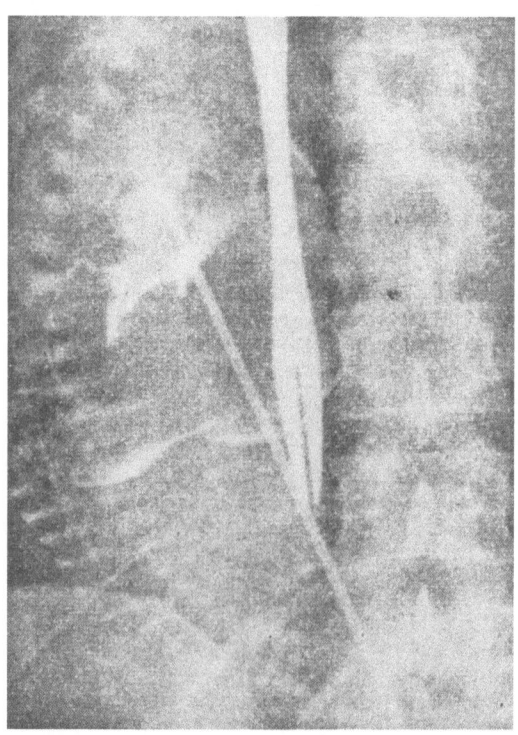

Contrast medium and the coiled catheter in the foetal peritoneal cavity. The Tuohy needle has been withdrawn and lies on the mother's abdominal skin.

exchange transfusion 48 minutes later had an Hb of 6.2 g./ 100 ml. Fractionation by the method of Singer, Chernoff, and Singer (1951) showed Hb F 43%, Hb A 57%.

The exchange transfusion of 155 ml./kg., using O, Rh-negative blood, occupied one and one-quarter hours. Shortly after delivery a respiratory distress syndrome of moderate severity appeared, but the baby's breathing improved steadily over the next 20 hours. X-ray examination showed no evidence of bowel damage. A tapered course of A.C.T.H. was begun. With a rising serum bilirubin a second exchange transfusion was carried out at 19 hours, using 14 ml. of concentrated serum albumin and 170 ml. of blood/kg. Serum bilirubin averaged 17, 14, 12, and 11 mg./100 ml over the next four days. Apart from being slow to feed and to regain his birth weight, the baby has given no further concern to the age of 4 weeks.

COMMENT

It could be asked whether this baby might have survived without foetal transfusion. Although the previous obstetric history is strongly suggestive of progressive haemolytic disease there were no haemotological or post-mortem examinations of these stillborn infants. Moreover, a mildly affected infant is always a possibility even after stillbirth early in the third trimester. However, the size of the pigment peak in the amniotic fluid leaves little room for doubt that this foetus was very severely affected. In our experience a peak of this size has been accompanied invariably by a foetus dead or hydropic before 34 weeks' gestation and usually before 33 weeks. Further, the high fraction of Hb A in the baby at delivery at 34½ weeks suggests that roughly half the circulating blood was donor blood, for the normal proportions of Hb F and Hb A are not altered by haemolytic disease (Ponder and Levine, 1949).

This case is the fourth pregnancy on which this procedure has been performed. In the first two the foetus was already hydropic and death occurred within 24 hours of the transfusion. In the third case two transfusions were performed by the described technique at 31 and 33 weeks. Death occurred within a few hours of the second transfusion, and a mildly hydropic foetus was delivered.

It is apparent that timely discovery and selection of these cases is critical, and only amniotic-fluid analysis can provide the necessary precision. Amniography can exclude gross ascites, and the persistence of swallowed dye in the foetal gut provides a convenient permanent marker which enables solid viscera to be avoided. There was no sign of trauma to abdominal viscera at post-mortem examination on the first three babies. In the absence of ascites the detection by needle of planes free from resistance to injection of saline has proved a simple method of locating the peritoneal cavity. The prompt introduction of a catheter with generous slack and withdrawal of the needle removes any risk of trauma from foetal or maternal movement or Braxton Hicks contractions.

Reports on intraperitoneal transfusions in neonates and infants (Macdougall, 1958 ; Mollison, 1961 ; Scopes, 1963) suggest that both the rate of absorption and total proportion absorbed into the circulation are not entirely predictable. In foetal transfusion further uncertainty is added by a lack of knowledge of the combined blood volume of the foetus and placenta, and the possibility of some leakage from the puncture site on withdrawal of the catheter. For these reasons it cannot be expected that the procedure will restore the foetus to normal. The aim of the exercise is simply to arrest deterioration if possible and gain a few extra weeks of gestation so that the skilled paediatric care of severe haemolytic disease is not nullified by gross prematurity.

My thanks are due to Dr. C. H. Thompson, of Hastings, for his co-operation, to Professor G. H. Green and Mr. G. C. Liggins for their assistance and obstetric management, to the Rh Committee for their support and encouragement, and to the staff of the x-ray department and laboratory for technical assistance. This work was supported in part by the Medical Research Council of New Zealand.

A. W. LILEY, Ph.D., M.B., B.Med.Sc., Dip.Obst.,
Senior Research Fellow
National Women's Hospital,
Auckland, New Zealand.

REFERENCES

Bevis, D. C. A. (1956). J. Obstet. Gynaec. Brit. Emp., 63, 68.
Liley, A. W. (1961). Amer. J. Obstet. Gynec., 82, 1359.
—— (1963). Ibid., 86, 485.
Macdougall, L. G. (1958). Brit. med. J., 1, 139.
Mackay, E. V. (1961). Aust. N.Z. J. Obstet. Gynaec., 1, 78.
Mollison, P. L. (1961). Blood Transfusion in Clinical Medicine, 3rd ed. Blackwell, Oxford.
Ponder, E., and Levine, P. (1949). Blood, 4, 1264.
Scopes, J. W. (1963). Lancet, 1, 1027.
Singer, K., Chernoff, A. I., and Singer, L. (1951). Blood, 6, 413.
Walker, A. H. C. (1957). Brit. med. J., 2, 376.

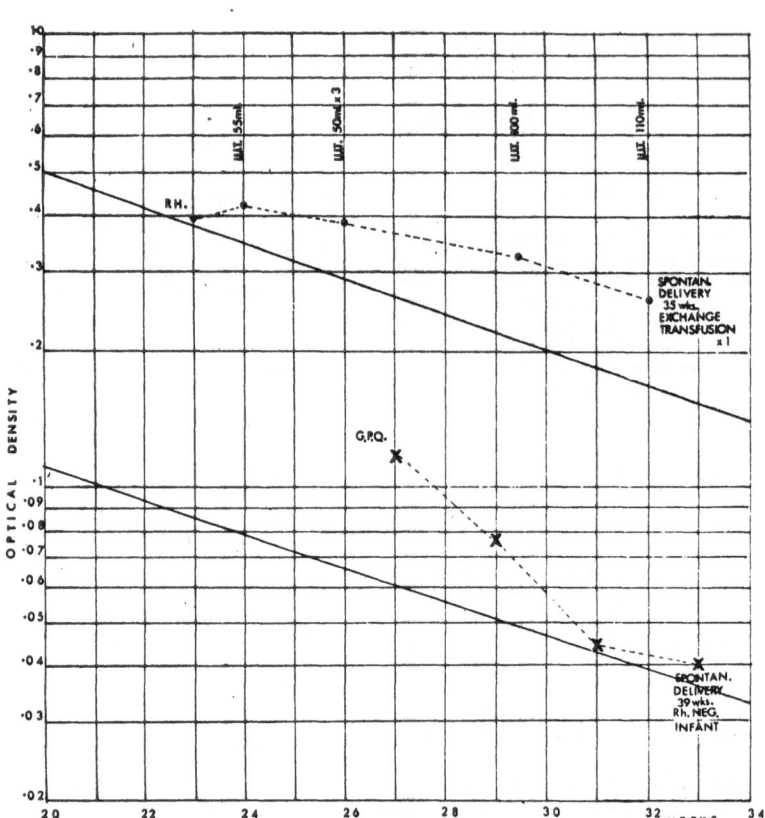

Fig. 107. LILEY'S CHART relating optical density of the liquor against maturity and effect on the fetus.

The chart is divided into three zones—upper, middle and lower. Hydrops fetalis would be expected in the upper zone; a severely affected baby in the upper middle zone; a mildly affected infant in the lower middle zone, and an unaffected baby in the lower zone.

The optical density of the 450 mµ peak is plotted at various stages during pregnancy in the two cases already described. Case G.P.Q. (X————X) had a healthy Rhesus negative infant. Case P.H. (●————●) required six intrauterine transfusions; the infant, delivered at 34 weeks, had one exchange transfusion and subsequently did well.

Mrs. P. H. gravida 6, with a homozygous Rhesus positive husband had one living child, her first, born in 1956. Her second child in 1958 died during the third exchange transfusion. In 1959 she had a stillborn hydrops at 37 weeks; in 1961 she was delivered by Cæsarean section at 34 weeks of a hydropic infant which died at 15 minutes during exchange transfusion; in 1964 she had a stillborn hydrops at 30 weeks.

In the current pregnancy she was found to have a high titre of antibodies and spectrophotometry of the liquor amnii at 23 and 24 weeks showed a very severly affected infant. Intra-uterine transfusion was performed at 25 weeks—55 ml. of packed cells (Rh. negative) given. At 26 weeks 50 ml. of blood was given on three occasions at intervals of 48 hours via an indwelling catheter. At 29½ weeks a further 100 ml. of blood was given, and at 32 weeks 110 ml. was transfused.

Spontaneous labour began at 34 weeks and she had an assisted breech delivery of a 5 lb. 8 oz. boy which required one exchange transfusion at 3 hours and a "top up" transfusion at 2 months.

At birth the infant was Rhesus negative with less than 0·5 per cent fetal blood in his circulation—the remainder was donor blood.

Follow up at 10 months has revealed a normal infant who is now Rhesus positive.

Mrs. G. P. Q. gravida 4. Group O Rhesus negative, Husband Group O Rhesus positive Heterozygous (cDe/cde).

1959 & 1961. Normal pregnancies and deliveries.

1965. Rhesus antibodies first detected. Surgical induction at 39 weeks, infant showed severe hæmolytic disease of the newborn and required three exchange transfusions.

1967. Rhesus antibodies at 15 weeks present in higher dilutions than in previous pregnancy. Amniocentesis at 27 weeks showed a bilirubin 450 mµ peak of 0·115—this could suggest a moderately affected infant being in the mid-zone of Liley's Chart. Further amniocenteses at 29 weeks, 31 weeks and 33 weeks showed a progressive fall in the peaks and the correct prediction of a Rhesus negative infant was made. Normal delivery at 39 weeks of a healthy, 7 lb. 15 oz. male infant.

OTHER THERAPEUTIC PROCEDURES IN ESTABLISHED HDN

Transfusion (exchange and intrauterine) is the sheet anchor in the treatment of established HDN, but two other procedures may also be useful.

The first is phototherapy, which stemmed from the observation of a ward sister who noted the fading of the jaundice in babies who had been exposed for a short time to the sunlight. Though there seems no doubt that this is true, the concensus of opinion seems to be that the therapy is of more use in the jaundice associated with prematurity than in that due to Rh disease. The primary paper on the topic is by Cremer, R. J., Perryman, P. W. and Richards, D. H. (1958). Influence of light on the hyper-bilirubinaemia of infants. *Lancet, i,* 1094–7.

The second ancillary line of treatment consists in giving phenobarbitone, either to the mother a few days before delivery, or to the newborn baby, or both. Serum bilirubin concentration is decreased in the baby, probably due to induction of enzymes in liver microsomes. The exact usefulness of the drug is still being assessed. The primary reference on the topic is by Trolle, Dyre, (1968). Decrease of total serum bilirubin concentration in newborn infants after phenobarbitone treatment. *Lancet, ii,* 705–8.

The third, which is more controversial, is the use of intensive plasmapheresis during pregnancy to lower the antibody titre in the mother. The results are difficult to evaluate statistically, as other methods of treatment are given. It is possible, however, that repeated plasmapheresis lowers the affinity of the Rh antibody (Stratton, personal communication) and this may explain the apparent success of the procedure.

Clarke, C. A., Bradley, J., Elson, C. J., Donohoe, W. T. A., Lehane, D. and Hughes-Jones, N. C. (1970) Intensive plasmapheresis as a therapeutic measure in Rhesus-immunised women. *Lancet, I,* 793-798.

Fraser, I. D., Bennett, M. O. Bothamley, J. E. (1974) ante-natal plasmapheresis in severe Rhesus Iso-immunization. *Brit, J. Haemat., 28, 147.*

Section III

Prophylaxis

Paper 21

21.   Nevanlinna, H. R. and Vainio, T. (1956). The influence of mother-child ABO incompatibility on Rh immunisation. *Vox. Sang, 1*, 26.

Commentary

As has been pointed out earlier (Paper 6), Levine in 1943 found that immunisation to Rh during pregnancy is much less common when the father is ABO incompatible (e.g. mother O, father A) than when he is compatible (e.g. mother O, father O), and possible explanations for this are given by Race and Sanger (Paper 7).

Nevanlinna and Vainio (1956) set out to study two points:

(1) The ABO group of the immunising fetus.

(2) The severity of Rh haemolytic disease in ABO compatible as compared with ABO incompatible affected babies.

The authors deliberately selected families where babies with Rh haemolytic disease had been born in spite of the fact that the protective mechanism of ABO incompatibility between mother and father was apparently present, i.e. the mother could not safely have been transfused with the husband's blood. The authors showed that the healthy Rh-positive child immediately preceding the first affected Rh-positive child was much more commonly ABO compatible than incompatible. This of course could be because the father, though typing as A or B, might easily have been heterozygous AO or BO, in which case the healthy child could be compatible with the mother (e.g. OO) and therefore act as the immunising fetus.

Nevanlinna and Vainio also found that after immunisation had occurred affected children were equally likely to be ABO incompatible as compatible, that is to say the protective effect was no longer operative. Furthermore, in affected infants the ABO incompatibility or compatibility of the child with the mother had no effect on the severity of the disease.

Nevanlinna and Vainio's work also explained one of the outstanding features in the natural history of Rh HDN—namely the rarity of its occurrence in a first-born child. This is because maternal immunisation requires not only the passage into the mother of Rh-positive fetal cells but also their continuing presence in her circulation for some considerable time. Since Rh antibodies do not develop for many weeks the immunising fetus is usually unaffected because it is delivered before the antibodies appear.

The Influence of Mother-Child ABO Incompatibility on Rh Immunisation *

H. R. NEVANLINNA and T. VAINIO

State Serum Institute and Finnish Red Cross Blood Transfusion Service, Helsinki

The observation by *Levine* in 1943 [6], almost classic now, was that a considerably smaller proportion of the husbands of Rh immunised patients were ABO incompatible with their wives as compared with the normal population of husbands. This has been corroborated in various parts of the world so often that it would be superfluous to add to the long list of materials [3, 1, 13, 15, 6, 10, 2, 9, 12].

Most authors confine themselves to computing the relative number of ABO incompatible *husbands* in Rh immunisation. It goes without saying that incompatibility between the child and the mother is involved: briefly, *the A and B properties of the foetus, if lacking in the mother, reduce the chance of her being immunised by foetal Rh antigen.* Put differently, an ABO compatible foetus does not reduce the probability of maternal Rh immunisation. It follows naturally from this that among ABO incompatible husbands selection takes place towards heterozygotes (AO, etc.), a fact to which we drew attention a few years ago [8, 9]. The degree of selection is dependent on the strength of the inhibitory effect: if the foetal A and/or B properties always inhibit immunisation none of the husbands of Rh immunised patients are A and B homozygous. *Reepmaker* with his co-workers[11, 12] recently found that the distribution of both ABO incompatible husbands and children of Rh immunised women into the different ABO groups is similar to that arrived at if all the husbands are assumed to be heterozygous to the A and/or B factor. This no doubt supports the above conclusion but naturally reveals nothing about the mechanism of the inhibitory action.

The way in which foetal A and B properties reduce the probability of maternal Rh immunisation is as yet not clear. It is customary in this connection to quote three hypotheses [5, 14, 10], of which *Race*'s is doubtless the most logical. However, in our opinion no observation supports this theory; also, why a rapidly eliminated red cell should act as a poorer antigen than a red cell that remains longer in the maternal circulation remains an open question. The contrary explanation might serve just as well. The fact that selection towards heterozygotes (AO, etc.) takes place among the AB incompatible husbands of Rh immunised women does not seem to support *Race*'s theory in any way, as has been claimed [11, 12]: the same selection follows whether the ultimate reason for the inhibitory effect be the early elimination of incompatible foetuses or the competition of antigens.

To clarify the mechanism of the inhibitory effect of the foetal A

---

* Aided by a grant from the "Sigrid Juselius Foundation".

and B properties it seems important to know at which stage of the immunisation, i.e. during which pregnancy the inhibitory effect exists. Different possibilities may be considered in this connection:

(1) An incompatible foetus acts as a weaker stimulus than a compatible independent of whether or not immunisation has already taken place. The result would be, apart from a reduction in the number of incompatible children, an alleviation in the severity of their disease. This is indicated in the literature [4].

(2) The inhibitory effect persists until serologically (and clinically) detectable immunisation has occurred due to either an ABO compatible foetus or blood transfusion. Subsequently the foetal A and B properties will either cease to prevent the foetal Rh antigen from acting as a stimulus or, at the most, they will just weaken it.

(3) The inhibitory effect exists only in relation to the first (primary, sensibilisation) stimulus, i.e. before the immunisation proper. After the change in the mode of reaction, or sensibilisation, has taken place due to a compatible foetus or blood transfusion, the A and B properties are no longer capable of affecting in any way the immunisation proper or its strengthening the following pregnancies.

We have previously [8, 9] endeavoured to explain the rarity of pregnancy immunisation by means of factors which inhibit immunisation or, more correctly, sensiblisation. We gave the foetal A and B antigens as examples of such factors whose effect, in our opinion, merely amounted to sensibilisation preceding the immunisation proper, i.e. sensibilisation never develops in Rh negative women if the foetus has the A/B antigens lacking in the mother. For various reasons we considered that the sensibilisation stimulus was decisive in the development of immunisation: where the sensibilisation stimulus came from blood transfusion or an Rh positive foetus, manifest immunisation would follow in any case from the next positive foetus. We cannot go into the details of this problem here; reference is made to the investigations reported above.

Finally, the possibility that the inhibitory effect of the foetal A and B properties fails to come into play in all cases must be taken into account; hence there may be exceptions to the rules under items (2) and (3). This would imply, in the first place, that the A and B properties alone, without the presence of some other (primarily hereditary) property, are incapable of inhibiting immunisation or sensibilisation.

The main object of the present work is to study two points:

(1) Whether foetal A or B incompatibility has an alleviating influence on the severity of the haemolytic disease.

(2) The way in which the relative number of A or B incompatible children is dependent on the seniority in the family of the child compared with the date of maternal immunisation.

Material and Results

The material covers a total of 429 families in which the ABO groups of the Rh immunised mother and her husband are known. Patients who had received blood transfusions or blood injections were excluded. In 114 cases, 26.6%, the husband was ABO incompatible. In this connection it must be pointed out that, due to the relatively high incidence of A and B, Finland has relatively more incompatible marriages than many other European countries. In the normal population the percentage of incompatible marriages is approx. 40; in the Netherlands the figure is approx. 34% [11, 12]. Similarly calculated the proportion of incompatible children in the normal population in Finland is approx. 24% [8, 9], in the Netherlands only 19.8% [12].

(1) Does foetal A or B incompatibility exert an alleviating influence on the severity of the haemolytic disease?

To study this question, 67 children were selected from the above material; their fathers were ABO incompatible and *Rh immunisation had been established in their mothers before the children were born.* Another 67 children with ABO compatible fathers were selected as a control material. The cases were selected so that the *diseased child's seniority in the family was the same in both groups* (see discussion).

A comparison of the severity of the disease in the children revealed no appreciable difference between those by incompatible and those by compatible fathers (Table I).

TABLE I   *Outcome of the Disease in Children of ABO-Compatible and Incompatible Fathers*

Outcome of the disease	Father compatible				Father incompatible			
	Order of sick children				Order of sick children			
	I	II	III	Tot.	I	II	III	Tot.
Recovered	24	16	15	55	22	13	13	48
Exchange transfusion .	15	14	14	43	17	11	12	40
No transfusion	9	2	1	12	5	2	1	8
Died	1	5	6	12	3	8	8	19
Exchange transfusion .	1	3	3	7	—	1	1	2
No transfusion	—	—	—	—	1	1	2	4
Stillborn	—	2	3	5	2	6	5	13
Total	25	21	21	67	25	21	21	67

Table II compares the type of disease of the compatible and incompatible children by incompatible fathers. No differences are observed between them, though it is true that the material is regrettably small.

TABLE II   *Outcome of the Disease in Compatible and Incompatible Children of ABO-Incompatible Fathers*
(13 Stillbirths where ABO Group is Unknown are Excluded)

Outcome of the disease	Child compatible				Child incompatible			
	Order of sick children				Order of sick children			
	I	II	III	Tot.	I	II	III	Tot.
Recovered	10	7	6	23	14	5	7	26
Exchange transfusion .	7	6	6	19	10	5	6	21
No transfusion	1	2	—	3	—	1	2	3
Died	1	1	1	3	—	1	2	3
Exchange transfusion .	—	1	—	1	—	—	1	1
No transfusion	1	—	1	2	—	1	1	2
Total	11	8	7	26	14	6	9	29

(2) What is the dependence of the relative number of ABO incompatible children on the seniority of the children compared with the date of maternal immunisation?

The material includes 70 of the above-mentioned 114 incompatible couples; the cases in which the date of immunisation, due to obviously unreliable or incomplete medical history, was difficult to determine were excluded. Similarly omitted were the cases in which abortion preceded immunisation.

The distribution of the patients' and her husbands' ABO combinations was as follows (Table III).

The 70 mothers under review had a total of 266 children, 15 of them Rh negative. 114 children were healthy, 137 children were considered to have haemolytic disease of the newborn on the basis of clinical or serologic findings or, in a number of cases, merely from medical history data. The make-up of the material is illustrated in Table IV.

For statistical treatment, the 251 children of the material were divided into four groups: (1) First sick child; (2) other sick children; (3) last healthy child; (4) other healthy children. The children found

TABLE III *Distribution of ABO Groups in 70 Cases of Rh Immunisation. Cases with Blood Transfusion or Abortion Preceding the First Sick Child are Excluded*

Patient	Husband	
O	A	20
O	B	5
O	AB	2
A	B	14
A	AB	9
B	A	16
B	AB	4
Total		70

TABLE IV *Distribution of ABO Incompatibility and Compatibility among 251 Children of 70 Rh Immunised Mothers with Incompatible Husbands. Known Rh Negative Children are Excluded.*

Incompatible	56 (39.4%)
Compatible	86 (60.6%)
Death, no sample	69
No sample for other reasons	40
Total	251

to be Rh negative were not taken into account in determining the groups. Table V shows the distribution of compatible and incompatible children between these groups.

The numbers of incompatible and compatible children were equal among the group first sick child and the group other sick children, i.e. *incompatibility evidently has not inhibited the manifestation of immunisation.* Assuming that the majority, if not all, of the husbands were heterozygous to A and B factor, it was in fact to be expected that the numbers of incompatible and compatible children should be approximately equal in these groups.

TABLE V *Distribution of ABO Incompatibility and Compatibility among Four Different Groups of 251 Children of 70 Rh Immunised Mothers with Incompatible Husbands.*

	Incompatible	Compatible	Unknown	Total
First sick child	17	15	38	70
	33	30		
Other sick children	16	15	36	67
Last healthy child	11	39	20	70
	23	56		
Other healthy children	12	17	15	44
Total	56	86	109	251

The relative number of incompatible children is lowest among the group last healthy child, as is shown in Fig. 1 in which the results of Table V are plotted. Hence *the inhibitory effect of A and B properties has acted upon the so-called sensiblisation stimulus.*

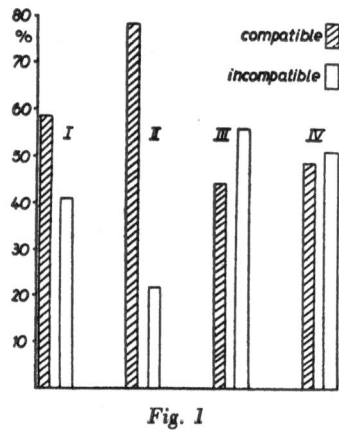

Fig. 1

I = Healthy children preceding the last healthy child.
II = Last healthy child.
III = First sick child.
IV = Other sick children.

It must be noted that the group last healthy child included 11 incompatible children: in other words, there are exceptions to the rule. In part this may be due to the fact that the time of immunisation was in reality one pregnancy earlier or later. On the other hand, the material includes a number of cases in which all the children born before immunisation were definitely incompatible. We have claimed before [8, 9] that the foetal A and B properties alone are incapable of inhibiting Rh sensibilisation and that the foetuses should simultaneously be secretors. 9 of the above 11 incompatibles from the group last healthy child were examined from this point of view: 4 were secretors, 5 non-secretors. The small number of the cases makes definite conclusions impossible.

Discussion

When the severity of the disease of children with haemolytic disease is studied it is to be expected that, on an average, the disease would be less severe in ABO incompatible than in compatible children. Such observations have in fact been reported [4]. However, the matter is not so simple. Considering the inhibitory effect of A and B properties we must take into account, in addition to the cases in which the mother is not immunised at all, those in which immunisation has occurred. Immunisation in these cases is no doubt "delayed". In most-cases the father is heterozygous to the inhibitory factor, and sensibilisation occurs only from a compatible foetus. In the first pregnancy, 50 % of the children are incompatible, and sensibilisation is inhibited. In the second, 50 % of the balance (or a total of 25 %) are again incompatible, and sensibilisation is again inhibited. The calculation can be continued. The conclusion is that in incompatible marriages with heterozygous husbands the development of immunisation requires an average of twice as many Rh positive children as in compatible marriages. It follows that the number of (diseased) children born after immunisation is smaller in the incompatible marriages. The more senior the diseased child the less severe is the disease; this is a fact established often enough.

For these reasons the severity of the disease of incompatible children was compared with that of compatible children who had equally many diseased siblings. This made it possible to eliminate the improving influence on prognosis of the delay in Rh immunisation due to ABO incompatibility, and no further differences were found.

According to the present material, the inhibitory effect of A and B properties merely acts on the sensibilisation stimulus prior to immunisation. We have already drawn attention to the importance of the sensibilisation phenomenon in the overall development of immunisation. It seems quite probable that in Rh immunisation manifest immunisation occurs always when sensibilisation has occurred, due to either an Rh positive foetus or blood transfusion. Without going into greater detail, it may be pointed out that in a sample [9] of Rh negative parturients who had previously received blood transfusions, 21 gave birth to an Rh positive child after blood transfusion. 19 of them were found to be Rh immunised.

It may be mentioned in conclusion that we know of a total of 44 Rh immunised patients to whom blood transfusions or blood injections had been given prior to the manifestation of immunisation. The husbands of 17 (40 %) of these patients were incompatible: the inhibitory influence was not observable after sensibilisation through blood transfusion.

The inhibitory effect on sensibilisation of the foetal A and B properties sheds some light on the mechanisms of the factors generally accounting for the rarity of pregnancy immunisation. We believe that in investigating these factors attention must be focussed on the stimulus preceding immunisation.

Acknowledgment: The authors are greatly indebted to Dr. *R. R. Race* for reading the manuscript and for valuable corrections and criticism.

Summary

(1) Assuming that the foetal A and B properties reduce the Rh immunisation probability of an Rh negative patient, selection towards A and B heterozygotes must take place among ABO incompatible husbands of Rh immunised women. Such selection, to be expected theoretically and also verified in clinical material, in our opinion does not expressly support the theory advanced by *Race* to explain the mechanism of the inhibitory influence.

(2) A study of the severity of the disease of the ABO incompatible and compatible children of Rh immunised patients revealed no difference between them.

(3) The inhibitory effect of the foetal A and B factors applies merely to the sensibilisation stimulus preceding manifest immunisation.

(4) The inhibitory influence is lacking in approximately a fifth of the cases. It is possible that the absence of the secretor property in them accounts for the absence of the inhibitory influence.

(5) The importance of focussing attention on the sensibilisation stimulus in investigating the factors responsible for the rarity of pregnancy immunisation, is emphasised.

Résumé

1⁰ Si l'on admet que les propriétés fœtales A et B ont un effet inhibiteur sur la probabilité d'une immunisation Rh chez les mères Rh-négatives, on peut conclure que chez les maris de femmes immunisées au Rh il doit y avoir sélection vers l'hétérozygotie dans le groupe A et B. Une telle sélection, bien que vérifiée en pratique, ne confirme pas, à l'avis des auteurs, la théorie formulée par *Race* pour expliquer l'effet inhibiteur mentionné ci-dessus.

2⁰ Une étude des enfants de femmes immunisées au Rh a montré que le fait qu'ils soient ou non compatibles avec leurs mères par rapport au système ABO, est sans influence aucune sur la gravité de leur maladie hémolytique.

3⁰ L'effet inhibiteur des facteurs A et B chez le fœtus se rapporte uniquement à la stimulation sensibilisante, et non pas à l'immunisation manifeste qui s'ensuit.

4⁰ L'effet inhibiteur est absent dans un cinquième des cas: il est possible que ceci soit dû à l'absence de la propriété de sécrétion dans ces cas.

5⁰ Les auteurs soulignent l'importance qu'il faut accorder à la stimulation sensibilisante parmi les facteurs qui ont une influence sur la rareté de l'immunisation au Rh pendant la grossesse.

Zusammenfassung

1. Da die fötalen Blutgruppeneigenschaften A und B bei ABO-in-kompatiblen Rh-negativen Müttern das Risiko einer Rh-Isoimmuni-sierung vermindern, ist anzunehmen, daß eine größere als statistisch zu erwartende Zahl von ABO-inkompatiblen Ehemännern von Rh-sensibilisierten Müttern in bezug auf ihre Blutgruppe heterozygot sind. Diese theoretisch zu erwartende und durch klinische Beobach-tungen gestützte Annahme vermag die *Race*'sche Theorie dieses Im-munisierungshemmungsmechanismus nicht zu stützen.

2. ABO-kompatible und ABO-inkompatible Rh-positive Kinder von Rh-sensibilisierten Müttern zeigen keine Unterschiede hinsicht-lich des Schweregrades ihres Morbus haemolyticus.

3. Die Hemmwirkung der fötalen Blutgruppeneigenschaften A und B beschränkt sich somit auf den ersten Sensibilisierungsstimulus und ist ohne Einfluß auf das nach diesem Stimulus folgende Immunisie-rungsgeschehen.

4. In ungefähr einem Fünftel versagt die Hemmwirkung. Dies läßt die Vermutung aufkommen, daß sie an die Anwesenheit der Sekre-toreneigenschaft gebunden ist.

5. Es wird auf die Bedeutung des ersten Sensibilisierungsstimulus zur Erklärung der relativen Seltenheit von schwangerschaftsbeding-ten Isoimmunisierungen hingewiesen.

References

[1] *Bessis, M.:* Etudes statistiques (cliniques et sérologiques) sur 50 familles at-taintes de maladie hémolytique du nouveau-né. Rev. Hémat. *1/2*, 167, 1946.

[2] *Brendemoen, O. J.:* Some Factors Influencing Rh Immunization during Preg-nancy. Acta path. microbiol. scand. *31*, 579, 1952.

[3] *Broman, B.:* The Blood Factor Rh in Man. Acta paed. scand. Suppl. 2, 178, 1944.

[4] *Donohue, W. L., M. A. Mullinger, E. G. Cook* and *C. E. Snelling:* A Survey of the Rh Problem in Toronto, 1947–1952. Amer. J. Obstet. Gynec. *67*, 233, 1954.

[5] *Fisher, R. A.:* Quoted by *Race* [10].

[6] *Levine, P.:* Serological Factors as Possible Causes in Spontaneous Abortions. J. Hered. *34*, 71, 1943.

[7] *Malone, R. H.:* ABO Incompatibility between Husband and Wife and its Relation to Rh Immunization. Brit. J. soc. Med. *3/4*, 228, 1949.

[8] *Nevanlinna, H. R.:* Rh: Serology and Clinic., Acta path. microbiol. scand. Suppl. *93*, 402, 1951.

[9] *Id.:* Factors Affecting Maternal Rh Immunization. Ann. Med. exp. Biol. Fenn. Suppl. 2, *31*, 1953.

[10] *Race, R. R.,* and *R. Sanger:* Blood Groups in Man. 2nd ed. Blackwell, Oxford, 1954.

[11] *Reepmaker, J., L. E. Nijenhuis* and *J. J. van Loghem:* Note on the Influence of ABO Blood Group Incompatibility on Rhesus Immunization in Pregnancy. Vox Sanguinis 4, 117, 1954.

[12] *Reepmaker, J.:* ABO antagonisme en Morbus Haemolyticus neonatorum. Thesis, Leyden, 1955.

[13] *Van Loghem, J. J.,* and *J. Spaander:* L'influence de l'incompatibilité du système ABO sur l'antagonisme Rh. Rev. Hémat. *3*, 276, 1948.

[14] *Wiener, A. S.:* Competition of antigens in iso-immunization by pregnancy. Proc. Soc. exp. Biol. Med. *58*, 133, 1945.

[15] *Wiener, A. S., I. B. Wexler* and *J. G. Hurst:* The Use of Exchange Transfusion for the Treatment of Severe Erythroblastosis due to A-B Sensitization; with Observations on the Pathogenesis of the Disease. Blood 4, 1014, 1949.

Authors' address:

Dr. *H. R. Nevanlinna,* Finnish Red Cross Blood Transfusion Service,
Topeliuksenk. 5., *Helsinki* (Finland)

Paper 22

22. Kleihauer, E., Braun, H. and Betke, K. (1957). Demonstration von fetalem Hämoglobin in den Erythrocyten eines Blutausstrichs. *Klin. Wschr., 35* 637-8.

Commentary

Before this paper it had not been possible to demonstrate individual fetal erythrocytes in an adult red cell population, although there had been several ways of detecting fetal haemoglobin by chemical means. The method described here (the acid elution technique) enabled this to be done, since by using an appropriate buffer, adult haemoglobin could be eluted from the red cells so that they appeared as ghosts, whereas the fetal cells stood out as dark refractile bodies, fetal haemoglobin being unaffected by the buffer.

The authors were interested in the possibility that some red cells might contain both types of haemoglobin, and this they found to be the case. They were not concerned with fetal cells in the maternal circulation in relation to feto-maternal haemorrhage.

Jg. 35, Heft 12
15. Juni 1957
ENNO KLEIHAUER, HILDEGARD BRAUN und KLAUS BETKE: Demonstration von fetalem Hämoglobin . 637

DEMONSTRATION VON FETALEM HÄMOGLOBIN IN DEN ERYTHROCYTEN EINES BLUTAUSSTRICHS

Von

ENNO KLEIHAUER, HILDEGARD BRAUN und KLAUS BETKE

Aus der Universitäts-Kinderklinik (Direktor: Prof. Dr. W. KELLER) und dem Radiologischen Institut (Direktor: Prof. Dr. H. LANGENDORFF) der Universität Freiburg i. Br.

Obwohl fetales menschliches Hämoglobin von bleibendem Hämoglobin in vielerlei Hinsicht beträchtlich differiert, konnte man es bisher nicht in einzelnen

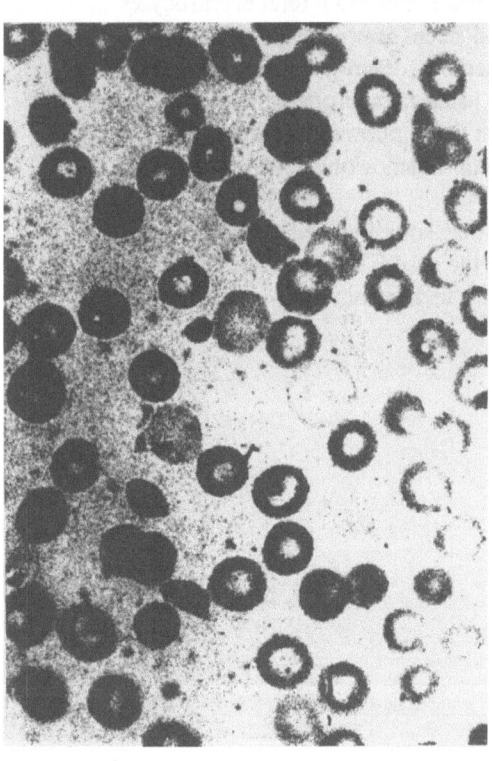

a   b

Abb. 1a u. b. In Alkohol fixierte Blutausstriche, bei p_H 3,5 in Citronensäure-Phosphat-Puffer extrahiert und nach MAY-GRÜNWALD-GIEMSA gefärbt. a Blut eines jungen Säuglings mit 74,5% fetalem Hämoglobin. Gut hämoglobingefüllte Zellen neben einzelnen mehr oder weniger schwächer gefärbten. b Erwachsenenblut. Man erkennt nur schattenhaft die Erythrocytenumrisse. Oben ein Lymphocyt

Erythrocyten kenntlich machen. Alle Bestimmungsmethoden (Alkalidenaturierung, Salzfällung, spektrophotometrische Analyse im Ultraviolett) gründen sich auf die Untersuchung von Blutfarbstofflösungen. Bei Verdauungsversuchen von fixierten Blutausstrichen konnten wir feststellen, daß mit Pepsin der Blutfarbstoff aus Erwachsenen-Erythrocyten schneller gelöst wird als aus Neugeborenenerythrocyten[1]. Die weitere Untersuchung dieses Phänomens zeigte, daß Pepsin nicht erforderlich ist, sondern daß es genügt, in Alkohol fixierte Blutausstriche mit Citronensäure-Phosphatpuffer vom p_H 3,4—3,6 zu extrahieren. An Filtrierpapierstreifen, die mit Hämoglobinlösungen getränkt und in Alkohol fixiert wurden, ließ sich die raschere Extraktion von bleibendem Hämoglobin in gleicher Weise

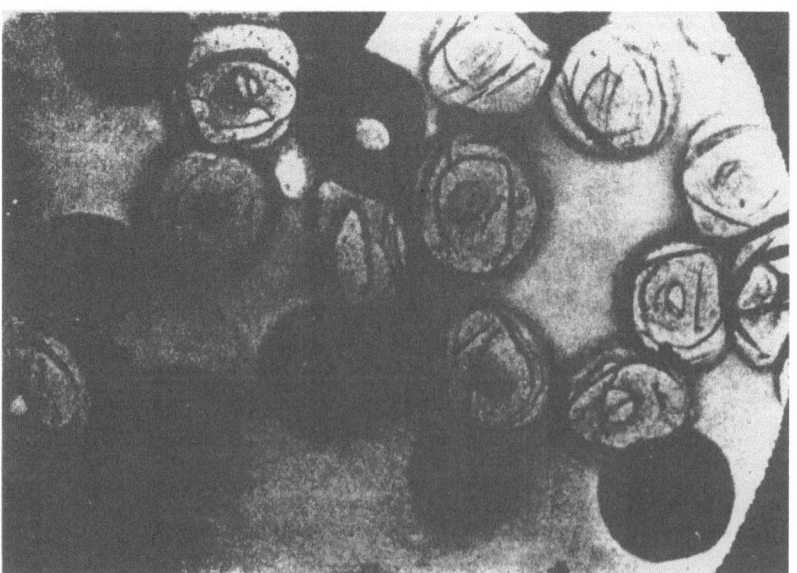

Abb. 2. Blutausstrich einer Mischung der beiden Blutarten von Abb. 1 nach Fixation und Extraktion. Man erkennt die noch Hämoglobin enthaltenden Säuglingserythrocyten neben den leeren Membranen der Erwachsenenerythrocyten. Ungefärbt, elektronenoptisch

demonstrieren. Das Phänomen hängt also offensichtlich vom Blutfarbstoff ab und nicht etwa von einem differenten Verhalten der fixierten Erythrocytenmembran bei Neugeborenen- und Erwachsenenerythrocyten.

Abb. 1 und 2 illustrieren die Ergebnisse an licht- und elektronenoptischen Bildern. Bei geeigneten Versuchsbedingungen (Extraktion bei p_H 3,5 und 37^0) werden Erwachsenenerythrocyten völlig hämoglobinfrei, während in Neugeborenenerythrocyten noch reichlich Hämoglobin vorhanden ist. Das Verfahren bietet eine Möglichkeit, zu entscheiden, ob der im Blut von Neugeborenen und jungen Säuglingen neben fetalem Hämoglobin vorhandene Prozentsatz an bleibendem Hämoglobin in einer getrennten Population von Erythrocyten vorliegt, oder ob es auch Erythrocyten gibt, die beide Hämoglobine enthalten. Nach unseren Ergebnissen ist das letztere der Fall. Außerdem hat man damit eine neue Methode für das elektronenoptische Studium der Erythrocytenstromata in der Hand: Bisher mußte man die Erythrocyten vor der Fixation immer erst hämolysieren, wenn man sie durchstrahlen wollte, und es war fraglich, ob durch die Hämolyse Strukturveränderungen auftraten. Die Möglichkeit, das Hämoglobin nachträglich aus fixierten Erythrocyten zu lösen, dürfte eine wertvolle Ergänzung des Studiums der Stromamorphologie anbieten.

Literatur. [1] BETKE, K.: Symposion über Struktur und Funktion der roten Blutzellen. Berlin Januar 1957.

Paper 23

23. Zipursky, A., Hull, A., White, F. D. and Israels, L. G. (1959). Foetal erythrocytes in the maternal circulation. *Lancet, i*, 451-2.

Commentary

In this short but very important paper Zipursky and his colleagues applied the acid elution technique (Paper 22) to detecting fetal red cells in the maternal circulation.

Before doing this a known volume of fetal cells was given to volunteers, so that the proportion of fetal to adult cells in the peripheral circulation could be ascertained. Using this information, and looking at the blood of post-partum women they concluded that 'transplacental haemorrhage of fetal blood is rather common'.

It was this paper more than any other which stimulated the Liverpool group to go ahead with their ideas on preventing immunisation, since here was a method of assessing the success or otherwise of getting rid of Rh-positive fetal cells from the circulation of a volunteer or a mother. Few or no cells would be expected when the mother and baby were ABO incompatible, and this is what has been found by many workers.

From A. Zipursky, A Hull, F. D. White and L. G. Israels (1959). Lancet, i, 431-2. Copyright (1959), by kind permission of the authors and The Lancet Ltd

FŒTAL ERYTHROCYTES IN THE MATERNAL CIRCULATION

ALVIN ZIPURSKY
M.D. Manitoba
RESEARCH FELLOW IN DEPARTMENT OF PÆDIATRICS

ALAN HULL
B.Sc. Manitoba
RESEARCH ASSISTANT, DEPARTMENT OF BIOCHEMISTRY

F. D. WHITE
Ph.D. Edin., F.R.I.C.
PROFESSOR OF BIOCHEMISTRY

L. G. ISRAELS
M.D., M.Sc. Manitoba, F.R.C.P.(C.)
ASSISTANT PROFESSOR OF BIOCHEMISTRY

From the Faculty of Medicine, University of Manitoba, Winnipeg, Canada

Kleihauer et al. (1957) recently reported that the hæmoglobin of adult red cells in a fixed smear was readily eluted by an acid phosphate buffer whereas the hæmoglobin of fœtal cells was not. We have applied this observation to the detection of small numbers of fœtal cells in the blood of newly delivered women.

Venous blood was collected with ammonium-potassium oxalate as anti-coagulant, and diluted 1 in 3 with normal saline. Smears were made of this saline suspension, dried, and fixed in absolute ethyl alcohol for 2 minutes. After fixation and drying, the slides were washed for 90 seconds in citrate phosphate buffer ($0.16M$ K_2HPO_4 and $0.18M$ citric acid, pH 3.4–3.6 at 37°C). They were stained with May-Gruenwald and then washed until practically no stain was visible to the naked eye. After drying, they were examined microscopically under low power. Fœtal cells appeared as pink-staining refractile cells in a field of erythrocyte ghosts (figs. 1–4).

In-vitro mixtures of fœtal and adult blood were made and smears prepared as described above (fig. 1). Arbitrarily, each smear was scanned for 2 minutes under low power. The numbers of fœtal cells seen in a 2-minute scan of smears of various dilutions were:

Fœtal cells/adult cells	No. of fœtal cells seen
1/25,000	2
1/10,000	7
1/5000	10
1/1000	21

When three adults were given 3, 5, and 15 ml. of compatible placental blood intravenously, the fœtal cells were demonstrated in the expected concentration in their blood (figs. 2 and 3). In the adult receiving 15 ml., the fœtal cells were still demonstrable 6 weeks after infusion.

The blood of 90 blood-donors (males and non-pregnant females) was examined. No fœtal cells were found.

The blood of 42 mothers, selected at random without reference to the blood-groups of mother and child, was examined on the 2nd to 6th day post partum with the following results:

No. examined (2-minute scan)	No. of fœtal cells	Estimated amount of fœtal blood in maternal circulation (ml.)
33	0	0.0
2	1	0.1
3	2	0.2–0.3
3	3–4	0.4–0.7
1	16	2.0–3.0

A fœtal erythrocyte in a maternal smear is shown in fig. 4.

The finding that 11 out of 42 (21%) postpartum women had fœtal cells in their circulation suggests that trans-

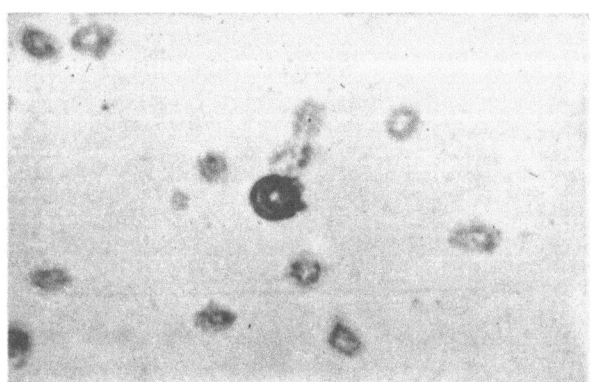

Fig. 1—In-vitro mixture of fœtal and adult red cells. The fœtal cell appears as a relatively intact refractile cell in a field of adult "ghost" erythrocytes.

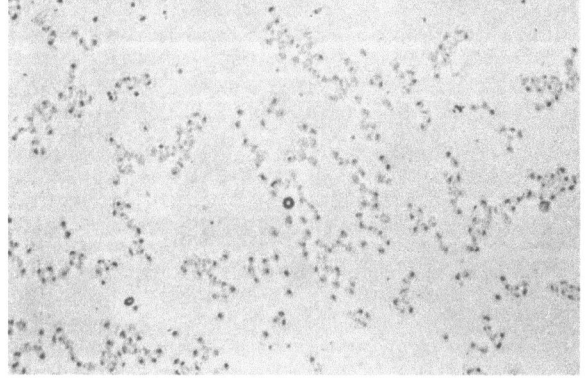

Fig. 2—Low-power photomicrograph of a fœtal cell in an adult, 3 weeks after injection of 15 ml. placental blood.

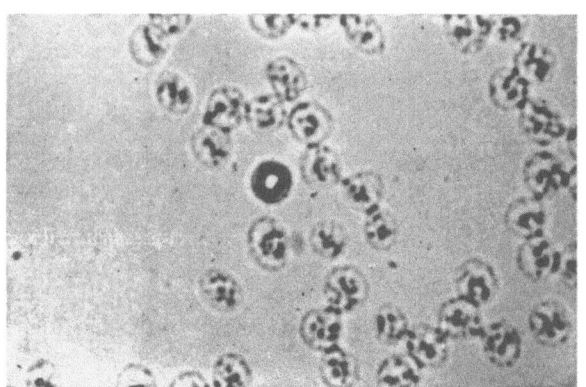

Fig. 3—High-power view of the same.

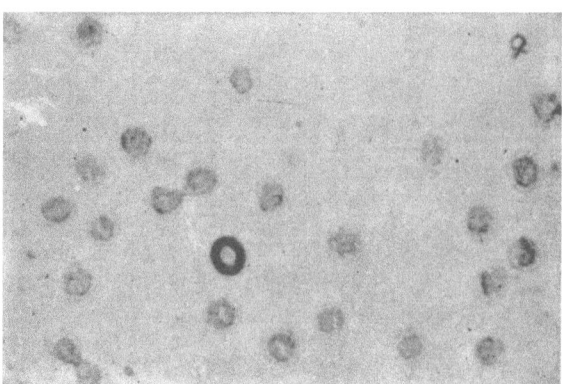

Fig. 4—Fœtal cell in a postpartum mother.

placental passage of fœtal blood is rather common. This finding, obtained by a relatively simple technique, is in agreement with those suggested by the more complex methods of Creger and Steele (1957) and of Hosoi (1958). This method has the advantage of not being dependent on the blood-groups of the mother or fœtus.

This study was aided by grants from the Playtex Park Research Foundation and the National Cancer Institute of Canada. We wish to express our thanks to Dr. B. Chown and Dr. J. Hoogstraten for help and advice.

REFERENCES

Creger, W. P., Steele, M. R. (1957) *New Engl. J. Med.* **256,** 158.
Hosoi, T. (1958) *Yokohama med. Bull.* **9,** 61.
Kleihauer, E., Hildegard, B., Betke, K. (1957) *Klin. Wschr.* **35,** 637.

Paper 24

24. Jewkes, J., Sawers, D. and Stillerman, R. (1969). The prevention of Rhesus haemolytic disease. In: *The Sources of Invention* (2nd ed.). pp 348-351. Macmillan: London. (Extract).

Commentary

The idea of the Liverpool group of giving anti-D to prevent immunisation was based on the hypothesis that it would destroy any Rh-positive fetal cells which had leaked into the maternal circulation of the Rh-negative mother. The American workers tackled the problem from a different point of view, and the story of the two approaches is accurately given in the extract from the book by Jewkes and his colleagues (Paper 24).

As they state in the preface, they derived their information from Mrs A. G. Clarke (no relation to the editor), from Professor P. M. Sheppard and Dr J. G. Gorman.

From J. Jewkes, D. Sawers and R. Stillerman (1969). The Sources of Invention, 2nd. ed., 348-351.
Copyright (1969), by kind permission of the authors and Macmillan and Co Ltd

THE SOURCES OF INVENTION

THE PREVENTION OF RHESUS HAEMOLYTIC DISEASE

THE first recorded description of haemolytic disease of the newborn was in 1609 but until the discovery of the human blood groups during this century, and in particular the description of the group known as the Rhesus (Rh.) factor in 1939, no treatment was possible. The American physician and research scientist, Dr. P. Levine, discovered and described the hitherto unknown antibody (later named the Rhesus factor by Drs. Wiener and Landsteiner, then at Wisconsin University) when he established that the disease occurs when a Rh. negative mother produces a Rh. positive baby, who inherits this blood type from its father. Since the baby's cells usually, although not always, invade the mother at delivery the first baby is not normally affected; such foreign foetal cells entering her circulation may cause her to react, as the body does to any foreign material, by producing antibodies to destroy them. The presence of these antibodies becomes a permanent factor in the mother's blood stream and, as the level of antibodies may rise after each birth, subsequent Rh. positive children's cells are attacked with increasing severity. Although about eight per cent of all pregnancies may give rise to antibodies, only about 1 in 180 babies in western countries are affected because the child may not be Rh. positive, may be a first child, or may be protected by one or other of several factors. In the milder form of the disease anaemia and jaundice develop; increasing severity leads to stillbirth, to infant death or to brain damage of the surviving children. After the discovery of the cause of the disease, the only remedy available was the drastic one of immediate blood transfusion of the newborn to clear the antibodies; later a technique was developed of changing the blood of unborn babies repeatedly until labour could be safely induced, but this also involves dangers to the mother and child.

An entirely new method, that of prevention rather than treatment, arose almost simultaneously in England and the United States. In England it had an unusually fascinating beginning. During the 1950's, Dr. Philip Sheppard, an Oxford geneticist, was working on the behavioural genetics of the butterfly *Papilio machaon* and advertised in the Amateur Entomological Society Journal for some living specimens. Dr. C. A. Clarke, a consultant physician in Liverpool, who took an amateur interest in butterflies, was able to supply some hybrids he had bred. These surprised Sheppard as, scientifically, he would have expected them to look intermediate between the two species; instead they all resembled just one of their parents. So in 1953 they began to investigate the butterflies genetically. Inheritance of genetic variability occurs essentially in the same way in all animals – in human populations hair and eye colour and blood groups are examples of inherited variants.

In 1956 Dr. Sheppard went to Liverpool in order to work more closely with Dr. Clarke, taking with him a small grant of £2,000–£3,000 which he had received from the Nuffield Foundation*for his research on butterflies. Dr. Clarke suggested they should study similar systems of inheritance in humans and a year later, together with Dr. R. B. McConnell they set up an heredity clinic. The Rh. complex with its system of closely linked genes particularly attracted their attention.

Dr. Levine had first observed in 1943 that another factor influenced the incidence of Rh. haemolytic disease. He noticed that in the majority of families with a history of the disease the mother belonged to the same ABO group as the father and that when the opposite was the case Rh. antibodies were not usually formed. Further supporting evidence came in 1956 from the work of H. R. Nevanlinna and T. Vainio. The explanation of why ABO incompatibility gives protection is that when foreign foetal cells enter the mother's circulation they are immediately eliminated and consequently she is not stimulated to form anti-Rh. antibodies. In 1957 Sheppard and Clarke and two other doctors at Liverpool, Dr. McConnell and Dr. R. Finn became greatly interested in the interaction between the rhesus and ABO blood systems. A large family study was carried out and an article describing the results was published in 1958. These and further studies have confirmed that ABO incompatibility reduces the risk of Rh. haemolytic disease by about one-fifth.

Early one morning Mrs. C. A. Clarke woke up her husband to suggest he might use the antibody formed against the Rhesus factor to prevent the occurrence of rhesus haemolytic disease; this idea was discussed in the Department and at a Liverpool symposium in 1960 Dr. Finn tentatively put forward the view that it

---

* A later grant of £400,000 from the Nuffield Foundation to the University of Liverpool enabled the Nuffield Unit of Medical Genetics to be built in 1963. (C.A.C.)

might be possible to destroy foetal blood cells in the maternal circulation following delivery by means of suitable antibody, thus mimicking the natural protection afforded by ABO incompatibility.

During the next four years the Liverpool workers carried out experiments. Male volunteer blood donors with Rh. negative blood, who had previously received injections of Rh. positive red blood cells, were given injections of anti-Rh. antibody. After some initial failures, improvements in the type and dose of antibody led to the effective clearance of foreign blood cells before active antibodies could be formed against them. The trials were carried out in co-operation with the Liverpool Regional Blood Transfusion Service under the direction of Dr. D. Lehane. This organisation approached the Lister Institute, a non-profit-making body, which agreed to produce the antibody serum. The results of the first experiments of the Liverpool workers were published in an article in the British Medical Journal in May 1961. In 1964 they started strictly controlled clinical trials in Liverpool's five maternity units; teams in Sheffield, Leeds, Bradford and in Baltimore (where Dr. Finn went for a year) also ran similar trials. Another group experimented at Freiburg.

Meanwhile Dr. J. G. Gorman of Columbia University, an Australian who had emigrated to the United States in 1955, was assigned to the blood bank at Columbia Presbyterian Hospital, New York and there came into contact with Dr. V. J. Freda, an obstetrician. In 1959, Gorman and Freda, together with Dr. W. Pollack, an English immunologist of the Ortho Research Foundation in the United States, made an approach to the study of this disease which was direct, as contrasted with that of the English scientists. Gorman first learnt of the principle of passive antibody mediated immuno-suppression from Florey's textbook on General Pathology which he 'happened to read only because I was presented with a free copy by the publisher'. Of the many research schemes they discussed, this seemed the most promising avenue and there was no theoretical reason why it should not work if applied to Rh. negative mothers. They had mapped out a project almost identical with that of the Liverpool workers, although based on a slightly different line of reasoning, when the B.M.J. article, together with a hopeful editorial on the subject, appeared in May 1961. Although their first reaction was 'dismay at being scooped for publication by Liverpool, the effect in New York was to give a tremendous boost to our own plans. We were now suddenly working on a feasible and reputable research project whereas before we had been largely talking to deaf ears.' But even before the article appeared, they had been successful in receiving a grant from the Health Research Council of New York City and afterwards the Ortho Pharmaceutical Foundation contributed considerable funds for the research. The Company was responsible for producing, as early as 1961, the gamma globulin which, as an antibody, was superior to the raw serum because of its purity and freedom from hepatitis. Ortho Pharmaceuticals is the only American producer of this gamma globulin.

The American research workers carried out trials for three years on male volunteers at Sing Sing Prison. There was free exchange of information between them, the Liverpool workers and others in the field, in particular when some trials revealed there was an enhancement rather than the desired suppression of immunity with the passive antibody. It was discovered that the danger was dose-related: small doses might increase the risk of immunisation, large doses were safe and completely immunosuppressive. Clinical trials were started on American women at risk in 1964 and by 1967 some 3,000 mothers had been treated.

An unusually interesting case of individual initiative was revealed in 1967 when an American doctor, Eugene Hamilton of St. Louis, stood up at one of Dr. Gorman's lectures and announced that he had started clinical trials in April 1962. He had read the B.M.J. article of May 1961 giving the first results of the Liverpool workers, and had been impressed with the logic of the approach. He carefully prepared his own plasma from Rh. negative mothers who were severely sensitised and had delivered stillborn foetuses but had no history of hepatitis or other communicable disease. Unknown to others working in the field, he had for five years given protection with successful results to three times as many mothers as any other of the clinical trials, thus doubling the world figures of proven effectiveness of the treatment.

In Australia, since August 1967, about fifty per cent of women at risk have been given the treatment through the agency of the Red Cross; in Germany, due to the work of Schneider and Preisler, who started trials on male volunteers in 1962, the anti-Rh. gamma globulin is available and is being used. The United States and British health authorities have been cautious in approving the treatment; in the former it was passed for general use in June 1968; in Britain it has been available for selected, high-risk cases from the beginning of 1968.

This is a case where the important discoveries were made by scientists in Britain and the United States who became acquainted with each others' work through the free publication of results. In England the work began with the study of butterflies and a method of thought originating in one branch of science was successfully applied to another, apparently unconnected, area of study. A practising doctor in America, operating independently, carried out early clinical trials with extraordinary success. One pharmaceutical company in the United States was interested in the work from the start and made substantial grants for research. But in the early stages of this remarkable discovery, especially in England, the funds available or needed were comparatively small.

REFERENCES

1. Clarke, C. A., Finn, R., McConnell, R. B., and Sheppard, P. M., 'Intern. Arch. Allergy', *Applied Immunology*, 13 (1958), pp. 5–6.

2. Finn, R., *Lancet*, I (1960), pp. 526–7.

3. Finn, R. *et al.*, *British Medical Journal* (1961), pp. 1468–90.

4. Finn, R. *et al.*, *Nature*, 190 (1961), pp. 922–3.

5. Freda, V. J., and Gorman, J. G., *Bulletin of the Sloane Hospital for Women*, 8 (1962), pp. 147–58.

6. Clarke, C. A. *et al.*, *British Medical Journal*, I (1963), pp. 979–84; and (1965) pp. 279–83.

7. Clarke, C. A., and Sheppard, P. M., *Lancet* (Aug. 14, 1965), p. 343.

8. Clarke, C. A., *Vox Sang*, II (1966), pp. 641–55.

9. Freda, V. J., Gorman, J. G., and Pollack, W., *Science*, 151 (1966), p. 828.

10. Gorman, J. G., Freda, V. J., Pollack, W. J., and Robertson, J. G., *Bulletin of the New York Academy of Medicine* (June 1966).

11. McConnell, R. B., *Annual Review of Medicine*, 17 (1966), pp. 291–306.

12. Smith, C. H., *Blood Diseases of Infancy and Childhood*, 2nd edition (The C. V. Mosby Co., St. Louis, 1966), pp. 121–65.

13. Hamilton, E. G., *Rh. Isoimmunization: A Simple Method of Prevention using Anti-D Antibody* (unpublished paper).

14. Correspondence and interview with Professor P. M. Sheppard.

15. Correspondence with Dr. J. G. Gorman.

Paper 25

25. Finn, R. (1960). Erythroblastosis. *Lancet, i,* 526. (Extract).

Commentary

It is not often that in the proceedings of a local medical society there is a reference which becomes of outstanding importance as regards priority. In 1960 the editor of this book organised a symposium which dealt with the various lines of genetic research being carried out in the Department of Medicine in the University of Liverpool, and he sent a report to the *Lancet* part of which is shown in Paper 25. Under 'Erythroblastosis' Dr Ronald Finn put forward the view that the protection afforded by ABO incompatibility against Rh haemolytic disease might be mimicked where the mother and fetus were ABO compatible by the giving of an antibody to destroy the Rh-positive fetal cells in the circulation of the Rh-negative mother. This had previously been discussed by members of the Department in Liverpool following our confirmatory work on the ABO blood group of the immunising fetus (see Clarke *et al.* 1958*, and Paper 21), but there is no doubt that the reference in Paper 25 is the first time that the suggestion appears in print.

* Clarke, C. A., Finn, R., McConnell, R. B. and Sheppard, P. M. (1958). The protection afforded by ABO incompatibility against erythroblastosis due to Rhesus anti-D. *Int. Arch. Allergy, 13,* 380.

MARCH 5, 1960   MEDICAL SOCIETIES   THE LANCET

Medical Societies

LIVERPOOL MEDICAL INSTITUTION

A SYMPOSIUM on the Role of Inheritance in Common Diseases was held on Feb 18, under the chairmanship of Dr. E. N. Chamberlain, the president.

Erythroblastosis

Dr. RONALD FINN said that only 1 in about 20 rhesus-negative women married to a rhesus-positive husband becomes sensitised to the rhesus factor. Probably, therefore, protective mechanisms existed for 19 out of 20 such matings.

P. Levine was the first to suggest that ABO incompatibility was protective against erythroblastosis fœtalis. In a Liverpool series of 164 families with erythroblastosis the proportion of incompatible matings was 24%, and the immunising fœtus (when it could be determined with certainty) was always found to be compatible.

Using a modification of the Zipursky method for the detection of fœtal red cells, Dr. Finn had investigated the blood of 50 mothers within seventy-two hours of delivery. Fœtal cells were found in about a third of the compatible matings, but were never found in incompatible matings. This finding further supported the hypothesis that ABO incompatibility is protective.

Dr. Finn tentatively suggested that it might be possible to destroy any fœtal red cells found in the maternal circulation following delivery by means of a suitable antibody. If successful, this would prevent the development of erythroblastosis, so mimicking the natural protection afforded by ABO incompatibility.

Paper 26

26. Finn, R., Clarke, C. A., Donohoe, W. T. A., McConnell, R. B., Sheppard, P. M., Lehane, D. and Kulke, W. (1961). Experimental Studies on the prevention of Rh haemolytic disease. *Brit. Med. J. i,* 1486-1490.

Commentary

In this paper the Liverpool team produced data which gave further support for the relevance of ABO incompatibility in preventing immunisation.

Much more important, however, was the finding that using the Kleihauer technique the higher the fetal cell scores at delivery in a series of mothers investigated, the more likely they were to become immunised (Table 2).

The first steps were also taken to test the hypothesis that it might be possible to prevent immunisation by giving anti-D to Rh-negative male volunteers after the injection of Rh-positive red cells. It was demonstrated that 50 to 60% of these ^{51}Cr tagged Rh-positive cells were removed from the circulation within 48 hours, the anti-D which was administered being of the complete or 19S type and given in the form of plasma. The reason for giving 19S rather than the incomplete 7S was because the naturally occurring anti-A and anti-B is of the former type and an attempt was being made to mimic the protective effect associated with ABO incompatibility.

From R. Finn et al. (1961). Brit. Med. J., i, 1486-1490. Copyright (1961), by kind permission of the authors and The Lancet Ltd

EXPERIMENTAL STUDIES ON THE PREVENTION OF Rh HAEMOLYTIC DISEASE

BY

R. FINN, M.B., Ch.B., M.R.C.P.

C. A. CLARKE, M.D., F.R.C.P.

W. T. A. DONOHOE, A.M.I.L.T.

R. B. McCONNELL, M.D., M.R.C.P.

Department of Medicine, University of Liverpool

P. M. SHEPPARD, M.A., D.Phil.

Sub-Department of Genetics, University of Liverpool

D. LEHANE, M.B., B.Ch.

Liverpool Regional Blood Transfusion Service

AND

W. KULKE, M.B., Ch.B., D.M.R.T.

Radio-isotope Unit, Liverpool Radium Institute

ABO Incompatibility

In the context of haemolytic disease of the newborn, ABO incompatibility means that the father's blood is unsuitable for transfusion into the mother, and our interest in this stems from the work of Levine (1943), who noted a deficiency of such mating types in the parents of affected children. He deduced, therefore, that ABO incompatibility affords a degree of protection against Rh haemolytic disease, and this has been confirmed by many workers. Of particular interest are the experiments of Stern et al. (1956), who showed that male volunteers could be much more easily sensitized to Rh if the injected blood were ABO compatible.

Nevanlinna and Vainio (1956) emphasized the importance of the sensitizing foetus and showed by means of a family study that once sensitization had occurred there was no evidence that ABO incompatibility between mother and foetus afforded any further protection. We carried out a somewhat similar survey in order to determine the ABO group of the Rh-sensitizing foetus, and in 14 ABO incompatible matings in which the sensitizing foetus could be determined with certainty its ABO group was always compatible with the mother (this can happen because of heterozygosity in the father—for example, a group O woman married to an AO man can produce a group O child). The probability of our results being found by chance alone was less than 1 in 500 (Clarke et al., 1958). Nevertheless, the sensitizing foetus is not invariably ABO-compatible, and we have recently found one which is incompatible.

One of us (R. F.) has investigated a series of 85 families with Rh-negative mothers where four or more children have been born and yet no haemolytic disease or Rh sensitization occurred. In 22 the husband was also Rh negative, but in the remainder the percentage of ABO incompatible matings was 42.9% ± 6.23 compared with 33.6% in the general population (as judged by phenotype frequencies) and 22.0% ± 2.83 in the investigated families with haemolytic disease (Finn, 1961).

The most obvious explanation for the protection afforded by ABO incompatibility is that suggested by

Race and Sanger (1950). They point out that if Rh sensitization is due to foetal red cells entering the maternal circulation, it seems possible that they may be eliminated before they have time to act as Rh antigens—for example, foetal cells containing A antigen would be removed by a maternal serum containing anti-A.

Foetal Cells in Maternal Circulation

" Massive " transplacental haemorrhage from the foetal into the maternal circulation was first postulated by Wiener (1948), who described a probable case. Chown (1954) proved the point by means of differential agglutination and by tests for foetal haemoglobin, but neither of these techniques is sensitive enough to detect small foetal bleeds such as may be responsible for most cases of Rh sensitization. Kleihauer et al. (1957) described a method which is very suitable, the principle being the differential elution of adult and foetal haemoglobin. This is effected by means of a citric-phosphate buffer on an ordinary blood smear, the adult cells appearing as ghosts while the foetal cells stand out as dark refractile bodies (see Fig. 1). Zipursky

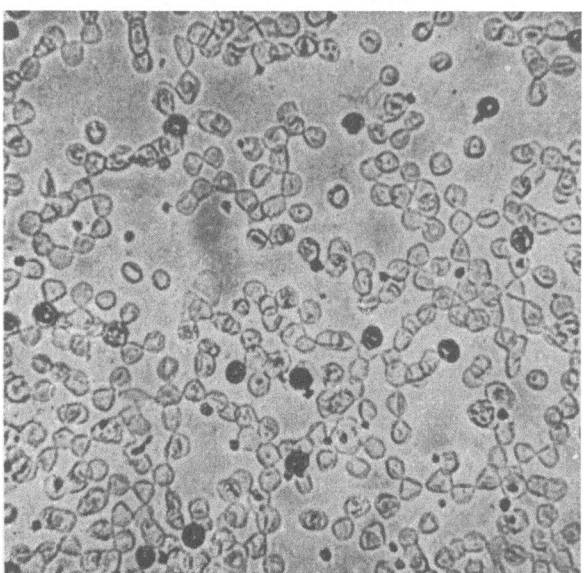

FIG. 1.—Large numbers of foetal red cells in the maternal circulation demonstrated by the phosphate elution technique.

et al. (1959) used this method to demonstrate foetal red cells in the blood of women after delivery. They studied 42 cases and detected foetal red cells in 11 (21%).

We decided to use a modification of this technique in a large series of Rh-negative women to find out: (a) the incidence of transplacental foetal bleeding, (b) the correlation between circulating foetal cells and the production of Rh antibodies, (c) the role of the placental barrier in protection against Rh sensitization, and (d) the time of foetal bleeding.

Technique

The Kleihauer technique has been used, the only modification being that the blood smear has not been stained. To establish its sensitivity, one of us (R. F.) examined blood from 50 men along with an equal number of specimens from post-partum women, the observer being unaware of the source of the material. Two smears from each of the subjects were made, and each was examined twice for three minutes, the number of refractile cells found being counted. Each individual was given a quantitative figure (foetal score) by taking the average of the number of refractile cells counted in the four scans. No male score was found to exceed 0.5. To give a wide margin a figure of 2 or more has therefore been accepted as indicating definite transplacental foetal bleeding. In the application of the technique to the series of post-partum bloods from 206 Rh-negative women, only one smear was made and the foetal score is the average of two three-minute counts.

In order to arrive at a correlation between foetal scores and quantity of foetal blood in the maternal circulation, mixtures of adult and foetal blood were made at varying dilutions. Thus at 1 in 5,000 the score was 5 (SD $\pm$ 1.5). On the assumption of a maternal blood volume of about 5 litres, a score of 5 would therefore represent about 1 ml. of foetal blood in the maternal circulation.

Incidence of Transplacental Haemorrhage

Examination has been made of 256 specimens of post-partum blood, all the patients being unselected for ABO group and for parity. The first 50 were also unselected for Rh, but the remainder were all Rh-negative. The only other selection was that none of the women had a history of haemolytic disease nor any demonstrable Rh antibody. Table I shows the

TABLE I.—*Foetal Scores in 256 Mothers After Delivery*

Foetal Score	No. of Women
0	205
1	21
2	7
3	5
4	5
5-9	7
10-19	2
20 and over	4
Total	256

results of the foetal cell scores. It can be seen that foetal bleeding, as judged by our definition, has been detected in only 30 (11.7% $\pm$ 2.01) of the women. The blood groups of the baby were tested in 135 of the Rh-negative women. In none of the 21 cases in which foetal cells were detected in the maternal system was the foetus incompatible with the mother on the ABO system. In the 114 cases in which no foetal cells were detected in the mother the foetus was incompatible with the mother on the ABO system in 26 cases. These two groups are significantly distinct (P=0.013). Clearly, 11.7% is an underestimate of the frequency of foetal bleeding, since the 256 specimens examined must have contained a number of incompatible foetuses, and the presence of bleeding is almost certainly not detectable in such cases.

In most of the cases in which foetal cells were detected—that is, scores which were above 2—the quantity of foetal blood in the maternal circulation seems to be 1 ml. or less. Our data do not reveal any definite division into small and larger bleeds, but rather progressively smaller numbers of women with increasing quantities of foetal blood. Only four women had foetal scores indicating that they had received about 5 ml. or more of foetal blood. It would appear, therefore, that about 2% of women have what might be called " large " transplacental foetal haemorrhage (the bleeds of 50-100 ml., which cause anaemia of the infant, being called " massive ").

Correlation of Circulating Foetal Cells and Rh-antibody Production

We have followed up 85 of the Rh-negative women who had Rh-positive foetuses, and tested their serum for antibodies two or three months after delivery. The series is not random, in that it includes as many women as possible in whom foetal cells had been detected. The results are shown in Table II. It will be seen that of the

TABLE II.—*Transplacental Haemorrhage and the Development of Antibodies in the Puerperium*

Foetal Score	No. of Women	Antibody Present
Less than 2	75	1
2-19	7	—
20 and over	3	2
Totals	85	3

75 whom we had scored as having had no transplacental bleed, only one has developed an antibody. This, curiously enough, is an anti-C, even though the baby's Rh genotype was CDe/cde, and repeated testing has failed to reveal any anti-D. Of the women with " small " bleeds (foetal scores 2-19) none has developed an antibody. Of the three women scored as having had a " large " bleed, two have developed anti-D, active both in saline and in albumin, while the third has produced no antibody. There is a significant association between " large " foetal bleeds and antibody formation (P=0.025).

Role of Placental Barrier in Protecting Against Rh Sensitization

There are various factors which can play a part in preventing Rh-negative women mated to Rh-positive men from developing Rh antibodies. Our results suggest that the placental barrier is the most important, always provided that foetal bleeding is necessary for maternal sensitization. If this be so our data imply that about 85% of women are thus protected by the placental barrier. Two other known factors—ABO incompatibility in the mating and Rh heterozygosity in the husband—are much less important, though by no means negligible in a small-family society such as is found in this country. There is also the possibility that immunological tolerance plays a part in a small number of cases (see Race and Sanger, 1958).

Time of Foetal Bleeding

It seems probable that most though not all (see Discussion and Weiner *et al.*, 1958), foetal bleeds occur during labour. We are examining the blood of women at the 36th week of pregnancy to determine the precise incidence of ante-partum transplacental haemorrhage.

Experimental Protection Against Rh Sensitization

The weight of evidence given above strongly supports the hypothesis that circulating foetal cells are necessary to cause Rh sensitization. This raises the possibility that Rh sensitization might be prevented if such foetal cells could be destroyed or their antigen sites blocked. The mechanism by which ABO incompatibility protects, and the agglutination of foetal cells which we effected *in vitro* in a case of " massive " foetal bleeding (Finn *et al.*, 1960), made us consider methods which could be carried out *in vivo*. We decided to inject radioactive-chromium (Cr-51)-tagged Rh-positive cells into a number of Rh-negative male volunteers, and shortly afterwards to give half of them anti-D serum. Initially, only six men were used in order to give us information on whether (*a*) the Rh-positive cells become coated with anti-D, and (*b*) the Rh-positive cell survival time was the same in the two groups. The results of this experiment are described here.

We are also studying whether or not Rh sensitization is similar in these six men and in a larger series injected later.

Method

The volunteers were male blood donors who were fully informed of the nature of the experiments. They were all of blood group A cde/cde. The donor of the Rh-positive blood injected into the men had previously given 8 pints (4.6 litres) of blood that was believed never to have caused jaundice in any of the recipients. His blood groups were A CDe/cde. Cross-matching tests between these cells and the volunteers' sera has not revealed any incompatibilities.

The donor was bled two days before the experiment, and this blood was tagged with Cr-51 on the day of the experiment. The amount of the Rh-positive blood injected intravenously was 5 ml., this volume being decided upon because it was known to be large enough to cause Rh sensitization, and yet not so large as to require a large volume of anti-D; it was also consistent with the amount concerned in the sensitization of the two women in our investigation who produced anti-D.

The anti-D serum had a titre with the donor's cells, both in saline and in albumin, of 1 in 64. We injected 10 ml. of it intravenously into three of the men chosen at random, half an hour after the Rh-positive blood injection.

Samples of blood were withdrawn from each of the six men, 2, 5, and 14 days later, and the following tests carried out.

1. The proportion of radioactive cells was estimated.

2. Samples were tested by the technique of Jones and Silver (1958) for the detection of minor cell populations. The method, as applied here, is to add incomplete anti-D to the blood so that any D-positive cells (but not D-negative cells) persisting will be coated with the antibody; the cells are then washed to remove excess antibody. Next, anti-human globulin (A.H.G.) is added, and this will attach itself to the antibody coating the D-positive cells. Because any D-positive cells will be sparsely distributed, agglutination (as in the indirect Coombs test) cannot occur. The cells are now washed to remove free A.H.G., and an equal volume of D-positive cells coated with incomplete anti-D are added. These will attach themselves to the anti-D plus A.H.G. coated cells to give "rosettes," each indicating the presence of a single original D-positive cell in the D-negative population. It is possible to count the number of rosettes per unit area and compare the figure with the number of unagglutinated cells (presumably the method could also be used for detecting an extremely weak anti-D).

3. Samples were tested as above, but omitting the initial treatment of the cells with incomplete anti-D. It will be appreciated from the method that no rosettes will be found unless the cells have been coated with anti-D *in vivo*.

4. Samples were tested for the presence of anti-D in the serum in saline, in albumin, and by the indirect Coombs test.

Results

Table III and Fig. 2 show the remaining percentage radioactivity at various times after the injection of the labelled cells. It will be seen that there is a great difference in the proportion of cells remaining in the circulation according to whether antibody had or had not been given. The administration of antibody seems at least to halve the number of circulating cells in the first two days, but thereafter the differential decline is less pronounced. The difference between the two groups in the first sampling is highly significant (P = <0.02).

Table IV gives the number of rosettes—that is, Rh-positive cells—counted at various times after the initial injection. Even though this test is qualitative and of unknown precision, it will be seen that the numbers are less in the volunteers who had received anti-D than in those untreated.

Table V gives the results of tests carried out as described in No. 3 above (in which the initial treatment with incomplete anti-D is omitted). It will be seen that rosettes were present only in those persons who had received the anti-D injection. This demonstrates conclusively that at any rate a good proportion of the Rh-positive red cells have been coated by the anti-D administered 30 minutes after the injection of the tagged red cells.

None of the volunteers' sera contained detectable anti-D, even though three of them had been injected

TABLE III.—*Percentage of Cr-51-labelled Cells Remaining at Various Times After Their Injection*

Volunteers		2 Days	5 Days	14 Days
Unprotected	{	106 94 98	88 85 87	69 67 77
Anti-D given	{	48 40 13	33 30 6	22 21 4·6

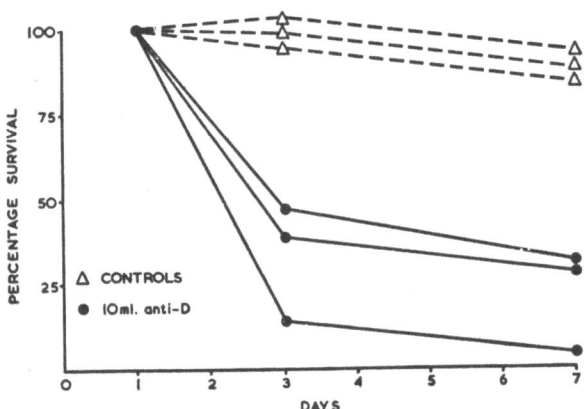

FIG. 2.—Remaining percentage radioactivity at various times after injection of 5 ml. of Rh-positive blood tagged with Cr-51 into 6 Rh-negative male volunteers.

TABLE IV.—*Number of Rosettes—that is, Rh-positive Cells—Per Unit Volume of Recipient Blood at Various Times After Injection of 5 ml. Rh-positive Blood*

Volunteers		2 Days	5 Days	14 Days
Unprotected	{	10 12 11	8 9 9	9 8 9
Anti-D given	{	8 9 9	5 6 4	5 5 4

TABLE V.—*Number of Anti-D Coated Rh-positive Cells Per Unit Volume of Recipient Blood at Various Times After Injection of 5 ml. Rh-positive Blood*

Volunteers		2 Days	5 Days	14 Days
Unprotected	{	0 0 0	0 0 0	0 0 0
Anti-D given	{	4 2 5	Not counted " " " "	4 4 4

with it two days previously. This was to be expected in view of the dilution of the anti-D by the recipient's serum.

Discussion

The results of our investigation into ABO incompatibility and foetal cells in the maternal circulation lend further weight to the hypothesis that sensitization against the D antigen is caused in most cases by circulating foetal cells in the maternal system. The results also suggest that if these cells were destroyed rapidly, as they are when the cells are incompatible with the mother on the ABO system, sensitization would be avoided. It therefore seems obvious that a way to prevent sensitization in an ABO-compatible mother would be to destroy the foetal cells rapidly by some other means. Since the cells are by definition D-positive, the injection of anti-D would be the first thing to try.

Our results show quite conclusively that the administration to Rh-negative male volunteers of 10 ml. of a particular anti-D has, firstly, coated at least a good proportion of previously injected Rh-positive cells, and, secondly, as judged by radioactive tagging, caused the elimination of at least 50% of them in two days. These results are very encouraging, particularly in view of two previous investigations. Thus, Jandl *et al.* (1957) showed that red cells fully coated with incomplete anti-D *in vitro* were rapidly removed from the circulation by the spleen, and that the proportion of cells destroyed depended on the completeness of the coating. Again, Stern and Berger (1960) have demonstrated that if Rh-positive cells are coated with anti-D before injection into Rh-negative men the formation of antibodies is prevented.

If rapid elimination of all foetal cells is necessary to prevent sensitization, our 50% destruction may mean that we did not give enough anti-D, and that a second dose was needed. On the other hand, most of the remaining Rh-positive cells have picked up antibody and have some blocking of their antigen sites, and this, together with the 50% destruction, may have been enough for complete protection. The matter is somewhat complicated because we used an antiserum which contained both complete and incomplete antibodies, and it is obviously necessary to try antisera of the incomplete type only before deciding on the most efficient type of anti-D. For protection with different antisera different doses may be needed.

The 5 ml. of Rh-positive blood which we injected into the volunteers introduces fewer red cells than the 5 ml. of foetal blood which we took as our dividing line between "small" and "large" foetal bleeds because of the higher number of cells per unit volume in foetal blood. If we are successful in reducing or eliminating sensitization in the three protected male volunteers, it would be important to give cells of different Rh-positive genotype because of the known differences in their ability to lead to haemolytic disease. Furthermore, the question of using foetal blood will have to be considered.

An important problem remains unsolved. We are uncertain what proportion of foetal bleeds occur before labour, and until we have more evidence on this point it is impossible to know how many women would be protected from sensitization by the giving of anti-D after delivery. The case in which an antibody was produced without our having detected any foetal cells in the mother's post-partum blood may possibly have

been associated with foetal bleeding many weeks before term. On the other hand, the case was anomalous in that anti-C without any anti-D was produced in spite of the foetus being of Rh genotype CDe/cde. We are unconvinced by the paper of Taylor and Kullman (1961) who, using the Kleihauer technique, found 18% of 40 ante-partum mothers and 17% of 58 post-partum mothers to be positive for foetal erythrocytes. Kleihauer *et al.* 1960), using a modification of their original technique, report that in 111 pregnancies, foetal cells were found before delivery in 37% and after in 71%. In the majority, however, they found only one foetal cell per 5–20 million maternal cells—that is, at dilutions which we would score as "no foetal bleed."

Despite the unsolved problems, we feel that the signs are very hopeful, though the final proof of the feasibility of protection will have to await the results of tests for sensitization in these first six and many other volunteers. Waiting for antibodies to appear is inefficient, and a way of detecting sensitization may be to give, after about two months, a small provocative dose of Rh-positive cells to all the volunteers, whether they have received anti-D or not. Alternatively, repeated injections of Rh-positive blood could be given, the protected volunteers each time receiving further anti-D.

Should these experiments lead to an efficient method for preventing Rh sensitization, there ought to be no difficulty in detecting the women who need it, since the technique of screening for the presence of circulating foetal cells could be applied in any hospital laboratory. If it can be shown that incomplete anti-D is fully effective, the numbers of women requiring prophylaxis (about 2% of all pregnancies if all detectable foetal bleeds were treated) are not likely to be too large for available supplies of antiserum.

Summary

The various factors responsible for the occurrence of Rh haemolytic disease in only 1 in 20 of the families at risk are discussed. Of these we have investigated ABO incompatibility and the ability of the placenta to prevent the passage of foetal cells into the maternal circulation.

Our data give further support for the importance of ABO incompatibility and for the view that Rh sensitization is caused by the circulation of foetal red cells in the mother. Using a simple slide technique, we have found foetal cells in the blood of 11.7% of 256 post-partum women. It is estimated that most of the foetal bleeds had been of 1 ml. or less, but that in about 1.5% it had been "large"—that is, 5 ml. or more.

Rh antibodies developed in two of three women who had had "large" foetal bleeds and in 1 of 75 women in whom no foetal cells had been detected. This association of antibody formation with "large" foetal bleeds is statistically significant, and we conclude that the placental barrier is the most important of the factors preventing Rh sensitization.

Foetal cells were never found when the foetus was ABO incompatible with the mother, and ABO incompatibility probably protects because the foetal cells are rapidly eliminated by maternal anti-A or anti-B. It seemed possible that circulating Rh-positive foetal cells might be similarly eliminated by the administration of anti-D, thus preventing Rh sensitization of the mother.

To test this hypothesis we have injected Rh-positive

blood tagged with Cr-51 into six Rh-negative male volunteers, and given three of them 10 ml. of anti-D intravenously 30 minutes later. In the men not given anti-D the Rh-positive cells have survived normally, whereas in the three who received the antibody at least 50% of the injected cells had disappeared within two days. Using a modification of the technique of Jones and Silver (1958) for the detection of minor cell populations, we demonstrated that a proportion of the surviving foetal cells had been coated with the anti-D. This blocking of the antigen sites may protect from sensitization, and we are studying the men to see if the blocking and the 50% destruction prevent the production of Rh antibodies. On the other hand, a larger dose of anti-D will be needed if 100% elimination of foetal cells is necessary.

Our results suggest that it may be possible to prevent most cases of Rh sensitization, and thus in time eliminate Rh haemolytic disease. There remain, however, several problems, the chief being that of the women into whom the foetus bleeds before delivery.

We would like first to thank the six blood donors who volunteered for the experimental studies and who have so willingly attended for venesection on many occasions. We are much indebted to Professor T. N. A. Jeffcoate and Mr. C. H. Walsh for giving us every facility to enable us to investigate their obstetric patients. We are also grateful to Dr. R. R. Race, Dr. Ruth Sanger, Dr. A. E. Mourant, and Dr. I. Dunsford for invaluable advice and for supplies of antisera. Our thanks are due to Miss Sheila M. Manning for the part she played in the field work and for her untiring secretarial assistance. This work has been made possible by grants from the Research Committee of the United Liverpool Hospitals, under the chairmanship of Lord Cohen of Birkenhead, the Medical Research Council, and the Nuffield Foundation.

ADDENDUM.—A further 12 volunteers have been studied, and the radioactivity results confirm that about 60% of the injected Rh-positive cells are removed from the circulation by the administration of anti-D. It is now apparent that the major part of the fall occurs within a few hours.

REFERENCES

Chown, B. (1954). *Lancet*, 1, 1213

Clarke, C. A., Finn, R., McConnell, R. B., and Sheppard, P. M. (1958). *Int. Arch. Allergy*, 13, 380.

Finn, R. (1961). M.D. Thesis submitted to University of Liverpool.

Clarke, C. A., Donohoe, W. T. A., McConnell, R. B., and Sheppard, P. M. (1960). Letter submitted to *Nature (Lond.)*.

Jandl, J. H., Jones, R. A., and Castle, W. B. (1957). *J. clin. Invest.*, 36, 1428.

Jones, R. A., and Silver, S. (1958). *Blood*, 13, 763.

Kleihauer, E., and Betke, K. (1960). *Der. Internist*, 1, 292.

Braun, H., and Betke, K. (1957). *Klin. Wschr.*, 35, 637.

Levine, P. (1943). *J. Hered.*, 34, 71.

Nevanlinna, H. R., and Vainio, T. (1956). *Vox sang (Basel)*, 1, 26.

Race, R. R., and Sanger, R. (1950). *Blood Groups in Man*, 1st edition. Blackwell, Oxford.

—— (1958). Ibid., 3rd edition. Blackwell, Oxford.

Stern, K., and Berger, M. (1960). Abstract from American Association of Blood Banks, program, p. 39.

Davidsohn, I., and Masaitis, L. (1956). *Amer. J. clin. Path.*, 26, 833.

Taylor, W. C., and Kullman, G. (1961). *J. Obstet. Gynaec. Brit. Com.*, 68, 261.

Weiner, W., Child, R. M., Garvie, J. M., and Peek, W. H. (1958). *Brit. med. J.*, 2, 770.

Wiener, A. S. (1948). *Amer. J. Obstet. Gynec.*, 56, 717.

Zipursky, A., Hull, A., White, F. D., and Israels, L. G. (1959). *Lancet*, 1, 451.

Papers 27 & 28

27. Stern, K. and Berger, Maya. (1960). Experimental isosensitization to hemo-antigens in man. Paper given at the 13th Annual meeting of the American Association of Blood Banks, San Francisco.

28. Stern, K., Goodman, H. S. and Berger, M. (1961). Experimental isoimmunization to hemoantigens in man. *J. Immunol.*, *87*, 189–198.

Commentary

At a meeting of the American Association of Blood Banks in 1960 Kurt Stern and Maya Berger gave a paper on experimental isoimmunisation in man (Paper 27). In it they showed that Rh-negative volunteers failed to make Rh antibodies when they were injected with Rh-positive cells coated *in vitro* with anti-D, even after repeated injections of the antigen. The abstract of the paper was given to the Liverpool team by Dr Ruth Sanger, who had attended the meeting, and it is mentioned in Paper 26 (page 157). Paper 27 encouraged us to try the incomplete (7S) antibody when we found that the complete (19S), though it cleared the cells, did not protect against immunisation.

Paper 28, published in 1961, gives much fuller details of the work of Stern and his colleagues, and it is interesting that it did not apparently occur to them to apply their findings to the practical situation of HDN.

In Tables I—V, and in Figure 1, the protective effect of ABO incompatibility is amply confirmed. Moreover, when immunisation did take place with ABO incompatible cells the titre was generally lower than when ABO compatible cells had been the stimulus. Furthermore it was demonstrated that the non-formation of antibodies was not 'constitutional' in these subjects. Thus Rh antibodies were often made when the subsequent injections were of ABO *compatible* Rh-positive blood.

Another extemely interesting experiment concerns specificity. Stern *et al.* coated Rh-positive A cells with incomplete anti-A and found that there was no significant interference with Rh immunisation. In the discussion of the paper, however, the authors point out that this might be due to the fact that coating with anti-A is not as heavy as with anti-Rh and that anti-A is easily washed off the cells. This might explain why the findings are in contrast with those in the anti-Kell experiment carried out in Liverpool. These showed conclusively that coating Rh-positive, Kell-positive red cells with anti-Kell protects against Rh immunisation.

From the point of view of prophylaxis of HDN, by far the most important experiment in Paper 28 is given on page 164. None of the Rh-negative men who were injected repeatedly with Rh-positive cells coated *in vitro* with anti-Rh produced antibodies. This result was entirely different when some of the same volunteers were injected with non-coated cells (Table VII).

If any paper demonstrates the gap between a scientific and a medical viewpoint, this surely is it, for why did it have to be left to non-immunologists to put two and two together?

13th Annual Meeting AABB, San Francisco 1960

EXPERIMENTAL ISOSENSITIZATION TO HEMOANTIGENS IN MAN

KURT STERN AND MAYA BERGER

It was shown previously that experimental Rh isosensitization in man as well as formation of hemoantibodies in rabbits are inhibited in hosts possessing preformed antibody for another antigen of the sensitizing red cells. Additional studies were carried out in order to obtain more insight into the mechanisms of isosensitization in man.

The three types of experimental designs and their results were: 1) Injection of Rh-positive ABO-compatible cells, coated *in vitro* with anti-A antibody, into Rh-negative recipients: this procedure did not interfere with development of Rh antibodies. 2) Injection of Rh-negative recipients with Rh-positive ABO-compatible red cells previously coated *in vitro* with Rh antibody: this failed to produce Rh sensitization even after repeated exposures to the antigen. 3) Injection of Kell-negative recipients with Kell-positive red cells. Recipients and immunizing red cells were selected in such a manner that two groups were created in one of which Kell was the only major incompatible antigen whereas in the other there was also incompatibility for Duffy (Fy^a). Greater liability to Kell sensitization was observed in the first group.

The implications of these observations will be discussed. A tentative explanation will be offered which is derived from the clonal selection theory of antibody formation proposed by Jerne and Burnet.

From K. Stern H. S. Goodman and M. Berger(1961),J. Immunol., 87, 189-198. Copyright (1961), by kind permission of the authors and the Williams and Wilkins Co

EXPERIMENTAL ISOIMMUNIZATION TO HEMOANTIGENS IN MAN[1]

KURT STERN,[2] HAROLD S. GOODMAN[3] AND MAYA BERGER

From the Blood Center, Mount Sinai Medical Research Foundation and Hospital, and the Department of Pathology, Chicago Medical School and Mount Sinai Hospital, Chicago, Illinois

Received for publication December 2, 1960

In 1955 we reported that ABO-incompatible Rh-positive blood injected into Rh-negative men was much less likely to induce formation of Rh antibodies than ABO-compatible Rh-positive blood (1). This study confirmed experimentally the well established clinical observation, first reported by Levine (2), on the much higher incidence of Rh sensitization in Rh-negative women with ABO-compatible (homospecific) pregnancies as compared with ABO-incompatible (heterospecific) pregnancies (for review of literature, cf. (3)). Obviously, exposure of pregnant Rh-negative women to ABO-incompatible Rh-positive red cells of their fetus in heterospecific pregnancies is a situation comparable to injection of ABO-incompatible Rh-positive red cells into Rh-negative men. In addition to data confirming and expanding the original observations, this paper presents results of experiments which were designated to furnish some insight into the mechanism(s) of interference of ABO-incompatibility with Rh sensitization, and also some tentative generalizations concerning factors influencing immune responses to red cell isoantigens.

MATERIALS AND METHODS

The subjects were healthy, 21- to 58-year-old male inmates of the Joliet branch of the Illinois State Penitentiary.[4] Before start of isosensitization the ABO, Rh, and frequently other blood

[1] Supported (in part) by Grant RG-5539 from the National Institutes of Health, Bethesda, Maryland.

[2] Present address: University of Illinois College of Medicine, Department of Pathology, 1853 West Polk Street, Chicago 12, Illinois.

[3] Present address: University of Chicago Department of Medicine, 5801 South Ellis Avenue, Chicago 37, Illinois.

[4] The authors are greatly indebted to Warden Joseph E. Ragen and his staff for their most helpful cooperation.

types of the men were determined and their sera screened with suitable panel red cells for presence of irregular red cell antibodies. Screening for and titration of Rh antibodies were done with papainized red cells (4) of suitable type; antiglobulin techniques were employed when antibodies for Kell and Duffy were searched for

or titrated. All titrations were done in serial 2-fold dilutions prepared volumetrically, with addition of 0.1 ml of 2% suspensions in saline of suitable red cells to 0.1 ml of the proper serum dilution. After incubation in a water bath of 37°C for 30 min (papainized red cells) or 2 hr (antiglobulin technique) agglutinations were recorded. The titers given are the reciprocal of the highest serum dilution in which macroscopic agglutination was observed. Whenever titers of successive specimens of the same subject were compared with each other, all specimens were titrated simultaneously with the same red cell specimens. This was made possible by storage in the deep freeze of all serum specimens until use.

Blood used for isosensitization was obtained from healthy donors meeting the "Minimum Requirements" of the National Institutes of Health (5) and the recommendations of the American Association of Blood Banks (6). Five milliliters of equal parts of blood and ACD (acid citrate dextrose) solution (solution B) were injected intravenously within 24 to 48 hr after blood collection. Intervals between injections ranged for the most part from 8 to 10 weeks; occasionally intervals were as long as 5 months because of temporary unavailability of the subjects. Injections subsequent to development of antibodies when given, were reduced to 2 ml of the blood-ACD mixture. Only in rare exceptions did men experience transient discomfort—flushing, dizziness—after any of the injections; none of them developed any serious sequelae of the immunization procedure.

Rh sensitization. The blood administered to Rh-negative men was of type Rh_1hr'-negative (CCDe). Different donors were used for consecutive injections but on each occasion men of control and experimental groups to be detailed below, received blood from the same donor at the same time.

Coating in vitro of A Rh-positive blood with anti-A. The serum selected was that of an acceptable donor of group O with anti-A titer of 1:128; "incomplete" anti-A was present as shown by failure of antibody neutralization by group-specific substance (7). To a 20-fold dilution of this serum in saline, one-fourth of the serum volume of ACD-blood of type A_1Rh_1

(CDe) (*e.g.*, 40 ml of ACD-blood to 160 ml of diluted serum) was added drop by drop and the mixture was incubated in a water bath at 37°C for 1 hr; in some instances, the mixture was then transferred to 4°C overnight. As a control, another portion of the same ACD-blood was treated in the same manner, except that serum of a person of group AB was used instead of the group O serum. Both portions of blood were spun in a refrigerated centrifuge (International, PR 1), the supernatant was removed, and the red cells were resuspended in saline to the original volume of blood. This material was used for injection. All operations were carried out aseptically and bacteriologic examination of the final product revealed no contamination. Aliquots of the blood "coated" with anti-A gave strongly positive direct antiglobulin tests, thus demonstrating the success of the "coating" procedure. The "coated" blood suspensions were free of visible agglutinates although occasional small clumps were noted on microscopic examination.

Coating in vitro of O Rh-positive blood with Rh antibodies. The serum used was that of an acceptable donor of group AB rh (cde) with titers of anti-Rh$_0$(D) of 1024 and of anti-rh'(C) of 256. To a 5-fold dilution in saline of the serum, approximately one-seventh volume was added drop by drop of ACD-blood of type O Rh$_1$ (CDe) (*e.g.*, 30 ml of blood to 215 ml of serum dilution). Another portion of the same blood was exposed to diluted AB serum in an analogous manner. The cell-serum mixtures were incubated in a water bath at 37°C for 1 hr and then treated as described for blood coated with anti-A. Strongly positive direct antiglobulin tests were obtained with aliquots of the blood exposed to serum with Rh antibodies; agglutination was not present in the "coated" blood suspension.

Isoimmunization to Kell (K). Blood of the same acceptable donor was used for the entire experiment; her blood type was O rh(cde) Kell-negative (kk) Fy^a-positive.

RESULTS

ABO-compatibility and Rh sensitization. In Tables I to III, data previously reported (1) are combined with the recent observations. As shown in Table I, Rh antibodies developed in 5 of 32 Rh-negative men injected with ABO-incompatible Rh-positive red cells, or in less than 16%. In Table II this incidence of Rh sensitization is compared with Rh sensitization resulting from immunization with ABO-compatible blood in 17 of 24 men, or 70%. The numbers of injections

TABLE I

Formation of Rh antibodies in Rh-negative men injected with ABO-incompatible blood

Blood Group of:		Number of Men:	
Recipient	Injected blood	With Rh antibodies	Total
O	A	2	13 ⎫ 16
B	A	0	3 ⎭
O	B	2	7 ⎫ 16
A	B	1	9 ⎭
Total.......		5	32

TABLE II

Incidence and time of appearance of Rh sensitization

Immunized with Blood	No. of Men	Rh Antibodies	Tested after Injection No.:							Total
			1	2	3	4	5	6	7	
ABO-compatible	24	Present	2	5	8	1	1			17
		Absent		1	2	1		2	1	7
ABO-incompatible	32	Present		3		1	1			5
		Absent		2	1	11	6	7		27

TABLE III

Rh antibody titers in men immunized with ABO-incompatible blood

ABO Group of			Rh Antibody Titer after Injection No.:				
Case no.	Recipient	Injected blood	2	3	4	5	6
14357	O	B	0	0	1	1	2
14398	O	B	8	32	32	32	32
19394	A	B	0	0	0	8	
14324	O	A	4	8	8	8	8
19036	O	A	2	2	2	2	2*

* Remained at same level after seventh and eighth injection.

required for inducing antibodies were similar in the 5 men with Rh sensitization following injection of ABO-incompatible blood and the 17 men injected with ABO-compatible blood. It should be noted that all but 3 of the 27 men injected with ABO-incompatible blood who failed to develop Rh antibodies, received at least four injections, a form of treatment sufficient to induce antibodies in 16, or two-thirds, of 24 men injected with ABO-compatible blood.

In our first report (1) we noted that titers of Rh antibodies in two men immunized with ABO-incompatible blood were lower than titers of antibodies induced by ABO-compatible blood. Table III contains Rh antibody titers of five men immunized with ABO-incompatible blood, four of whom received additional injections of ABO-incompatible Rh-positive blood after development of Rh antibodies. In none of them was there any significant rise in antibodies, including subject no. 19036 who received eight subsequent injections. The relationship between Rh antibody titer and the number of additional injections given after initial development of antibodies is also illustrated in Figure 1. In view of the consistently higher titers observed in men injected with ABO-compatible blood as compared with the titers in the four men injected with ABO-incompatible blood, ABO-incompatible blood may represent an inferior stimulus not only for primary immunization, but also for secondary responses. In order to investigate this question further, antibody responses were compared in previously Rh-sensitized men after stimulation with ABO-incompatible and ABO-compatible blood, respectively. As shown in Table IV, only 4 of 13 men so tested exhibited significant rises in antibody level, that is, increase in titer of at least two dilutions. In two of these men only ABO-compatible blood, in one both ABO-compatible and ABO-incompatible blood, and in one only ABO-incompatible blood induced the rise in titer.

TABLE IV

Secondary responses of Rh-negative men to injection of Rh-positive blood

Recipient		Injection		Rh Antibody Titer*		
		No. 1	No. 2			
No.	Group	With blood of group:		Before injection No. 1	After injection No. 1	After injection No. 2
19383	O	A	O	1	*64*	*256*
19411	O	B	O	32	32	*512*
14349	A	B	O	64	64	*256*
14144	A	B	O	8	*128*	256
19380	O	A	O	16	32	32
19125	O	A	O	64	32	64
19161	O	A	O	128	128	256
19136	O	B	O	32	32	64
19382	A	B	O	2	4	8
14183	A	B	O	4	4	4
14395	A	B	O	16	16	32
14361	A	B	O	64	64	64
19159	A	B	O	64	128	256

* Figures in italics represent rises in antibody titers of at least two serum dilutions.

Additional experiments concerned the question as to whether men who did not respond with Rh antibody formation after injection of ABO-incompatible blood would be capable of forming

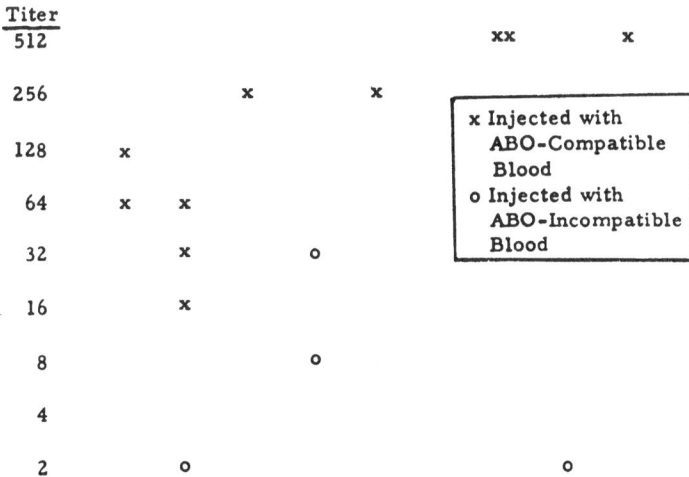

Figure 1. Effect of continued stimulation on Rh antibody titers

TABLE V

Rh sensitization induced by injection of ABO-compatible blood subsequent to injection of ABO-incompatible blood

ABO-Incompatible Blood: Antibodies Absent		ABO-Compatible Blood				
		Antibodies present after injection no.:			Total number of men:	
After injection no.:	No. of men	2	3	4	With anti-bodies	Without anti-bodies*
4	7	1	1	1	3	4
5	2		1		1	1
6	1					1
Total	10	1	2	1	4	6

* After five injections of ABO-compatible blood.

TABLE VI

Rh sensitization induced by A Rh-positive blood coated in vitro with anti-A

Recipients		Injected with	Rh Antibodies				
			Present after injection:				Absent after injection 5
Group	No.		2	3	4	5	
Arh	5	Noncoated blood	1	3		1	0
Arh	8	Blood coated with anti-A	4	2			2

TABLE VII

Rh sensitization induced by injection of "noncoated" blood subsequent to injection of "coated" blood

Injection No.	No. of Men with Antibodies Present or Absent	
	Present	Absent
1	2	2
2	1	1
3	1	1
4	1	1
Total	5	5

antibodies when subsequently injected with ABO-compatible blood. Table V summarizes findings in 10 men so treated. After receiving from four to six injections of ABO-incompatible blood without developing Rh antibodies, four of the 10 men developed Rh antibodies after two, three or four injections of ABO-compatible blood, whereas the remaining six failed to develop antibodies; thus incidence of Rh sensitization was 40% in this experiment.

Immunization with "coated" red cells. The lesser ability of ABO-incompatible blood to induce Rh sensitization might possibly be attributed to the almost instantaneous coating by the incompatible isoagglutinin of red cells entering the circulation of the recipient, e.g., anti-A becoming immediately attached to red cells of group A injected into a recipient of group O. This fixation of anti-A to corresponding antigenic sites on the red cell surface might in some way impair the immunogenicity of the Rh antigen. In order to test this possibility A Rh-positive red cells coated *in vitro* with anti-A antibody, as described in the preceding section, were injected into A Rh-negative recipients. Simultaneously, A Rh-negative recipients of a control group were injected with "noncoated" blood of the same A Rh-positive donor. As shown in Table VI, six of eight A Rh-negative men injected with "coated" A Rh-positive blood and all five men injected with noncoated blood developed Rh antibodies. Thus there was no significant interference with Rh sensitization as a result of the "coating" *in vitro* with anti-A antibody of ABO-compatible Rh-positive blood.

In view of these results it became of interest to investigate the effect of "coating" of Rh-positive cells *in vitro* with Rh antibodies on their ability to induce Rh sensitization. Sixteen O Rh-negative men were injected with blood of type O Rh_1 (CDe) "coated" *in vitro* with anti-Rh_o' (anti-CD). Fourteen men received five injections each whereas two received only four. None developed Rh sensitization, in striking contrast to the results obtained with "noncoated" blood administered under comparable conditions. As seen from Table VII, of 10 men first injected with "coated" Rh-positive blood five developed Rh antibodies after subsequent injection of "noncoated" blood.

In one instance the ability to induce secondary immune responses to Rh antigen of "coated" Rh-positive blood was tested. A group O Rh-negative (rh, cde) man with low-titered antibodies for Rh_o (D) and rh' (C) was given five injections of such "coated" blood (O Rh_1, CDe)

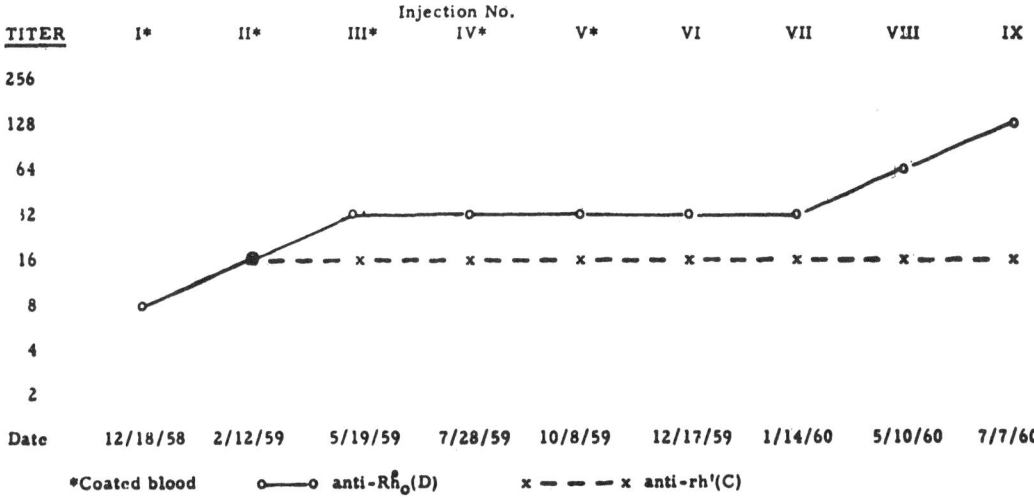

Injection No.

TITER	I*	II*	III*	IV*	V*	VI	VII	VIII	IX

256
128
64
32
16
8
4
2

Date   12/18/58   2/12/59   5/19/59   7/28/59   10/8/59   12/17/59   1/14/60   5/10/60   7/7/60

*Coated blood   o——o anti-Rh₀(D)   x — — — x anti-rh'(C)

Figure 2. Secondary responses to "coated" and "non-coated" Rh positive blood

within a period of 11 months. As shown in Figure 2, only slight rises of anti-Rh₀ (D) occurred after the first and second injections, and three subsequent injections failed to change the titer. On the other hand, two additional injections of "noncoated" blood of type O Rh₁ (CDe) elevated the anti-Rh₀ (D) titer whereas the anti-rh' (C) titer was not affected.

Isosensitization to K, Fyᵃ and hr' (c). This experiment was designed to study the effect on isosensitization of differences in more than one blood factor between immunizing blood and recipients who do not possess circulating antibodies for any of the factors in question. Twenty-nine Kell-negative (kk) men were subjected to repeated injections of Kell-positive blood derived from a sngle donor with the blood formula O rh (cde) Kell-positive (Kk) Fyᵃ-positive. As seen from Table VIII, the men injected with this blood could be divided into four groups determined by their blood types: men in groups I and II were Fyᵃ-positive, whereas men in groups III and IV were Fyᵃ-negative; furthermore, hr'(c) was present in men of groups I and III but was absent in groups II and IV. Thus the blood of men in group I differed from the injected blood in, and was susceptible to isosensitization to, at least one factor, K; men in group II, at least two factors, K and hr'; men in group III, at least two factors, K and Fyᵃ; men in group IV, at least three factors, K, Fyᵃ and hr'. Although 21 of the 29 men received the full course of five injections, antibodies were detectable in only two men of group II, both of whom showed anti-K antibodies after the second injection, with a rise in titer produced by an additional injection. One of these men also developed anti-hr'(c) after the third injection.

DISCUSSION

Data presented in this communication have corroborated our earlier results (1) on the lesser ability of ABO-incompatible Rh-positive blood to induce Rh sensitization as compared with ABO-compatible Rh-positive blood. Furthermore, ABO-incompatible Rh-positive blood also appears to be an inferior stimulus for secondary responses to the Rh factor, inasmuch as titers in men injected with ABO-incompatible Rh-positive blood remained at lower levels than those found in men given ABO-compatible Rh-positive blood.

When Rh-negative men who failed to develop Rh antibodies after exposure to ABO-incompatible Rh-positive blood were subsequently challenged with ABO-compatible Rh-positive blood, some of them did respond with formation of Rh antibodies. The incidence of Rh sensitization in 40% of the rather small series probably does not represent a significant difference from the 70% observed in our main series, or reported in similar studies by other investigators (8–10). These results are important for two reasons: a) they remove the possible objection that failure of antibody development after injection of ABO-incompatible blood may reflect nonspecific immunologic unresponsiveness of the men tested; b) they appear to eliminate the possibility that preceding injection with ABO-incompatible blood may permanently change responsiveness to Rh antigen in a manner comparable to that of "immunologic tolerance."

Since Levine (2) called attention to the protective effects of ABO-incompatibility on Rh sensitization in pregnancy, various explanations have been offered to explain this phenomenon. In our opinion, none is convincing. Thus, there seems to be no tangible evidence for the assumption that "competition of antigens" (11) accounts for the observed suppression of Rh sensitization since injection into Rh-negative recipients of Rh-positive ABO-incompatible blood is not followed by formation of large amounts of anti-A and anti-B (Stern, K., and Goodman, H. S., unpublished data). Another commonly proposed hypothesis, namely, that ABO-incompatible red cells are rapidly eliminated (12) can hardly be considered a valid explanation since antibody formation takes place in tissue and not intravascularly. Concerning the concept that intravascular hemolysis of ABO-incompatible red cells deprives the Rh antigens of the ability for inducing antibodies, one may refer to the fact that not all anti-A and anti-B antibodies are hemolytic. In this context a recent report by Cohen and co-workers (13) is significant. By means of fluorescent antibody the authors demonstrated presence of Rh-positive fetal red cells in blood of pregnant Rh-negative women, including one instance of ABO-incompatible Rh-positive red cells. This indicates the possibility of prolonged intravascular persistence of such incompatible red cells. Application of this technique to further experimental work might disclose whether intravascular survival of red cells is correlated with development of isosensitization.

One of the possibilities considered was that anti-A or anti-B antibody attached to the red cell surface might interfere with the immunogenic integrity of the Rh antigen and thus be responsible for the decreased incidence of Rh sensitization. This hypothesis found no support from the results of our experiments in which Rh-positive ABO-compatible red cells were "coated" *in vitro* with anti-A. When such material was injected into Rh-negative recipients, there was no indication of any interference of this "coating" with Rh immunization. Admittedly, these negative results may not be conclusive for several reasons. Coating with anti-A, although capable of producing positive antiglobulin tests, is not as heavy as coating with Rh antibodies. The anti-A antibodies attached to the A cells may be readily eluted after injection into recipients of group A. In this connection, observations of Loutit and Mollison (14) are of great interest: when blood of group A was mixed *in vitro* with anti-A serum prior to transfusion into A recipients, the transfused cells showed normal survival curves.

Recently we reported (15) that rabbits immunized to factor A formed significantly less anti-N when injected with AN red cells than did comparable animals injected with ON red cells.[5] As a possible explanation for these findings in animals and for the results of the present study, we wish to propose that they reflect a phenomenon that might be designated as *"clonal competition for antigen."* This hypothesis is based on the clonal selection theory of antibody formation of Burnet (16, 17) and similar concepts as proposed by Jerne (18), Talmage (19) and Lederberg (20).

The basic concept of this theory presupposes the presence of clones of antibody-forming cells, each of which produces a specific globulin which is identical with an antibody for a specific antigen. Exposure to antigen results in proliferation of the corresponding clone which then synthesizes large amounts of this globulin and thus brings about appearance of circulating antibody. The theory explains differences between responses to primary and secondary exposures to the antigen. In the first case, the small number of cells of a specific clone initially present accounts for the delayed and lower antibody response whereas in secondary responses antigen meets large numbers of cells derived from the proliferated clone.

Applying this concept to immune responses involving red cell antigens, certain hypothetical situations can be considered as they would result from exposure of a host to red cells containing two isoantigens, X and/or Y. In the simplest situation, red cells containing either X or Y may be introduced into a host who lacks this antigen and who may respond to this stimulation with proliferation of the corresponding clone designated as x or y capable of synthesizing and releasing into the circulation anti-X or anti-Y. Examples of this situation would be isoimmunization of persons of type O rh(cde) following injection of O Rh-positive blood, or of Kell-negative (kk) individuals to K after exposure to otherwise compatible Kell-positive red cells. In a second situation, red cells containing antigens X and Y may enter a host having X(or Y) antigen in his red cells; since he therefore lacks the x(or y) clone, immunization can take place only to X(or Y). This situation would apply, *e.g.*, to A rh(cde) persons immunized with A Rh-positive blood. A third, more complex situation may concern a host lacking both X and Y antigens in his red cells but who possesses anti-X antibodies, indicative of previous stimulation and proliferation of his x clone, and who is immunized with red cells containing X and Y. Obviously in this

[5] A detailed report of this work is in preparation.

host a much greater number of cells of clone x are available than of cells of the clone y which had not been previously stimulated. It is therefore reasonable to expect that red cells containing both X and Y will, according to the "mass law," be taken up by the more numerous cells of the x clone so that there will be little or no opportunity for them to come in contact with and stimulate the few cells of the y clone. This would be the situation when ABO-incompatible Rh-positive blood is introduced into Rh-negative men or women.

The validity of the hypothesis of clonal competition for red cell isoantigens is predicated on two conditions: a) antibody formation must be assumed to require availability of intact red cells to the antibody-forming tissue; b) it must be postulated that each antibody-forming cell is capable of producing antibody of only one specificity. As to the first point, no information directly proving or disproving this contention seems to be available. Obviously, clonal competition for antigens cannot operate in situations in which intact cells are either not required for, or are not capable of inducing, development of antibodies.

Strong evidence for the second assumption, *i.e.*, individual cells producing only one type of antibody, has been brought forth by the work of Nossal (21), Coons (22), and White (23) although there are exceptions to this rule: Attardi and associates (24) demonstrated by means of a phage inhibition technique formation of two types of antibodies in about 2% of cells.

The clonal selection theory of antibody formation may also explain the lack of antigenicity of O Rh-positive red cells after they were coated with Rh antibodies *in vitro*. In order to induce proliferation of the respective clone the intact antigen must presumably act upon the antibody-forming cells in order to cause them to proliferate. When "coated" red cells were injected this interaction between red cell antigen and active cellular sites was apparently prevented. Significantly, preceding exposure to "coated" Rh-positive red cells did not permanently change the responsiveness of the men studied in this series, since 50% developed Rh antibodies when subsequently injected with untreated Rh-positive blood.

Inhibition of antibody responses to certain bacterial antigens introduced simultaneously with homologous antibody has been reported by several groups of workers. In 1935 Olitsky (25) observed suppression of agglutinin formation after immunization of rabbits with Proteus and Salmonella vaccines when excess of free antibody

and antibody attached to the antigen *in vitro* were used. Mason and associates (26) demonstrated marked inhibition of antitoxin response in guinea pigs passively immunized with diphtheria antitoxin prior to active immunization with this antigen. Although these results appear to parallel the observations made in our experiments with "coated" Rh-positive red cells, some other forms of immune responses are actually enhanced when antigen-antibody mixtures are utilized for active immunization, as demonstrated for rabbit antiovalbumin (27) and confirmed by several other workers (28, 29). Thus, there may be a significant difference in the ability of various antigen-antibody complexes to induce immune responses, a phenomenon that may be worthy of further investigation as a promising approach to study of immunologic mechanisms.

The final experimental series in which men were exposed to Kell sensitization was intended to test a further extension of the hypothesis of clonal competition for antigen. This refers to situations in which the host is potentially susceptible to immunization to more than one blood factor present in the immunizing red cells, without, however, having demonstrable circulating antibodies for any of these antigens. Conceivably in this situation the likelihood for isosensitization might be decreased because, when red cells are taken up randomly by different clones and, at the same time, are not endowed with a high immunogenic property, this "scatter" may critically depress the opportunity for antibody development.

The low incidence of Kell sensitization, occurring in 2 out of 29 men, is not too different from findings obtained in another study employing deliberate immunization of Kell-negative subjects: Kornstad and Heistö (30) found that 4 out of 160 Kell-negative recipients of one or more Kell-positive transfusions developed anti-Kell. Wiener and associates (31) did not observe any formation of anti-Kell in 10 Kell-negative subjects after they had received three injections of Kell-positive blood. Although it is not possible to draw any definitive conclusions from the small number of men tested in our experiment, it would be a rather unusual coincidence that Kell-positive Duffy-positive blood was entirely ineffective in inducing Kell antibodies in 14 Kell-negative Duffy-negative men (Table VIII, groups III and IV), whereas the same treatment produced Kell antibodies in 2 out of 15 Kell-negative Duffy-positive men (groups 1 and II). The main difference was that men in groups I and II were nonidentical with the injected blood only

TABLE VIII

Isosensitization to K, Fy^a, and hr'(c)

Recipients			Antibodies Absent after Injection No.:				Antibodies Present after Injection No.:		
Group	Blood type	Total	2	3	4	5	2 Anti-K*	3 Anti-K*	Anti-hr'†
I	KK Fy(a+) hr'-positive	7		2		5	I: 4	64	
II	kk Fy(a+) hr'-negative	8	2	1		3	II: 4	32	16
III	kk Fy(a−) hr'-positive	12	1		3	8			
IV	kk Fy(a−) hr'-negative	2				2			

* Titer with antiglobulin technique.

† Titer with papainized red cells.

in Kell but not in Duffy, whereas men of groups III and IV were nonidentical in Kell as well as Duffy. This would fit in with the assumption that presence of more than one difference in blood factors reduces likelihood for isosensitization. On the other hand, both men who developed Kell antibodies, were hr'-negative and hence differed also in this factor from the injected blood, with one man actually producing this additional antibody. One might speculate that sites of antibody formation for Kell and Duffy are derived from relatively similar clones and hence are more likely to compete with each other, whereas sites for formation of hr' may be present in different locations or are endowed with proliferative abilities making them independent of clones responsive to Kell antigen. Obviously in connection with any such tentative generalizations about the possible interference with isoimmunization of multiple blood factor incompatibilities, one must take into account the numerous instances of multiple isosensitization observed clinically after pregnancies or transfusions. Undoubtedly, complex mechanisms are involved in this phenomenon, probably including host factors inasmuch as patients with certain types of disease appear to be especially prone to form multiple isoantibodies. Another important determinant in this process may well be the chemical nature and structure of the respective hemoantigens.

Finally, reference should be made to pertinent studies carried out by several groups of workers on the fate *in vivo* of radioisotopically labeled red cells when exposed to various types and concentrations of incompatible hemoantibodies. Thus Jones and associates (32) observed that incompatible red cells survived intravascularly for significantly differing periods of time depending on kinds of antigen and antibody involved. They also established some correlation of intravascular disappearance of such red cells to the sites of their sequestration. Culp and Chaplin (33) in studying the posttransfusion survival of Rh-positive red cells coated with Rh antibody observed that they remained in the vascular compartment for less than 90 min with subsequent sequestration in the spleen. Jandl and Kaplan (34) established that coated red cells were first trapped in the spleen, and in direct proportion to the extent of damage and quantity of antibody the overflow of incompatible red cells was trapped in other reticuloendothelial tissues, particularly in the liver. In order to provide a more solid foundation for some of the hypothetical assumptions that we derived from our experiments on isosensitization it would undoubtedly be most desirable to utilize radioisotope-labeled red cells permitting estimates of their intravascular survival and tissue localization.

SUMMARY

1. Expanded data have been presented and analyzed concerning interference of ABO incompatibility with formation of Rh antibodies in Rh-negative men injected with Rh-positive blood. ABO-incompatible Rh-positive blood appeared to be also less capable of stimulating secondary responses to Rh antigen.

2. Forty per cent of the men who had failed to form Rh antibodies after injection with ABO-incompatible blood did form Rh antibodies after subsequent injection of ABO-compatible blood.

3. Injection into A Rh-negative recipients of A Rh-positive blood coated *in vitro* with anti-A was an efficient stimulus for formation of Rh antibodies.

4. Injection into O Rh-negative men of O Rh-positive blood coated *in vitro* with Rh antibodies was completely ineffective in inducing

Rh antibodies. Subsequent injection of such recipients with noncoated Rh-positive blood led to the development of Rh antibodies in 50%.

5. These data were interpreted as compatible with the hypothesis of "clonal competition for antigen," namely, that presence of large numbers of antibody-forming cells for one red cell factor may interfere with antibody response to another blood factor contained in the same red cell.

6. On the basis of preliminary experiments the possibility was considered that, even without preformed antibody in the host, presence of more than one difference in blood factors between recipient and donor may lessen likelihood for isoimmunization in certain circumstances.

REFERENCES

1. STERN, K., DAVIDSOHN, I. AND MASAITIS, L., Am. J. Clin. Path., **26**: 833, 1956.
2. LEVINE, P., J. Hered., **34**: 71, 1943.
3. LEVINE, P., Human Biol., **30**: 14, 1958.
4. KUHNS, W. J. AND BAILEY, A., Am. J. Clin. Path., **20**: 1067, 1950.
5. *Minimum Requirements: Citrated Whole Blood (Human)*, National Institutes of Health, 4th revision, March 15, 1955.
6. *Technical Methods and Procedures*, American Association of Blood Banks, revised edition, Ed. by J. B. Ross, p. 2, 1960.
7. WITEBSKY, E., Fed. Proc., **8**: 414, 1949.
8. HATTERSLEY, P. G., J. Lab. & Clin. Med., **32**: 423, 1947.
9. WIENER, A. S., Proc. Soc. Exper. Biol. & Med., **70**: 576, 1949.
10. WALLER, R. K., J. Lab. & Clin. Med., **34**: 270, 1949.
11. WIENER, A. S., Proc. Soc. Exper. Biol. & Med., **58**: 133, 1945.
12. RACE, R. R. AND SANGER, R., *Blood Groups in Man*, 3rd Ed., p. 315, Charles C. Thomas, Springfield, Ill., 1958.
13. COHEN, F., ZUELZER, W. W. AND EVANS, M. M., Blood, **15**: 884, 1960.
14. LOUTIT, J. F. AND MOLLISON, P. L., J. Path. & Bact., **58**: 711, 1946.
15. STERN, K., Fed. Proc., **19**: 200, 1960.
16. BURNET, F. M., *The Clonal Selection Theory of Acquired Immunity*, Nashville, Vanderbilt University Press, 1959.
17. BURNET, F. M., Perspect. Biol. & Med., **3**: 447, 1960.
18. JERNE, N. K., Proc. Nat. Acad. Sc., **41**: 849, 1955.
19. TALMAGE, D. W., Science, **129**: 1643, 1959.
20. LEDERBERG, J., Science, **129**: 1649, 1959.
21. NOSSAL, G. J. V., Brit. J. Exper. Path., **39**: 544, 1958.
22. COONS, A. H., J. Cell. & Comp. Physiol., **52**: (Suppl. 1): 55, 1958.
23. WHITE, R. G., Nature, **182**: 1383, 1958.
24. ATTARDI, G., COHN, M., HORIBATA, K. AND LENNOX, E., Bact. Rev., **23**: 213, 1959.
25. OLITSKY, L., J. Immunol., **29**: 453, 1935.
26. MASON, J. H., ROBINSON, M. AND CHRISTENSEN, P. A., J. Hyg., **53**: 172, 1955.
27. UHR, J. W., SALVIN, S. B. AND PAPPENHEIMER, A. M., J. Exper. Med., **105**: 11, 1957.
28. TERRES, G. AND WOLINS, W., Proc. Soc. Exper. Biol. & Med., **102**: 632, 1959.
29. LESKOWITZ, S., J. Immunol., **85**: 56, 1960.
30. KORNSTAD, L. AND HEISTÖ, H., 1957; cited by Mollison, P. L., Brit. M. Bull., **15**: 92, 1959.
31. WIENER, A. S., SAMWICK, A. A., MORRISON, H. AND COHEN, L., Exper. Med. & Surg., **13**: 347, 1955.
32. JONES, N. C., MOLLISON, P. L. AND VEALL, N., Brit. J. Haematol., **3**: 125, 1957.
33. CULP, N. W. AND CHAPLIN, H., JR., Blood, **15**: 525, 1960.
34. JANDL, J. H. AND KAPLAN, M. E., J. Clin. Invest., **39**: 1145. 1960.

Paper 29

29. Freda, V. J. and Gorman J. G. (1962). Current Concepts: Antepartum management of Rh hemolytic disease. *Bull. Sloane Hosp. Women, 8,* 147-158. (Extract).

Commentary

The early parts of this paper are concerned with the organisation of the Sloane Hospital erythroblastosis fetalis clinic, followed by a discussion of the role of amniocentesis and spectrophotometric scanning of amniotic fluid, which are omitted here. The interest of the paper for this book is that it is the first reference to the American ideas of the prevention of sensitisation by giving anti-Rh (anti-D).

The authors start from the known fact that if an excess of passive antibody is given to an individual, subsequent injections of antigen completely fail to sensitise. Applying this to the Rh system, they gave passive anti-Rh antibody (as high titre gammaglobulin) to Rh-negative prisoners, *followed by* injections of Rh-positive cells.

The authors, with the help of the Ortho Research Foundation, were anxious to produce anti-Rh antibody which would not cross the placenta (i.e. the 19S type) because their proposal, optimally, was to give the gammaglobulin during pregnancy. Nevertheless, they felt that 7S antibody might be useful given at the end of the second stage of labour, since they thought that most big fetomaternal bleeds occurred during labour.

No actual data on the prisoners is given, but the Liverpool work is mentioned and the difference of approach emphasised.

The authors note that the Liverpool group had adopted the Kleihauer method for estimating the amount of fetal blood escaping into the maternal circulation at different times during pregnancy, but they do not mention Zipursky *et al.* (Paper 23) for it was the Canadian workers who first used the Kleihauer method for this purpose and the Liverpool group learnt it from them.

From V. J. Freda and J. G. Gorman (1962), Bull. Sloane Hosp. Women, 8, 147-158. Copyright (1962), by kind permission of the authors

Current Concepts

Antepartum Management of Rh Hemolytic Disease

Vincent J. Freda, M.D.* and John G. Gorman, M.B., B.S.†

PREVENTION OF SENSITIZATION

Recently there has arisen the possibility of preventing sensitization altogether and thereby preventing new cases of E.F. from appearing. In 1909 Theobald Smith[21] showed that mixtures of diptheria toxin—antitoxin, in which a state of antibody excess was maintained, did not immunize (or was non-antigenic) when injected. In the years since, much data has accumulated and a general immunological phenomenon applicable to a wide range of antigens has become evident. If specific antibody is given passively to an individual, subsequent injections of antigen completely fail to sensitize. It was found that the circulating levels of passively administered antibody must be sufficient to maintain a state of antibody excess at all times and that this antibody excess is the key to prevention of sensitization.

Therefore, the present authors began a program to show that this inhibition phenomenon was equally applicable to the Rh antigen-antibody system. At present, a series of experiments on Rh negative prisoners at Sing Sing prison is in progress to see whether passively administered antibody followed by injections of Rh positive cells can prevent sensitization to the Rh factor.

First it was necessary to obtain anti-Rh antibody in a quantity capable of achieving good circulating titers when injected intramuscularly. For this study, William Pollack senior research scientist of the Ortho Research Foundation prepared an experimental batch of an extremely high titered anti-Rh containing gamma globulin. Five ml. of this reagent injected intramuscularly proved capable of eliciting within 24 hours anti-Rh circulating titers of 1:64 or better. Further advantages of this preparation are that it is free from the risk of transmitting serum hepatitis and also that it can be injected intramuscularly. Thus far, not enough antigenic stimulations have been performed in antibody-protected Rh negative individuals to provide statistically significant conclusions.

RELATED STUDIES BY OTHERS

Finn et al.[22] have also been actively working on the concept that passively transferred antibody might be a method of preventing initial sensitization of the mother to the Rh factor. Finn had adopted the Kleihauer method[23] for staining red cells for fetal hemoglobulin and has applied this to estimating the amount of fetal blood escaping into the maternal circulation at different times during pregnancy and labor. He believes that this method will detect fetal bleeds of as little as 1 ml. in the entire maternal circulation. He also noted that 4 of 256 maternal samples contained appreciable amounts of fetal cells, and from these preliminary data he has speculated that these are the mothers who run the risk of being sensitized by pregnancy. They then entertained the next logical step of wondering whether passively administered antibody would destroy this minor population of fetal cells in the maternal circulation so quickly that sensitization would be prevented, as occurs with ABO incompatible fetal cells in the maternal circulation. This protection against Rh sensitization provided by an incompatibility with the fetus in the

Departments of Obstetrics and Gynecology and Pathology, College of Physicians and Surgeons, Columbia University.
* Supported by the Health Research Council of the City of New York I-264; U-1307.
† Supported by the Health Research Council of the City of New York U-1154.

ABO system was first pointed out by Levine.[3] Finn et al.[22, 24] have also initiated experiments to see whether Rh negative volunteers can be protected from sensitization by passively transferred antibody. Their protocol differs from ours in that the English workers inject the Rh positive cells first, followed by antibody in the form of 50 ml of intravenous whole plasma containing anti-Rh antibody. None of their protected group has become sensitized, in contrast to 10 percent sensitization in the unprotected controls. Statistically significant data will be available shortly from their studies in both Liverpool and Baltimore and our own studies at the Sing Sing Prison.

Franklin and Kunkel discovered that while gamma globulins in maternal sera sediment into two classes, 7S and 19S, only 7S gamma globulin is found in cord sera. Kochwa, Rosenfield et al.[26] found that the anti-A and anti-B activities of thirty-three specimens of cord sera were restricted to the fraction containing principally 7S $gamma_2$-globulin (i.e. the first 0.02 M fraction eluted off the DEAE cellulose column). These molecules were found to occur in equilibrium on both sides of the placenta. Rosenfield[27] then speculated that the human placenta may have an active transport system for the $gamma_2$-globulin but not for the non-$gamma_2$-globulins. Thus placental permeability for an antibody would not be dependent on its molecular size (i.e. 7S versus 19S) but on the fact that it is a $gamma_2$-globulin molecule. The data obtained to date tends to support this hypothesis.

NEW EXPERIMENTAL PREPARATIONS

In co-operation with the Ortho Research Foundation we have devised a program for studying two new promising experimental preparations of anti-Rh antibody which should have the advantage of not being able to cross the placenta in appreciable quantity. These are a preparation of 19S, B_2 M globulin with anti-Rh specificity and 3.5 S $gamma_2$-globulin fractions (Porter fractions) with anti-Rh activity. Porter[28] has demonstrated that if the rabbit gamma-globulin antibody molecule is digested with papain it will split into three smaller constituent fragments separable by chromatography. Fractions I and II retain the antibody reactive sites, whereas fraction III does not; also only fraction III retains the antigenic activity of the original molecule. Brambell, Hemmings, Oakley and Porter[29] then made the very critical observation that despite the reduction in molecular size, only fraction III reaches the fetal circulation in the animal at the same rate as the whole molecule, whereas the immunologically reactive fractions, I and II, pass at only one tenth this rate.

Franklin[30] found that human 7S gamma globulin also yields similar fragments when digested with papain; employing chromatographic techniques somewhat different from Porter's, he was able to separate three fragments which he labeled A, B and C. Fragment B had a fast electrophoretic mobility, was rich in hexoses and was free of antibody reacting sites. Fragments A and C which showed slower electrophoretic mobility, contained the antibody reacting sites. Whether or not the serologically reactive fragments will also not cross the human placenta (as pertains to the rabbit) remains to be seen. The present authors have applied for a grant to study this very problem in man and to determine whether or not these serologically reactive "Porter fractions" will prevent sensitization to the Rh factor when administered passively. There is good evidence that the B_2 M globulins will not cross the human placenta and it is suspected that the serologically reactive "Porter fractions" also will not cross it.

It was first suggested by the author that these reagents may be of use in the management of mothers who are already sensitized. Passive injections of these products (which probably do not cross the placenta) might possibly cause a "back-action" or "feedback effect" which would suppress active endogenous production of the dangerous 7S gamma$_2$ antibody by the mother. The authors plan to test this concept by trial studies on sensitized male volunteers.

PROJECTED USE OF ANTIBODY IN rh NEGATIVE MOTHERS AT RISK

Before these preparations can be used in Rh negative mothers the fact that the antibody preparation is effective and safe in preventing sensitization must be established in Rh negative male volunteers. The following factors concerning the use of antibody to protect mothers must also be considered. The 7S gamma$_2$-globulin preparation passes readily through the placenta into the fetal circulation, probably by an active transport mechanism, and therefore cannot be given during pregnancy or labor because it would destroy the baby's red cells and actually cause hemolytic disease. However, if given at the end of the second stage of labor it may still be in time to prevent sensitization since it seems logical to presume that most of the significant fetal-to-maternal bleeds occur during labor and delivery rather than during pregnancy. It is possible that one of the other reagents mentioned above (i.e. 19S globulin antibody or Porter fractions, or perhaps another chemically modified antibody) which cannot pass the placenta may eventually become available for use during pregnancy itself, (provided that the inability of the preparation to reach the fetus has been satisfactorily proven in a significantly large number of cases).

It is apparent that the aim of this work is to prevent the initial sensitization to Rh. Once sensitization occurs passive antibody would be of no use unless a "back action" or "feedback" control can be demonstrated. This means that protection must be provided in the first pregnancy at risk, as well as in all succeeding pregnancies, so that active production of Rh antibody by the mother never develops.

If Finn's method of estimating significant fetal-maternal bleeds can be confirmed by others then this would prove very important, provided of course that it can also be shown that it is primarily these cases which result in maternal sensitization. If this event is the sole criteria for administering protective antibody then this would decrease considerably the number of mothers requiring protection and likewise decrease the expense of such a program. These special gamma globulin products are extremely expensive to manufacture but their cost would become less prohibitive if prepared in bulk.

It is essential that any future program designed to evaluate the use of these reagents must be entered into with the greatest caution and must be carefully planned and statistically controlled. Because only 10 percent of mothers at risk become sensitized to Rh in the natural course of events, fairly large numbers of mothers will have to undergo protection through several pregnancies before significant data as to their worth will be forthcoming.

The attack on erythroblastosis fetalis is gaining momentum and it is possible that in the next few years we may see a marked shift in emphasis from management of affected babies to prevention of the disease itself.

BIBLIOGRAPHY

1. ALLEN, F. H., Jr., AND DIAMOND, L. K.: Erythroblastosis Fetalis, Boston: Little, Brown and Company, 1958.
2. KELSALL, G. A., VOS, G. H. AND KIRK, R. L.: Med. J. Aust. *1:* 488, 1959.
3. LEVINE, P.: Human Biol. *30:* 14, 1958.
4. MOLLISON, P. L., MOURANT, A. E., AND RACE, R. R.: The Rh Blood Groups and Their Clinical Effects, Medical Research Council Memorandum No. 27, London: Her Majesty's Stationery Office, 1952.
5. MOLLISON, P. L. AND WALKER, W.: Lancet *1:* 429, 1952.
6. POTTER, E. L.: Rh, Chicago: The Year Book Publishers Inc., 1947.
7. "Premature Induction and Rh Antibody Titer", Leading article in Lancet *2:* 549, 1959.
8. ROBERTS, F.: Brit. Med. Bull. *15:* 113, 1959.
9. ROSENFIELD, R.: p. 391 in Medical, Surgical, and Gynecological Complications of Pregnancy, edited by A. F. Guttmacher and J. J. Rovinsky, Baltimore: The Williams & Wilkins Company, 1960.
10. SACKS, M. S.: p. 1042–1064 in Williams Obstetrics, edited by N. J. Eastman, 11th Edition. New York: Appleton-Century-Crofts, Inc., 1956.
11. TOVEY, G. H. AND VALAES, T.: Lancet *2:* 521, 1959.
12. WALKER, W.: Brit. Med. Bull. *15:* 123, 1959.
13. WALKER, W., MURRAY, S., AND RUSSELL, J. K.: J. Obst. & Gynaec. Brit. Emp. *64:* 573, 1957.
14. WIENER, A. S.: Rh-Hr Blood Types, New York: Grune & Stratton, 1954.
15. WIENER, A. S. AND WEXLER, I. B.: Heredity of the Blood Groups, New York: Grune & Stratton, 1958.
16. BEVIS, D. C. A.: J. Obst. & Gynaec. Brit. Emp. *63:* 68, 1956.
17. WALKER, A. H. C.: Brit. Med. J. *2:* 376, 1957.
18. CARY, W.: Med. J. Aust. *2:* 778, 1960.
19. MACKAY, E. V.: Aust. N. Z. J. Obst. & Gynaec. *1:* 78, 1961.
20. LILEY, A. W.: Am. J. Obst. & Gynec. *82:* 1359, 1961.
21. SMITH, T.: J. Exp. Med. *11:* 241, 1909.
22. FINN, R., CLARKE, C. A., DONOHOE, W. T. A., McCONNELL, R. B., SHEPPARD, P. M., LEHANE, D., AND KULKE, W.: Brit. Med. J. *1:* 1486, 1961.
23. KLEIHAUER, E., BRAUN, H., AND BETKE, K.: Klin. Wschr. *35:* 637, 1957.
24. FINN, R., CLARKE, C. A., McCONNELL, R. B., WOODROW, J. C., KULKE, W., LEHANE, D. AND SHEPPARD, D. M.: Nature *193:* 991, 1962.
25. FRANKLIN, E. C. AND KUNKEL, H. C.: J. Lab. & Clin. Med. *52:* 724, 1958.
26. KOCHWA, S., ROSENFIELD, R. E., TALLAL, L., AND WASSERMAN, L. R.: Clin. Invest. *40:* 874, 1961.
27. ROSENFIELD, R. E.: personal communication.
28. PORTER, R. R.: Biochem. J. *73:* 119, 1959.
29. BRAMBELL, F. W. R., HEMMINGS, W. A., OAKLEY, C. L., AND PORTER, R. R.. Proc. Roy. Soc. London (series B) *151:* 478, 1960.
30. FRANKLIN, E. C.: J. Clin. Invest. *39:* 1933, 1960.

Paper 30

30. Freda, V. J., Gorman, J. G. and Pollack, W. (1964). Successful prevention of experimental Rh sensitisation in man with an anti-Rh gamma$_2$-globulin antibody preparation. *Transfusion, 4,* 26-32.

Commentary

This is the first paper by the American group in which the results of their experiments in volunteers are reported.

The authors prepared a sterile anti-D gammaglobulin, entirely 7S, with an indirect antiglobulin titre of 1 : 64,000, containing no anti-A or anti-B. Nine unsensitised, group O, Rh-negative male volunteers at Sing Sing prison were challenged once a month for five successive months with intravenous injections of 2ml of Rh-positive whole blood. Five of this group acted as controls while the remaining four received the experimental antibody preparation. These four received each month, 24 hours *before* the injection of Rh-positive blood, an intramuscular dose of 5 ml of the antibody.

Saline and indirect antibody tests were carried out on the nine each month, the sample being taken just before the injection of Rh-positive blood. Following the last injection of the antibody in the fifth month, tests were carried out each month for an additional six months on both treated and control groups.

After the last injection of antibody in the treated group (in the fifth month) it required three additional months before all of the passive antibody had disappeared. At this time none of those treated had become immunised, but four of the five controls had, all of them after the fourth injection of Rh-positive cells. There were no untoward reactions, and all the bloods were screened for anti-gammaglobulin iso-antibody with negative results.

In an addendum to their paper, the authors report the results of an expanded study on volunteers. In this experiment they gave, on day 1, an intravenous injection of 10 ml of group O Rh-positive blood to 27 Rh-negative unsensitised volunteers. On day 4, 14 of these volunteers were given 4 ml of anti-D gammaglobulin, the remaining 13 acting as controls. After day 4 there were no additional injections either of blood or of gammaglobulin, and the blood of each of the 27 volunteers was tested at monthly intervals for six months.

At the time of writing, the study was in its seventh month and six of the thirteen controls were immunised as against none of the treated. The passive antibody had cleared by the fourth month and for the following three months no Rh antibody had been detected in the treated group either by the saline or indirect antiglobulin methods. There were again no untoward effects, and there seemed good grounds for hope that treatment of mothers 72 hours after delivery might succeed.

The authors felt that it was still not known for certain when the initial stimulus for Rh sensitisation usually takes place, and that therefore it would take three to five years for a clinical trial to show whether anti-D given *after* delivery protected, but they were hopeful that there would soon be a shift in emphasis from management of affected babies to prevention of the disease itself.

A most encouraging feature of the Rh prophylaxis research from the beginning was the striking similarity of the results from various centres, particularly those of a pioneering nature from Canada, Liverpool, Germany and the US. This was most reassuring to all concerned.

From V. J. Freda, J. G. Gorman and Pollack (1964). Transfusion, 4, 26-32. Copyright (1964), by kind permission of the authors, and J. B. Lippincott, Co

Successful Prevention of Experimental Rh Sensitization in Man with an Anti-Rh Gamma₂-Globulin Antibody Preparation:

A Preliminary Report

VINCENT J. FREDA,* JOHN G. GORMAN,** WILLIAM POLLACK

From the Departments of Obstetrics and Gynecology and Pathology, Columbia University, College of Physicians and Surgeons, New York City, and the Ortho Research Foundation, Raritan, New Jersey

An anti-Rh gamma₂-globulin antibody preparation has been developed which can be administered intramuscularly and appears to be both safe and effective in the prevention of experimental Rh sensitization. Nine unsensitized Rh-negative male volunteers were challenged once a month for five successive months with intravenous injections of 2 ml. of Rh-positive blood. Four of these nine volunteers were passively protected each month with intramuscular injections of 5 ml. of this antibody preparation, administered 24 hours prior to the antigenic challenge. Three months after the last injection the passively acquired Rh antibodies were no longer demonstrable (by either the saline or indirect antiglobulin technics) in any of the four protected subjects and there was no sign of active antibody production six months after the last injection, whereas four of the five controls were all strongly sensitized.

IN 1909 Theobald Smith showed that neutralized mixtures of diphtheria toxin and antitoxin containing an excess of antitoxin, did not immunize (or were non-antigenic) when injected. In the subsequent years evidence[1, 3, 4, 9, 17, 19, 22, 23, 25-27, 31-33, 35, 37, 38, 41, 43, 44] has been accumulated that, in general, if a particular specific antibody is administered passively to an individual, subsequent injections of the corresponding antigen usually fail to sensitize. It was found that the circulating levels of passively administered antibody must be sufficient to maintain a state of antibody excess at all times, and that it is this excess which is the key to prevention of sensitization.

Levine[21] has established that if the mother has an existing circulating antibody directed against the baby's red cells, e.g.,

anti-A as in group O, Rh-negative mothers with a group A, Rh-positive baby, then sensitization to Rh by pregnancy is extremely rare. Stern and his co-workers[39, 40] have shown that it is extremely difficult to sensitize Rh-negative volunteers to Rh with injection of ABO incompatible Rh-positive cells or with ABO compatible cells which have been coated *in vitro* with an excess of anti-Rh₀ antibody. It is suggested that these observations are similar to the phenomenon described above.

The concept that it might be possible to prevent initial sensitization of Rh negative mothers by administering the Rh antibody immediately following childbirth occurred independently to Finn et al.[10] and to the authors.[16] With this concept in mind, both groups independently set out to demonstrate that the inhibition phenomenon (*i.e.* suppression of a specific immune response with passively injected antibody of the same specificity) applies equally well to the Rh antigen-antibody system.

Our first step was to develop an experimental gamma globulin preparation (sterile) which contained sufficiently high levels of anti-Rh antibody so that a satisfactory circulating titer would result from a small intramuscular injection. This was considered necessary for the following reasons:

1) A small intramuscular injection of gamma globulin is considerably safer than large intravenous injections of whole plasma;

2) assured sterility;

3) freedom from risk of transmitting homologous serum jaundice;

4) ease of administration;

5) an available preparation with these

* Supported by the Health Research Council, N. Y. C. 1-264; U-1307.

** Supported by the Health Research Council, N. Y. C. U-1154. Present address: Dept. of Laboratories, Lennox Hill Hosp., N. Y. C.

Received for publication April 4, 1963; revised anl resubmitted August 16, 1963; accepted August 20, 1963.

characteristics would be absolutely essential before one could even begin to consider passive protection of mothers in the third stage of labor.

This preparation was employed throughout this study to achieve passive immunization as described below under methods and procedures.

The protocol for the study by Finn et al.[10] (including their expanded study reported on by Clarke et al.[5]) differed from that of the present study in that:

a) The Rh antibodies were used in the form of the original whole plasma;

b) the Rh antibody titers were much lower;

c) the plasma was administered intravenously;

d) the plasma was administered shortly after the experimental injection of the Rh-positive red cells.

One danger of such a procedure has been pointed out recently by Cohen and Allton,[7] who have shown on the basis of their studies in rabbits that significant enhancement of the antibody response can occur if antibody is not in excess. This same effect has been noted with underneutralized soluble antigen-antibody complexes (BSA—Anti-BSA).[42] Finn et al.[11] have also observed this enhancement in human volunteers when working with small amounts of passively administered antibody. Thus as stated earlier, antibody excess appears to be very important in any studies designed to demonstrate suppression of antibody response.

Methods of Procedure

Twelve liters of plasma were obtained by repeated plasmapheresis from four donors, each of whom had high anti-Rh titers by the indirect antiglobulin method. This was processed by a modification of the Cohn method into gamma$_2$ globulin, sterilized by filtration and packaged as a 16 per cent solution. Sterility checks were carried out as required by the National Institutes of Health for immune globulin before use. The final yield from the original 12 liters of plasma was 110 ml., which was distributed

into twenty-two 5 ml. ampoules, ready for injection. The Rh antibody (anti-Rh$_o$) in the final preparation was entirely 7S gamma$_2$ (as determined by immunoelectrophoresis and ultracentrifugation) and had an indirect antiglobulin titer of 1:64,000; there was no saline agglutination. There was no anti-A or anti-B isoagglutinin in the preparation by either the saline or acacia methods. An intramuscular injection of 5 ml. of this preparation resulted in a maximum circulating titer of 1:64 or 1:128 (indirect antiglobulin method) within eight hours.

Nine unsensitized group O, Rh-negative male volunteers at Sing Sing Prison were challenged once a month for five successive months with intravenous injections of 2 ml. of Rh-positive whole blood.* Five of this group acted as controls while the remaining four received the experimental antibody preparation. These four volunteers in the test group were passively protected each month with intramuscular injections of 5 ml. of the antibody preparation administered 24 hours prior to the injection of Rh-positive blood.

Anti-Rh titers by both the saline and indirect antiglobulin method were carried out each month on blood samples obtained from each of the nine volunteers just prior to the injection of Rh-positive blood. Titers were also carried out each month on blood samples obtained from the test group just before injecting the experimental antibody. Following the last injection of antibody in the fifth month, titers were obtained each month for an additional six months on both test and control groups.

The Rh-positive blood which was injected intravenously throughout this study was obtained, as required, from one donor (J.B.) who was type O Rh$_1$ Rh$_1$. This donor was known to the Presbyterian Hospital Blood Bank and had donated blood repeatedly over an adequate period of time with no evidence of jaundice occurring in any of the recipients of his blood (nine months follow-up). In all of the titrations

* On each day of injection, fresh donor blood was drawn—150 ml. was collected in 20 ml. ACD solution.

TABLE 1. *Anti-Rh Titer Results* in the Protected and Control Groups of Rh Negative Volunteers*

Rh negative volunteers	1st month		2nd month		3rd month		4th month		5th month	
	Day 1**	Day 2†	Day 1	Day 2	Day 1	Day 2	Day 1	Day 2	Day 1	Day 2
Protected group										
D. R.	neg	128	16	64	32	64	32	128	16	64
D. C.	neg	64	8	64	32	64	32	128	16	32
J. W.	neg	128	16	64	32	64	32	128	32	64
A. D.	neg	64	32	64	32	32	16	128	32	128
Control group										
J. F.	neg	—	neg	—	neg	—	neg	—	neg	—
J. W.	neg	—	neg	—	tr	—	128	—	256	—
H. C.	neg	—	neg	—	neg	—	1	—	128	—
J. C.	neg	—	neg	—	2	—	64	—	256	—
L. F.	neg	—	neg	—	16	—	16	—	64	—

* All titrations in this study were carried out by both the saline and indirect antiglobulin method. Since no saline titer above 2 units was encountered throughout this study, only the indirect antiglobulin titers are reported. A negative result ("neg") indicates that no antibody at all was detected by either method. All titration results are expressed as the reciprocal of the last dilution tube in which there was evident microscopic clumping (low power exam).

** Day 1 of 1st month reflects the unsensitized state for all nine volunteers. For each succeeding month Day 1 indicates the titers present just one month after the last injection of Rh positive red cells. After the specimens were drawn on Day 1 the experimental antibody preparation was given to the protected group.

that were carried out during this study, fresh washed red cells from this same donor (J.B.) were always employed as the test cells.

Prior to initiating this study the usual compatibility tests were carried out between the bloods of the donor and each volunteer and between the experimental antibody preparation and the red cells of each volunteer. These results were all negative and there was no atypical antibody present in any of the volunteers.

Results

There were no untoward reactions either to the intramuscular injections of the experimental gamma globulin or to the intravenous injections of Rh-positive blood. The protected group received 20 injections in all of the antibody preparation. Throughout this study each volunteer was specifically asked whether or not at any time he noted any undue discomfort and the answers were uniformly negative.

Representative samples from the entire series of blood specimens (both protected and control group) which were collected throughout this study were screened for anti-gamma globulin isoantibody by Doctors James C. Allen and Henry G. Kunkel

of the Rockefeller Institute. No antibodies of this type were found.

The titration results are summarized in Table 1. After the last passive immunization of the protected group in the fifth month, it required three additional months before all of the passively administered circulating antibody had disappeared. The indirect antiglobulin titers became negative in each of the four protected prisoners in the eighth and ninth months, thus indicating that none of the four had formed anti-Rh antibody of their own. The anti-Rh titers which were found each month in this group therefore reflect only antibody which was passively administered. On the other hand, four of the five control prisoners were strongly sensitized to Rh after the fourth injection of Rh-positive cells, indicating that the program of antigenic challenge employed in this study was adequate. All of the volunteers were in good health and all but one were in the same age group (20-35 years of age). One volunteer was 58 years old and he was the only control (J.F.) who was not sensitized.

Discussion

These preliminary results appear to indicate that the concentrated Rh antibody

TABLE 1—Continued

Anti-Rh Titer Results in the Protected and Control Groups of Rh Negative Volunteers

Rh negative volunteers	6th month Day 1	7th month Day 1	8th month Day 1	9th month Day 1	11th month Day 1
Protected group					
D. R.	32	8	neg	neg	neg
D. C.	32	16		neg	
J. W.	16	16	neg	neg	neeg
A. D.	64	16	neg	neg	neg
Control group					
J. F.	neg	neg	neg	neg.	neg
J. W.	128	256	128	128	128
H. C.	512	1,024	512	512	256
J. C.	512	1,024	256	256	512
L. F.	32				

† Day 2 for each month represents the time the Rh positive red cells were injected intravenously. Titers were carried out at this time on the protected group to show the rise in circulating titer due to the passively administered antibody given 24 hours earlier. The last protective injection was given in the 5th month and three months later there was no residual antibody.

preparation used in these studies was effective in preventing Rh sensitization when injected twenty-four hours prior to each antigenic challenge. It is easily administered and readily absorbed following intramuscular injection, and most important, it appears to be safe.

An expanded study with 30 Rh-negative volunteers is under way. One of the primary aims is to determine whether or not the antibody preparation can prevent sensitization when injected 72 hours after a challenge of Rh-positive blood. Also, the volume of Rh-positive blood has been increased from 2 to 10 ml. and the new donor is O Rh_2 Rh_2. The intervals between the injections has been increased from one month to four months in order to allow the passively administered antibody to disappear prior to a subsequent injection. These changes in protocol were essential in order to evaluate whether or not there is a possible projected risk of an enhancement phenomenon taking place. The results must be unequivocal on this important point before considering a projected study on unsensitized mothers. In general these studies will provide the necessary additional clinical experience in male volunteers, which is required before this preparation is tried in Rh-negative mothers. If there are no data forthcoming to show

conclusively that the delivery event is not an important factor in Rh sensitization by pregnancy, and if additional studies should confirm the safety and effectiveness of this experimental antibody preparation, then it would be ready for a prompt clinical trial.

It is essential that any future program designed to evaluate the use of this reagent in mothers must be approached with the greatest caution, must be carefully planned and statistically controlled. It appears that gamma$_2$ globulin (7S) passes readily through the placenta,[14, 15, 20, 34] probably by an active transport mechanism and therefore cannot be given during pregnancy or labor.* However, if given following the birth of the infant it may still be in time to prevent sensitization. This would be the logical method of employing this reagent in a trial study. Because only about 12 per cent of all mothers at risk become sensitized to Rh in the natural course of events, fairly large numbers of mothers will have to be *protected* through several pregnancies before data as to the value of the procedure becomes significant.

---

* There is good evidence that the gamma$_1$ M globulins will not cross the human placenta[13, 18, 36] and it is suspected from studies in lower animals that the serologically reactive 3.5S gamma$_2$ globulin fragments[2, 28, 29] also will not cross it. Studies of such preparations with anti-Rh specificity would be very worthwhile.

To the best of our knowledge, no one has ever provided conclusive evidence as to when the initial stimulus for Rh sensitization usually takes place—*i.e.,* during the antepartum period or at the time of labor and delivery. *Protection* with antibody following delivery can be of value only if this prime stimulus occurs about the time of delivery. A clinical trial with this specialized gamma-globulin could provide an answer within three to five years.

If one accepts the reasonable assumption that the placenta is no more efficient than the kidney in preventing red cells from passing through, then it follows that fetal red cells should be present routinely in the maternal circulation throughout pregnancy; whether or not they can always be demonstrated depends on the sensitivity of the technic employed and the volume of maternal blood examined. Cohen *et al.*[8] working with the fluorescent tagged antiglobulin method have demonstrated in some cases fetal red cells in the maternal circulation during gestation. These findings, however, do not prove that these small numbers of fetal red cells alone are effective antigenic stimuli — and indirect evidence can be proposed both *pro* and *con*. It is the opinion of the authors that the bulk of available clinical knowledge is contrary to the assumptions that these small numbers of cells are effective stimuli or that significant fetal-maternal bleeds occur routinely in the antepartum period alone. This issue is far from settled and much work remains to be done, particularly the following:

1) improved methods for quantitating minor populations of fetal red cells with determinations at all stages of gestation;

2) subsequent follow up on all cases from one pregnancy to another (beginning with the first pregnancy) to see which mothers actually do become sensitized later on.

The various studies on the subject of transplacental hemorrhage into the maternal circulation have been reviewed recently by Finn *et al.*[12] and data from their own study was presented. They concluded that *transplacental hemorrhage* is not a random phenomenon but is related to obstetric abnormalities and procedures. They also stress the importance of gaining more knowledge regarding the exact timing of sensitization by pregnancy; the present authors subscribe wholeheartedly to this aim.

The attack on erythroblastosis fetalis is gaining momentum and it is possible that in the next few years there may be a marked shift in emphasis from management of affected babies to prevention of the disease itself.

Acknowledgments

The authors are very grateful to Warden Wilfred L. Denno and his staff and to Dr. Harold Kipp for their most helpful cooperation.

Addendum

Data are now available from our expanded study at Sing-Sing with an additional 27 volunteers (ref. to text, under "Discussion"). In brief, the revised protocol for the expanded study is as follows: 1) On Day One of the study all 27 volunteers (Rh neg. and unsensitized) received intravenous injection of 10 ml. of O $Rh_2 Rh_2$ blood; 2) On Day Four of the study (3 days after the I.V. injections of Rh pos. blood) 14 of these volunteers were each protected with a single intramuscular injection of 4 ml. of specialized $gamma_2$-globulin; the remaining 13 volunteers acted as the control group; 3) after Day Four of the study there were no additional injections either of Rh pos. blood or of $gamma_2$-globulin and blood specimens were drawn from each of the 27 volunteers at monthly intervals for six months.

This study is now in its seventh month and the results to date are as follows: 1) Six of the 13 controls are now actively sensitized to Rh (earliest and latest intervals noted for first appearance of antibody were at 2 months and 4 months respectively); 2) not one of the 14 protected volunteers has become sensitized to Rh—the passively administered antibody had cleared by the fourth month and each month for the past three months no Rh antibody has been detected in this group either by the saline or indirect antiglobulin methods; 3) to date there have been no untoward reactions and no morbidity encountered either from the intravenous injections of Rh positive blood or from the intramuscular injections of the specialized gamma$_2$-globulin preparation.

References

1. Barr, M., A. T. Glenny and K. J. Randall: Diphtheria immunization in young babies. A study of some factors involved. Lancet 1: 6, 1950.
2. Brambell, F. W. R., W. A. Hemmings, C. L. Oakley and R. R. Porter: Proc. Roy. Soc. (Biol.) 151: 478, 1960.
3. Brodie, M.: Active immunization against poliomyelitis. J. Exp. Med. 56: 493, 1932.
4. Buxton, J. B. and A. T. Glenny: The active immunization of horses against tetanus. Lancet 2: 1109, 1921.
5. Clarke, C. A., W. T. A. Donohoe, R. B. McConnell, J. C. Woodrow, R. Finn, J. R. Krevans, W. Kulke, D. Lehane and P. M. Sheppard: Further experimental studies on the prevention of Rh hemolytic disease. Brit. Med. J. 1: 979, 1963.
6. Clayton, E. M., Jr., J. C. Robertson and W. Feldhaus: Antepartum and postpartum detection of fetal erythrocytes in maternal circulation. Obst. Gynec. 20: 608, 1962.
7. Cohen, C. and W. H. Allton, Jr.: Isoimmunization in the rabbit with antibody-coated erythrocytes. Nature 193: 990, 1962.
8. Cohen, F., W. W. Zuelzer and M. E. Evans: Identification of blood group antigens and minor cell populations by the fluorescent antibody method. Blood 15: 884, 1960.
9. Di Sant'Agnese, P. A.: Combined immunization against diphtheria, tetanus and pertussis in newborn infants. II. Duration of antibody levels. Antibody titers after booster dose. Effect of passive immunity to diphtheria on active immunization with diphtheria toxoid. Pediatrics 3: 181, 1949.
10. Finn, R., C. A. Clarke, W. T. A. Donohoe, R. B. McConnell, P. M. Sheppard, D. Lehane, and W. Kulke: Experimental studies on the prevention of Rh hemolytic disease. Brit. Med. J. 1: 1486, 1961.
11. Finn, R., C. A. Clarke, R. B. McConnell and J. C. Woodrow: Response to an article by Cohen and Allton (7). Nature 193: 991, 1962.
12. Finn, R., D. T. Harper, S. A. Stallings and J. R. Krevans: Transplacental hemorrhage. Transfusion 3: 114, 1963.
13. Foucaut, M. and M. Goudemand: Etude immuno-electrophoretique du serum des prematures. Rev. Franc. Etud. Clin. Biol. 6: 446, 1961.
14. Franklin, E. C. and H. C. Kunkel: Comparative levels of high molecular weight (19S) gamma globulin in maternal and umbilical cord sera. J. Lab. Clin. Med. 52: 724, 1958.
15. Freda, V. J.: Placental transfer of antibodies in man. Amer. J. Obst. Gynec. 84: 1756, 1962.
16. Freda. V. J. and J. G. Gorman: Antepartum management of Rh hemolytic disease. Bull. Sloane Hosp. Wom. 8: 147, 1962.
16a. Freda, V. J.: Unpublished data.
17. Glenny, A. T. and J. J. Sudmerson: Notes on the production of immunity to diphtheria toxin. J. Hyg. 20: 176, 1921.
18. Hitzig, W. H.: Die physiologische entwicklung der "immunoglobuline" (gamma-und beta$_2$-globuline). Helv. Paediat. Acta 12: 596, 1957.
19. Kalmanson, G. M. and J. Bronfenbrenner: Restoration of activity of neutralized biologic agents by removal of the antibody with papain. J. Immun. 47: 387, 1943.
20. Kochwa, S., R. E. Rosenfield, L. Tallal and L. R. Wasserman: Isoagglutinins associated with ABO erythroblastosis. J. Clin. Invest. 40: 874, 1961.
21. Levine, P.: The influence of the ABO system on Rh hemolytic disease. Hum. Biol. 30: 14, 1958.
22. Mason, J. H., M. Robinson and P. A. Christensen: The active immunization of guinea-pigs passively immunized with homologous antitoxin serum. J. Hyg. 53: 172, 1955.
23. Nagano, Y. and S. Takeuti: Études serologiques sur le bacteriophage, Japan. J. Exp. Med. 21: 427, 1951.
24. Nevanlinna, H. R.: Factors affecting maternal Rh immunization. Ann. Med. Exp. Fenn. Supp. 2, Vol. 31, 1953.
25. Osborn, J. J., J. Dancis and J. F. Julia: Studies of the immunology of the newborn infant. II. Interference with active immunization by passive transplacental circulating antibody. Pediatrics 10: 328, 1952.
26. Otten, L. and I. P. Hennemann: Combined (simultaneous) immunization against tetanus. J. Path. Bact. 49: 213, 1939.
27. Perkins, F. T., R. Yetts and W. Gaisford: Poliomyelitis immunization of infants in the presence of maternally transmitted antibody. Brit. Med. J. 1: 404, 1961.
28. Porter, R. R.: The hydrolysis of rabbit gamma-globulin and antibodies with crystalline papain. Biochem. J. 73: 119, 1959.
29. Porter, R. R.: Active fragments of antibody in protein structure and function. Brookhaven Symposia in Biology, No. 13, June 6-8, 1960, Assoc. Univ. Inc., pp. 203-209.
30. Queenan, J. T., R. Landesman, M. Nakamoto and K. H. Wilson: Postpartum immunization. Obst. Gynec. 20: 774, 1962.
31. Ramon, G. and C. Zoeller: Sur la valeur et la dures de l'immunite conferee par l'anatoxin tetanique dans la vaccination de l'homme contre le tetanos, Compt. rendu. Soc. biol. 112: 347, 1933.
32. Regamey, R. H. and W. Aegerter: La sero-anatoxitherapie experimentale du tetanos, Schweiz Z. allg. Path. u Bakt. 14: 554, 1951.
33. Rhoads, C. P.: Immunity following the injection of monkeys with mixtures of poliomyelitis virus and convalescent human serum. J. Exp. Med. 53: 115, 1931.

34. Rosenfield, R. E.: Personal communication.

35. Sawyer, W. A., S. F. Kitchen and W. Lloyd: Vaccination against yellow fever with immune serum and virus fixed for mice. J. Exp. Med. **55:** 945, 1932.

36. Scheidegger, J. J. and R. Martin Du Pan: Etude immuno-electrophoretique des proteines seriques du nouveau-ne et du nourrisson. Etudes Neo-Natales **6:** 135, 1957.

37. Smith, T.: Active immunity producel by so called balanced or neutral mixtures of diphtheria toxin and antitoxin. J. Exp. Med. **11:** 241, 1909.

38. Snell, G. D., H. J. Winn, J. H. Stimpfling and S. J. Parker: Depression by antibody of the immune response to homografts and its role in immunological enhancement. J. Exp. Med. **112:** 293, 1950.

39. Stern, K., I. Davidson and L. Masaitis: Experimental studies on Rh immunization. Am. J. Clin. Path. **26:** 833, 1956.

40. Stern, K., H. S. Goodman and M. Berger: Experimental isoimmunization to hemoantigens in man. J. Immun. **87:** 189, 1961.

41. Talmage, D. W., G. G. Freter and A. Thomson: The effect of whole body I radiation on the specific anamnestic response in the rabbit. J. Infect. Dis. **99:** 246, 1956.

42. Terres, G. and R. D. Stoner: Specificity of enhanced immunological sensitization of mice following injections of antigens and specific antisera. Proc. Soc. Exp. Biol. Med. **109:** 88, 1962.

43. Uhr, J. W. and J. B. Baumann: Antibody formation I. The suppression of antibody formation by passively administered antibody. J. Exp. Med. **113:** 935, 1961.

44. Uhr, J. W. and J. B. Baumann: Antibody formation II. The specific anamnestic antibody response. J. Exp. Med. **113:** 959, 1961.

Paper 31

31. Schneider, V. J. and Preisler, O. (1965). Untersuchungen zur Serologischen Prophylaxe der Rh-sensibilisierung. *Blut, XII*, no. 1, 4–8.

Commentary

The West Germans, who have maintained close contact with the Liverpool group throughout the research, were very quick (see Schneider 1963*) to begin experimental studies and clinical trials. In Paper 31 there are reports on both of these.

On the experimental side, the authors injected Rh-negative subjects with 0·5 to 1 ml Rh-positive cord blood intravenously. They then tested for red cell clearance using either; (a) intravenous anti-D serum, (b) intramuscular (high titre) anti-D gammaglobulin or (c) intramuscular low titre anti-D gammaglobulin. They found that the serum cleared the most rapidly, then the high titre gammaglobulin and then the low titre.

Their clinical trial was the first to be reported on in any country. They examined, three to six months after delivery, 73 Rh-negative women who had had a fetomaternal haemorrhage of from 0·05 to 3·5 ml after the birth of an Rh-positive baby. 46 of these women had been given, after delivery, from 10 to 20 ml anti-D serum intravenously, and 27 had not been treated. When the paper was written no woman of either group had made antibodies, but one untreated woman made them later and a note to this effect was added in proof.

*Schneider, J. (1963). Die quantitative Bestimmung fetaler Erythrocyten im mütterlichen Kreislauf und deren beschleunigter Abbau durch Anti-körperseren. *Geburtshilf. u. Frauenheilk.*, 23, 562-8.

English summary

The quantity of foetal erythrocytes entering the maternal circulation during labour has been estimated. Fetal erythrocytes entering the maternal circulation normally survive 90—120 days. However, when the passage of fetal erythrocytes into the maternal blood stream is coupled with the administration of an antiserum they are destroyed on average in two or at the most three days. Experiments are still in progress, similar to those of Finn, Clarke *et al.*, which should serve to show whether, in spite of the passage of Rh-positive cells in Rh-negative volunteers, sensitisation can be prevented if at the same time as Rh-antigen is injected a corresponding amount of antiserum is given.

Blut, Band XII, Seite 4–8 (1965)

ÜBERSICHT

Aus der Universitäts-Frauenklinik Freiburg/Br.
(Direktor: Prof. Dr. H. Wimhöfer)

Untersuchungen zur serologischen Prophylaxe der Rh-Sensibilisierung

Von J. Schneider und O. Preisler

Nach der Entbindung findet man im Kreislauf bei ca. $20^0{}_0$ aller Mütter quantitativ erfaßbare Mengen fetaler Erythrozyten. Meistens handelt es sich zwar um Mengen unter 1 ml, jedoch findet man gelegentlich auch Einschwemmungen von mehreren ml. Nach operativen Entbindungen findet man diese sogenannten „HbF"-Zellen häufiger (bis zu $40^0{}_0$), vor allem, wenn die Plazenta manuell gelöst oder durch Druck auf den Fundus uteri mit dem sogenannten *Kristeller*schen Handgriff exprimiert wurde [*Wimhöfer* et al.]. Bei Spontangeburten und nach Vakuumextraktionen erfolgen solche feto-maternen „Mikrotransfusionen" seltener ($10^0{}_0$—$15^0{}_0$), und sehr selten wird eine feto-maternale Transfusion von über 50 ml beobachtet, welche zu akuten klinischen Erscheinungen bei Kind und Mutter führen kann [2]. Der Übertritt erfolgt vorwiegend in der Austreibungs- und Plazentarlösungsperiode [3]. Am Ende der Schwangerschaft dagegen und vor Wehenbeginn findet man meßbare Mengen fetaler Erythrozyten im mütterlichen Kreislauf nur selten.

Der Nachweis der HbF-Zellen erfolgt am einfachsten und mit großer Sicherheit mit der Blutausstrich-Eluierungs-Methode [4]. Die verschiedentlich angegebenen Modifikationen scheinen keine Vorteile gebracht zu haben. Die Fluoreszenzmethode [5,6] scheint qualitativ keine wesentlichen Vorteile mit sich zu bringen, erfordert jedoch wesentlich mehr Arbeitsaufwand. Da die Verteilung der HbF-Zellen im mütterlichen Blut sehr groß ist, bereitet die quantitative Auszählung und Berechnung Schwierigkeiten. Von den verschiedenen angegebenen Methoden [1,7] sind nur relative Werte zu erwarten. Wir arbeiten mit einer Methode, die mit einer Fehlerbreite von $\mp 20^0{}_0$ jederzeit erlaubt, eingeschwemmte Mengen von 0,1—1,0—4,0 ml zu unterscheiden. was für die nachfolgend beschriebenen Untersuchungen von Bedeutung erscheint [8]. Unsicherheitsfaktoren bei den Berechnungen sind das Blutvolumen der Mutter, die Erythrozytenzahl im mütterlichen und im Nabelschnurblut, welche nur teilweise ausgeschlossen werden können. Die Auswertung eines Blutausstriches benötigt auch im Routinebetrieb 30 Min., so daß für Serienuntersuchungen erheblicher Zeitaufwand notwendig ist.

Wenn auch die Methode bei der generellen Bestimmung von Mikrotransfusionen aus obengenannten Gründen eine relativ große Fehlerbreite hat, so ist sie jedoch darüber hinaus für das Studium des Abbaus von HbF-Zellen bei der einzelnen Versuchsperson und z. B. für Bestimmungen der Überlebenszeit von HbF-Zellen im Kreislauf des Erwachsenen mit ausreichender Genauigkeit zu verwenden [9].

Es ist inzwischen gesichert, daß der gesunde Erwachsene in seine Erythrozyten teilweise HbF einlagert. Bei der Säureeluierung mit einem Puffer von pH 3,3 wird zwar alles HbA aus den Erythrozyten gelöst, das zunächst verbleibende HbF, welches dann angefärbt wird, kann jedoch in der Auswertung zu Fehlbestimmungen führen und echte fetale Zellen vortäuschen. Für den geübten Untersucher sind allerdings die blaßroten „HbF"-Zellen des Erwachsenen und die echten HbF-Zellen des Kindes, welche mit ca. 80% HbF gefüllt sind, leicht zu unterscheiden. Für die spezielle geburtshilfliche Fragestellung empfiehlt es sich, mit einem pH von 3,2 zu eluieren, da dann nur noch HbF in den „echten" vom Kinde stammenden Erythrozyten verbleibt. —

Wenn blutgruppenunverträgliche Erythrozyten in der normalen Zeit oder mit einer geringen Beschleunigung aus dem Kreislauf eliminiert werden, dann erfolgt der Abbau größtenteils in der Milz, und dort werden vermutlich die Antikörper gebildet. Wird der Abbau auf wenige Stunden beschleunigt, dann erfolgt er in der Leber, und die Bildung von Antikörpern wird weitgehend verhindert [10–13].

Wir führten zunächst experimentelle Untersuchungen bei rh-negativen antikörperfreien Personen durch, die Rh-positives Nabelschnurblut in einer Menge von 0,5 bis 1,0 ml i. v. injiziert bekamen. Der Spontanabbau dauert ca. 80, im Maximum 120 Tage. Durch i. v.-Nachinjektion von 1 ml Anti-D-Serum erreicht man eine Beschleunigung der Elimination auf 3 Tage [14,15]. Wenn man die Menge des Anti-D-Serums auf 10–26 ml erhöht, dann sind nach 3–12 Stunden alle Rh-positiven, fetalen Erythrozyten aus dem Kreislauf verschwunden [14]. Man kann an Stelle des i.v. gegebenen Anti-Rh-Serums auch ein hochtitriges Anti-D-Globulin oder Anti-D-γ-Globulin i. m. injizieren. Diese i. m.-Präparate benötigen zunächst eine Resorptionszeit von einigen Stunden, jedoch erfolgt die Totaleliminierung der injizierten Rh-Erythrozyten auch innerhalb von 48 Stunden. Der Titer dieser Fraktionen im Albumintest darf jedoch nicht unter 1:4000 liegen, ansonsten findet man die injizierten Erythrozyten noch bis zu 8 Tagen lang im Kreislauf. Durch Erhöhung der Menge des Anti-D-γ-Globulins kann ein niedriger Titer nicht voll kompensiert werden.

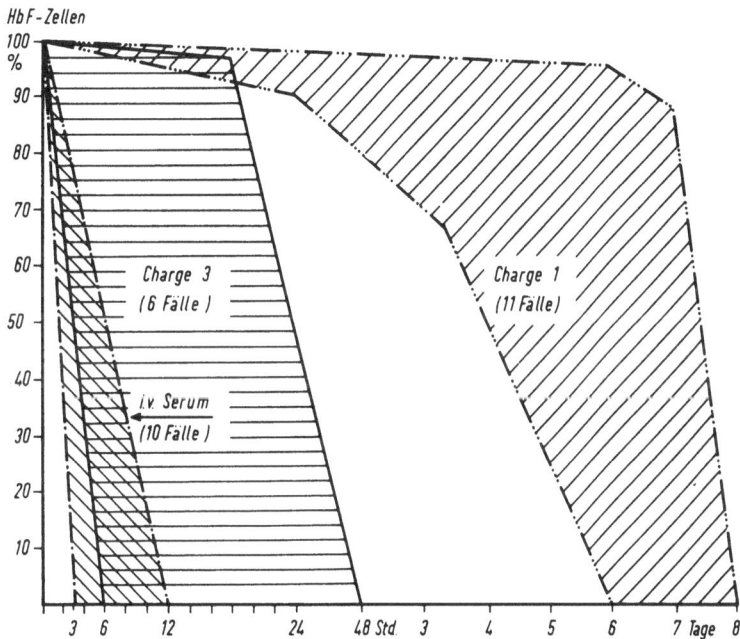

Abb. 1: Abbau von 1 ml Rh + Nabelschnurblut durch Anti-D-Serum i. v. und durch hochtitriges (Charge 3) und niedertitriges (Charge 1) Anti-D-Globulin i. m.

Nach Gabe von 0,5 ml Rh-unverträglichen Nabelschnurblutes werden etwa 20% der Frauen immunisiert. Wenn man Nabelschnurblut jedoch durch Tietfrieren und Wiederauftauen lysiert, so daß zwar das Rh-Antigen, aber nicht die intakten Rh-positiven Erythrozyten in den Kreislauf gelangen, wird die Sensibilisierungsrate herabgesetzt (1:17). Die Sensibilisierungshäufigkeit läßt sich nicht herabsetzen, wenn man nur 1 ml Anti-D-Serum i. v. nach 0,5 ml Rh-positivem Nabelschnurblut nachinjiziert. Injiziert man jedoch 10–26 ml eines Serums von einem Titer 1:128 bis 1:1000 im Albumintest, dann wird die Sensibilisierung immer verhindert.

Dabei kann die i. v.-Gabe des Serums bis zu 48 Stunden nach der unverträglichen Blutinjektion erfolgen. Mit hochtitrigen Rh-Globulinen, die i. m. gegeben werden, erreicht man die Verhinderung der Sensibilisierung in gleicher Weise. Auch sie können bis 48 Stunden nach der unverträglichen Blutinjektion

Gabe von Antigen und Antikörper und Abstand zwischen den Injektionen	Gesamt-zahl	Sensibilisiert ja	nein
2mal 0,5 ml Rh+ Nabelschnurblut i. v. im Abstand von 2 bis 5 Wochen	15	4	11
2mal 0,5 ml Rh+ kältelysiertes Nabelschnurblut i. v. im Abstand von 1 bis 7 Wochen	17	1	16
1mal 0,5 ml Rh+ Nabelschnurblut i. v. 1 Std. danach 1 ml Anti-D-Serum i. v.	20	5	15
1mal 1,0 ml Rh+ Nabelschnurblut i. v. 24 bis 48 Stdn. danach 10 bis 20 ml Anti-D-Serum i. v.	13	0	13
2- bis 3mal 0,5 ml Rh+ Nabelschnurblut i. v. im Abstand von 1 bis 6 Wochen, jeweils 1 bis 2 Stdn. danach 10 bis 26 ml Anti-D-Serum i. v.	13	0	13
1- bis 2mal 1,0 ml Rh+ Nabelschnurblut i. v., bei 2maliger Gabe im Abstand von 9 Tagen bis 4 Wochen, jeweils 12 bis 48 Stdn. danach 2 bis 8 ml Anti-D-Globulin oder Anti-D-γ-Globulin i. m.	16	1	15

Tab. 1: Sensibilisierung gegen den Rh-Faktor mit Rh+ Nabelschnurblut i. v. und die Verhinderung mit Anti-Rh-Serum i. v. und Anti-Rh-Globulinen i. m.

gegeben werden. Mit niedertitrigen Anti-Rh-Globulinen (1:128) wird die Sensibilisierungshäufigkeit zwar reduziert, aber nicht in jedem Fall verhindert.

Wir untersuchen bei jeder rh-negativen Frau mit einem Rh-positiven Kind 2–12 Stunden post partum, ob sie mehr als 0,05 ml fetales Blut eingeschwemmt hat. 73 von diesen Müttern mit Einschwemmungen von 0,05–3,5 ml konnten bisher 3–5 Monate post partum serologisch nachuntersucht werden. 46 Frauen hatten eine Prophylaxe mit 10–20 ml Anti-D-Serum i. v. erhalten und 27 Frauen nicht. Die Geschwindigkeit der Elimination der eingeschwemmten fetalen Erythrozyten ist auch nach Gabe von Anti-D-Serum i. v. abhängig von dem Titer des Serums, so wie bei den i. m. gegebenen Anti-D-Globulinen. Liegt er zwischen 1:256 und 1:16 000, dann sind sämtliche Erythrozyten in 2–24 Std. aus dem strömenden Blut verschwunden. Nimmt man aber ein Serum von einem Titer von nur 1:64, dann wird in 2–5 Tagen nur eine partielle Elimination der Erythrozyten erreicht. Auch hier kann der niedrige Titer durch eine größere Menge des injizierten Serums nicht ausgeglichen werden. Da wir annehmen müssen, daß ein Zusammenhang zwischen der Elimination der Erythrozyten aus dem strömenden Blut und der Sensibilisierung besteht, müssen die Seren immer hochtitrig sein. Auch steht zur Diskussion, ob die Gabe von zuwenig Antikörpern nach Antigen-Einschwemmung nicht die Sensibilisierungsrate entsprechend einer Simultanimpfung erhöht.

Zu unserer Überraschung konnten wir weder in der Gruppe der serumgeschützten Frauen noch bei den nicht geschützten bis jetzt eine aktive Bildung von Rh-Antikörpern nachweisen. Wir möchten daher annehmen, daß Rh-Antikörper normalerweise erst in der nachfolgenden Gravidität mit einem Rh-positiven Kind gebildet werden, wenn kleinste Erythrozyten-Mengen von der Frucht auf die Mutter übergehen, und es zu dem sogenannten Booster-Effekt kommt.

Da die Sensibilisierungsrate nach Erythrozyteneinschwemmung unter der Geburt aber nur 12% beträgt [1], wären in unserem Untersuchungsgut auch nur 3 sensibilisierte Frauen zu erwarten. Bei der kleinen Zahl ist unser Ergebnis noch im Bereich der Irrtumsmöglichkeit.*

Es ist anzunehmen, daß es eine Mindestmenge von Rh-Antigen gibt, die für die Sensibilisierung erforderlich ist. Ob dies jedoch allgemeingültig festzulegen ist, erscheint fraglich. 20 von den 73 genannten Müttern hatten unter der Geburt weniger als 0,1 ml eingeschwemmt und nur 14 mehr als 0,5 ml. Vielleicht ist das Ausbleiben der Sensibilisierung bei den nicht geschützten Frauen damit zu erklären, daß ein großer Teil von ihnen nur sehr kleine Mengen fetalen Blutes in ihren Kreislauf aufgenommen hat. In unseren Experimenten hatten wir mit 0,5 bzw. 1,0 ml Rh-positiven Nabelschnurblutes gearbeitet und damit einwandfrei Rh-Sensibilisierungen erzielt. Wir prüfen zur Zeit experimentell, ob auch noch nach Injektion von 0,1 ml Rh+ Nabelschnurblut eine Sensibilisierung gegen den Faktor D erfolgt ist. Es muß aber auch die Möglichkeit offenbleiben, daß der Organismus post partum anders reagiert als der der nichtschwangeren Frau. Deshalb wird der statistisch sichere Beweis, ob die vorgeschlagene und jetzt von uns durchgeführte Prophylaxe wirksam ist, erst dann erbracht sein, wenn ca. 600–700 Patientinnen der geschützten und der nichtgeschützten Gruppe wiederum ein Rh-positives Kind zur Welt bringen. In der nichtgeschützten Gruppe müßten sich ca. 12% Kinder mit einem Rh-bedingten Morbus haemolyticus neonarum finden, und in der mit Serum geschützten Frauengruppe dürfte bei den nächsten Kindern diese Erkrankung nicht auftreten. Nur unter dieser Bedingung kann man die Serum-Prophylaxe einer rh-negativen Mutter nach Geburt eines Rh-positiven Kindes empfehlen, falls sie bei der Entbindung die für eine Sensibilisierung erforderliche Mindestmenge fetaler Erythrozyten aufgenommen hat.

* Anm. b. Korrektur: Unterdessen wurde eine Sensibilisierung bei einer nicht mit Serum behandelten Frau in der nächsten Schwangerschaft nachgewiesen.

Literatur: 1 Woodrow J. C., C. A. Clarke, W. T. Donohoe, R. Finn, R. B. McConnel, P. M. Sheppard, D. Lehane, S. H. Russel, W. Kulke u. C. M. Durkin: Brit. Med. J. *1965/I*, 279. — 2 Kleihauer E. u. G. Brandt: Klin. Wschr. *42*, 458 (1964). — 3 Schneider J. u. G. Schoof: Zbl. Gynäk. *86*, 1829 (1964). — 4 Betke K. u. E. Kleihauer: Blut *4*, 241 (1958). — 5 Cohen F., W. W. Zuelzer u. M. M. Evans: Blood *15*, 884 (1960). — 6 Cohen F., W. W. Zuelzer u. D. C. Gustafson: Blood *23*, 621 (1964). — 7 Zipurski A., J. Pollock, P. Neelands, B. Chown, L. G. Israelis: Lancet *1963/II*, 489. — 8 Schneider J. u. G. A. Ludwig: Klin. Wschr. *41*, 563 (1963). — 9 Schneider J. u. H. Haefele: Klin. Wschr. (im Druck). — 10 Crome P. u. P. L. Mollison: Brit. J. Haemat. *10*, 137 (1964). — 11 Cutbush M. u. P. L. Mollison: Brit. J. Haemat. *4*, 115 (1958). — 12 Hughes-Jones N. C., P. L. Mollison u. N. Veall: Brit. J. Haemat. *3*, 125 (1957). — 13 Jandl J. H. u. M. E. Kaplan: J. Clin. Invest. *39*, 1145 (1960). — 14 Preisler O. u. J. Schneider: Geburtsh. u. Frauenheilk. *24*, 124 (1964). — 15 Schneider J.: Geburtsh. u. Frauenheilk. *23*, 562 (1963). —
Clarke C. A., W. T. Donohoe, R. B. McConnel, J. C. Woodrow, R. Finn, J. R. Krevans, W. Kulke, D. Lehane, P. M. Sheppard: Brit. Med. J. *1963/I*, 979. — Finn R., C. A. Clarke, W. T. Donohoe, R. B. McConnel, P. M. Sheppard, D. Lehane a. W. Kulke: Brit. Med. J. *1961/I*, 1486. — Finn R., D. T. Harper, S. A. Stallings a. J. R. Krevans: Transfusion *3*, 114 (1963). — Freda V. R., J. Gorman a W. Pollack: J. Immunol. Transfus. *4*, 26 (1964). — Krevans J. R.: 10. Kongr. d. intern. Ges. f. Bluttransf. Stockholm (1964). — Lewi S., T. K. Clarke, P. Guéritat, P. Walter et M. Mayer: Bull. Féd. Soc. Gynéc. Obstétr. *13*, 353 (1961). — Wimhöfer H., J. Schneider u. F. Leidenberger: Geburtsh. u. Frauenheilk. *22*, 589 (1962). —

Anschr. d. Verf.: Dozent Dr. O. Preisler und Dr. J. Schneider, Universitäts-Frauenklinik Freiburg im Breisgau, Hugstetterstraße 55.

Papers 32 & 33

32. Clarke, C. A., Donohoe, W. T. A., McConnell. R. B., Woodrow, J. C., Finn, R., Krevans, J. R., Kulke, W., Lehane, D. and Sheppard, P. M. (1963). Further experimental studies on the prevention of Rh haemolytic disease. *Brit Med. J., i,* 979-984.

33. Woodrow, J. C., Clarke, C. A., Donohoe, W. T. A., Finn, R., McConnell, R. B., Sheppard, P. M., Lehane, D., Russell, S. H., Kulke, W. and Durkin, C. M. (1965). Prevention of Rh-haemolytic disease: a third report. *Brit. Med. J., i,* 279-283.

Commentary

After the first suggestion, put forward by Finn in 1960, that it might be possible to prevent Rh immunisation by the giving of an appropriate antibody, three papers dealing with experiments in volunteers were produced by the Liverpool team. The first (Paper 26) dealt largely with clearance of Rh-positive cells by giving predominantly complete (19S) anti-D as serum, and the second (Paper 32) gave (a) the results of this procedure (Experiment 1) and (b) described Experiment 2, in which incomplete or 7S antibody was administered.

In Experiment 1, it was found that compared with control subjects, immunisation appeared to be *enhanced* rather than prevented, and it was surmised that this was because the clearance had been relatively poor, nearly half the injected Rh-positive cells surviving in the circulation for over a week. Subsequent follow-up of the control and treated cases, however, makes it more probable that although they did not succeed in protecting yet in all probability antibody formation was not enhanced.

In Experiment 2 a different approach was tried, namely giving incomplete (7S) anti-D, which it was hoped would block the D antigen sites on the red cells. The idea behind this stemmed from the work of Stern *et al.* (Papers 27 and 28).

The results from Experiment 2 gave a good indication that the Liverpool team was on the right lines, for significant protection occurred and the difference was ascribed to the much better clearance here than in Experiment 1. The injected cells in Experiment 2 were tagged with ^{51}Cr and were shown to go principally to the spleen, in contradistinction to the situation in ABO incompatibility in which the haemolysed cells are taken mainly to the liver, where there are few immunocompetent cells, and this is probably the main reason why ABO incompatibility is protective. Nevertheless, in spite of going to the spleen, the blocked Rh-positive cells did not usually immunise, and on later consideration this was thought to be because the macrophages which trapped them in the spleen were prevented by the coating from processing the cells normally.

In this paper was also described how, through the kindness of Drs W. Pollack, J. G. Gorman and V. J. Freda, the authors were able to test an Ortho anti-D gammaglobulin preparation (RhoGAM), given intramuscularly, and found that it cleared much better than their own high titre serum given intravenously.

Before they could be certain about protection in recently delivered women, they felt that it was important to use fetal blood experimentally, and also to be certain that women volunteers behaved immunologically in the same way as men. This was found to be the case, and the work is described in **Paper 33.**

In this third paper they also reported the fetal cell score in 200 primiparae (random for blood group) who were tested by the Kleihauer/Betke technique both before and after delivery. It was found that the majority of cases of transplacental haemorrhage took place either just before delivery or very shortly afterwards. This was important, because it meant that gammaglobulin given immediately after delivery (or within a day or two of it) was likely to be protective.

Furthermore, it was also found, in a new series of 216 Rh-negative primiparae, that there was a statistically significant relation between the detection of fetal cells in the

33. Commentary cont.

maternal circulation shortly after delivery and subsequent antibody production $(p = 0.005)$.

The outline of the proposed high risk clinical trial was given, and some early results suggested that the team was in fact picking the right cases, since at the time the paper was written three out of the eight controls and none of the six treated had made antibodies. Had the authors been selecting cases at random for fetal cell score it is unlikely that there would have beeen any antibodies at all in such a small number of controls.

The results of this high risk trial follow in the next paper.

From C. A. Clarke et al. (1963). Brit. Med. J., 1, 979-984. Copyright (1963), by kind permission of the authors and the British Medical Association

FURTHER EXPERIMENTAL STUDIES ON THE PREVENTION OF Rh HAEMOLYTIC DISEASE

BY

C. A. CLARKE, M.D., F.R.C.P.

W. T. A. DONOHOE, A.I.M.L.T.

R. B. McCONNELL, M.D., M.R.C.P.

J. C. WOODROW,* M.D., M.R.C.P.

Department of Medicine, University of Liverpool

R. FINN,† M.D., M.R.C.P.

J. R. KREVANS, M.D.

Divisions of Medical Genetics and Haematology, Department of Medicine, Johns Hopkins University and Hospital, Baltimore

W. KULKE, M.B., Ch.B., D.M.R.T.

Radio-isotope Unit, Liverpool Radium Institute

D. LEHANE, M.B., B.Ch.

Liverpool Regional Blood Transfusion Service

AND

P. M. SHEPPARD, M.A., D.Phil.

Department of Genetics, University of Liverpool

In a previous report (Finn *et al.*, 1961) we gave reasons for thinking that the rapid removal of Rh-positive foetal erythrocytes from the circulation of a mother who was Rh-negative would prevent her from becoming immunized and producing Rh antibodies. We have now investigated the matter further, and the present paper describes the completed results of the earlier work (Experiment I) and then gives details of some subsequent observations (Experiments II and III). The reasoning involved and the scope of the investigations are first discussed.

Levine (1943) demonstrated the marked degree of protection against Rh haemolytic disease afforded by ABO incompatibility between mother and foetus. We agreed with Race and Sanger (1950) that the probable mechanism lay in the rapid destruction of the incompatible foetal cells in the circulation by the anti-A and anti-B. Experiment I was therefore designed to determine whether immunization resulting from injection of ABO compatible Rh-positive blood into Rh-negative male volunteers could be prevented by the infusion of plasma containing high-titre saline-reacting (*complete*) anti-D antibodies, simulating the effect of anti-A and anti-B. Some initial results of this experiment have been briefly reported (Finn *et al.*, 1962). It was found that, compared with control subjects, antibody formation was enhanced rather than prevented and we noted that in some cases nearly half the injected cells survived in the circulation for over a week, though at that time free complete anti-D could be detected in the recipients' sera.

On the basis of these results a second approach which forms the substance of Experiment II was tried. Stern *et al.* (1961) had shown that prior *in vitro* coating of Rh-positive erythrocytes with *incomplete* anti-D would prevent antibody formation after subsequent injection

*Now Research Fellow, Johns Hopkins Hospital, Baltimore.
†Now Senior Medical Registrar, Sefton General Hospital, Liverpool.

into Rh-negative males. It was thought that the mechanism operating here might be the complete blocking of the D-antigen sites by incomplete antibody. Mollison (1959) had shown that this was associated with the rapid clearing of such cells from the circulation. Our experiment thus involved the use of plasma containing high titres of incomplete anti-D antibodies and a study of its effectiveness in preventing Rh immunization by previously injected Rh-positive blood.

Further studies were carried out in Baltimore (Experiment III) to elucidate the relationships between differing amounts and types of Rh antibody, the rapidity of clearance of injected Rh-positive cells, and subsequent immunization.

Materials and Methods

The experiments were carried out on groups of Rh-negative male volunteers. Those in Liverpool were blood donors and those in Baltimore were inmates of the Maryland State Penitentiary. The method of giving the blood and plasma was the same as that described in Finn *et al.* (1961).

In Experiments I and II the men were dealt with in groups of six; as a rule, three received 5 ml. of Rh-positive blood and then half an hour later were given the antibody-containing plasma, while the other three received only the Rh-positive blood and thus acted as controls. The details of what was given to each of the 24 men in Experiment I are shown in Table I and to each of the 42 men in Experiment II in Table II. It was the aim in the second experiment to use 50 ml. of plasma with a high titre of incomplete antibody, thus attempting to achieve rapid clearance of injected blood, but because of practical difficulties this dose was not always possible.

TABLE I.—*Details of Volume and Type of Anti-D Sera Used in Experiment I*

Group	Volunteer No.	1st Stimulus			2nd Stimulus		
		Volume (ml.)	Titre		Volume (ml.)	Titre	
			Saline	Albumin		Saline	Albumin
L.I	1, 2, and 3	10	128	128	10	1,024	1,024
	4, 5, and 6	Nil	—	—	Nil	—	—
L.II	1, 2, and 3	20	512	512	20	64	64
	4, 5, and 6	Nil	—	—	Nil	—	—
L.III	1, 2, 3, and 4	20	512	512	20	64	64
	5 and 6	Nil	—	—	Nil	—	—
L.IV	1, 2, and 3	20	0	16	15	64	64
	4, 5, and 6	Nil	—	—	Nil	—	—

Notes.—The volume of Rh-positive blood given at each stimulus was 5 ml. In L.I the Rh type was CDe cde and in L.II, III, and IV it was cDE cde. There was an interval of about three months between the two stimuli. L.III 4 did not receive a second stimulus. Groups L.III and IV received two doses of 10 ml. of antiserum with a week between the doses except for L.III 3, whose first dose was 5 ml. of antiserum.

In the further clearance studies of Experiment III the men were again dealt with in groups of six, but instead of matching " treated " subjects with controls three were given 10 ml. and the other three 50 ml. of the same plasma 20 minutes after the blood. Most of the subjects were given 5 ml. of Rh-positive blood, but 10 ml. was used in a few instances to see if this amount could be cleared as rapidly as 5 ml. The details of what each volunteer received are shown in Table III. The main purpose of these studies was to obtain information on how to clear Rh-positive cells from the circulation quickly, but the subjects were also tested for the development of immune antibodies to obtain more detailed information on the relationship between clearance and subsequent immunization.

TABLE II.—*Details of Rh Type of Blood Given to all Six Men in each Group, and Titre of Anti-D Sera Given to Three " Treated " Men in each Group at each Stimulus in Experiment II*

Group and Volunteer Nos.	1st Stimulus			2nd Stimulus			3rd Stimulus			4th Stimulus		
	Rh Type	Anti-D Titres		Rh Type	Anti-D Titres		Rh Type	Anti-D Titres		Rh Type	Anti-D Titres	
		Saline	Albumin		Saline	Albumin		Saline	Albumin		Saline	Albumin
L.V 1–6 ..	CDe'cde	0	8	CDe'cde	0	8	CDe cde	0	512	CDe cde	0	256
L.VI 1–6 ..	CDe cde	1	16	CDe'cde	1	2,048	cDE'cde	0	1,024	—	—	—
L.VII 1–6 ..	CDe cde	1	128	CDe cde	2	2,048	cDE cde	0	256	—	—	—
L.VIII 1–6 ..	CDe'cDE	2	1,024	cDE'cde	2	1,024	CDe cde	1	512	cDE'cde	0	1,024
L.IX 1–6 ..	CDe cDE	1	512	cDE'cde	4	512	CDe cde	2	1,024	cDE cde	0	512
B.I 1–6 ..	CDe cde	2	1,024*	CDe cDE	0	128*	CDe cDE	1	1,024*	CDe CDe	0	512*
B.II 1–6 ..	cDE'cde	2	512*	CDe.cDE	0	256*	CDe'cDE	0	2,048*	CDe.CDe	0	256*

* In groups B.I and B.II the incomplete titre was measured by the quantitative indirect Coombs test and not in albumin.

Notes.—The volume of Rh-positive blood given at each stimulus was 5 ml. The volume of anti-D given to the three " treated " men (Nos. 1, 2, and 3) in each group was 50 ml. at each stimulus until immune antibody developed, with the following exceptions: group L.VIII received 35 ml. at first stimulus; L.VII 1 received only 30 ml. at his second stimulus; L.VIII 3 received 36 ml. at his first stimulus; and B.II 2 received 44 ml. at his first stimulus. The time interval between stimuli varied from two to five months, but was usually three months, with the exception of groups B.I and B.II, where it was usually about one month.

TABLE III.—*Volume and Titre of Anti-D Given to Men in Experiment III*

Group	Volunteer Nos.	Volume of Anti-D (ml.)	1st Stimulus Anti-D Titre		2nd Stimulus Anti-D Titre		3rd Stimulus Anti-D Titre		4th Stimulus Anti-D Titre	
			Saline	I.C.T.	Saline	I.C.T.	Saline	I.C.T.	Saline	I.C.T.
B.III {	1, 2, and 3	50	8	1,024	1	512	0	1,024	0	256
	4, 5, and 6	10								
B.IV {	1, 2, and 3	50	0	8	0	64	64	1,024	4	1,024
	4, 5, and 6	10								
B.V {	1, 2, and 3	50	1	8	1	4	128	2,048	128	2,048
	4, 5, and 6	10								
B.VI {	1 and 2	50	2	512	0	256	0	2,048		
	3 and 4	10								
	5 and 6	Nil	—	—	—	—	—	—		
B.VII {	1, 2, and 3	50	32	512	1	1,024				
	4, 5, and 6	Nil	—	—	—	—				

Notes.—The Rh type of blood given was CDe'cDE in all groups and at each stimulus with the exception of B.III at the third stimulus, B.IV at the second and third stimuli, and B.VI at the first stimulus, when it was cDE/cde. The volume of Rh-positive blood injected was 5 ml. in groups B.III, B.IV, and B.V and 10 ml. in groups B.VI and B.VII. The time interval between stimuli varied from four to eight weeks, but was usually six weeks. Volunteers B.V 4 and 5 and B.VI 4 did not receive any anti-D serum at their second, third, and fourth stimuli. Volunteer B.VI 3 received 10 ml. anti-D at first stimulus and 50 ml. at second and third stimuli. Volunteers B.VI 1 and 5 received only the first stimulus. Volunteer B.V 2 received only two stimuli.

The anti-D-containing plasma was obtained either from immunized women or from our male volunteers who had become immunized during the course of the experiments. In all the Baltimore and many of the Liverpool studies, the Rh-positive cells were tagged with ^{51}Cr so that it was possible to tell how rapidly the cells had been removed from the circulation. At various times after an initial four-weeks period blood was taken and examined for the presence of immune anti-D. If it was not detected a further injection of Rh-positive blood was given followed by antibody in the " treated " groups of volunteers.

In some cases where the larger volumes of plasma containing high titres of incomplete antibody were used, the persistence of passive immunity was observed for many weeks. By following the titre of this antibody and by testing for the presence of saline antibodies it was always possible eventually to distinguish between passive and active immunization.

Results

Experiment I

Table IV shows the results in the four groups of men who received 5 ml. of Rh-positive blood followed by 10–20 ml. of plasma and in their controls. It can be seen that 8 out of the 13 volunteers receiving anti-D and 1 out of the 11 controls produced immune anti-D after two stimulations. One of the " treated " volunteers (L.III 4) withdrew after the first stimulus and before he could be followed up for antibody formation. Excluding this case, the data can be arranged as a 2×2 table, giving the number of volunteers who did and did not become immunized in the treated and control groups. Using Fisher's exact test for such tables and taking into account both tails of the distribution, we found that the

probability of getting by chance alone a difference between the two groups as great as or greater than that observed is 0.01.

Thus this experiment provides strong evidence that administering 10–20 ml. of these particular plasmas

TABLE IV.—*Immune Antibody Formation (A) in Experiment I, and Results of ^{51}Cr Studies Where These Were Carried Out (See Also Table I)*

Group and Volunteer Numbers	Percentage of Rh-positive Cells Surviving 48 Hours after Injection	
	1st Stimulus	2nd Stimulus
L.I { 1	13 A	
2	48 A	56 A
3	40 A	
4	98	100
5	94	89
6	106	77
L.II { 1	43	—
2	25	—
3	34	—
4	93	—
5	91	—
6	69	—
L.III { 1	53 A	
2	66	66 A
3	36 A	
4	37	*
5	93	—
6	98 A	
L.IV { 1	91	— A
2	91	
3	82 A	
4	79	—
5	82	—
6	90	—

* Volunteer L.III 4 did not receive a second stimulus and was not tested for immune antibody formation.

Note.—In groups L.I, L.II, and L.IV Nos. 1, 2, and 3 were given anti-D and Nos. 4, 5, and 6 were controls. In group L.III Nos. 1–4 were " treated " and Nos. 5 and 6 were controls.

enhances the likelihood of inducing immune antibody formation.

Experiment II

Table V shows the results in the men given 35–50 ml. of plasma containing predominantly incomplete anti-D and in their controls. Three of the 21 treated and 11 of

TABLE V.—*Immune Antibody Formation (A) in Experiment II (See Also Table II) and the Results of ^{51}Cr Studies Where These Were Carried Out. (In the Liverpool Series it Was the Usual Practice from Group L.V. Onwards Only to Tag One " Treated " and One " Untreated " in Each Group)*

Group and Volunteer Nos.	Percentage of Rh-positive Cells Surviving 24 Hours after Injection			
	1st Stimulus	2nd Stimulus	3rd Stimulus	4th Stimulus
L.V 1	3	2	—	4
2	1	0	—	0
3	4	1	—	19
4	98	—	—	—
5	84	—	—	—
6	85	—	— A	—
L.VI 1	43 A	—	—	
2	—	—	24	
3	—	—		
4	101 A	—	—	
5	—	— A		
6	—	—	—	
L.VII 1	2	1	9	
2	—	1	—	
3	—			
4	103 A	—		
5	—	— A		
6	—	— A		
L.VIII 1	2	1	3	1
2	—	—	—	1
3	—	—	—	2
4	98	76 A	—	—
5	—	—	—	73
6	—	—	—	82
L.IX 1	9	1	3	—
2	—	—	—	10
3	—	—	—	A
4	101	98	63	102
5	—	—	—	106
6	—	— A		
B.I 1	6	4	3	2
2	1	5	3	2
3	0	2	7	2
4	98	90	96	60 A
5	93	85 A	94	96
6	95	103	94	96
B.II 1	2	1	2	3
2	9	1	1	4 A
3	2	2	2	2
4	98	13	30	62
5	99	95	97	102
6	97	41	65	83 A

Note.—In all seven groups, Nos. 1, 2, and 3 were given anti-D and Nos. 4, 5, and 6 were controls.

the 21 controls were immunized. Here the exact test shows that the probability of getting by chance alone a difference between the two groups as great as or greater than that observed is 0.02.

This analysis thus indicates that individuals treated with 35–50 ml. of the types of plasma used here are significantly less likely to produce immune antibodies than their controls, in sharp contrast to the results of Experiment I.

Experiment III (Further Clearance Studies)

The results are given in Table VI. It can be seen that the injected cells were most rapidly cleared when the plasma contained predominantly incomplete antibodies.

Fate of Cleared Erythrocytes

In the case of L.V. second stimulus, detailed studies of the clearance rate for the three treated individuals during the first 24 hours were carried out. An antibody showing no saline activity and an albumin titre of 8 was

TABLE VI.—*Results of the ^{51}Cr Studies and Whether or Not Immune Antibodies (A) Had Developed Before the Next Stimulus in Experiment III*

Group and Volunteer Nos.	Percentage of Rh-positive Cells Surviving 24 Hours after Injection			
	1st Stimulus	2nd Stimulus	3rd Stimulus	4th Stimulus
B.III 1	3	0	7	4
2	1	0	15	4
3	1	0	4	3
4	47 A			
5	11	16	26	3 A
6	55	38	54	46 A
B.IV 1	5	1	29 A	
2	1	1	20	1
3	1	1	10	2
4	31	4	75 A	
5	34	5	73	4
6	26 A			
B.V 1	89	86	60	66
2	101	86	—	—
3	94	85	100	94
4	89	101	94	97
5	96	36	61 A	
6	89 A			
B.VI 1	8		2	
2	3	1		
3	11	2	3	
4	26	85	87	
5	106			
6	110	94	102	
B.VII 1	46 A	—		
2	62 A			
3	32	11 A		
4	92 A	—		
5	92	108 A		
6	98	103		

Note.—Details of anti-D dosage are given in Table III.

TABLE VII.—*Results of Studies of Splenic Radioactivity in Volunteers 1, 2, and 3 of Group L.V. at Time of Their Second Injection of 5 ml. Rh-positive Blood Followed by 50 ml. of Anti-D. Results of Heart and Spleen Counts are Expressed as Percentages of Heart Counts One Hour After Injection of Anti-D. Results are Also Given of Counts of Venous Blood Samples Taken at Same Time, These Being Expressed as a Percentage of the Venous Sample Count at Time of Anti-D Injection*

Time after Anti-D Injection	Organ	Volunteer No.		
		1	2	3
– 1 minute	Blood	100	100	100
1 hour	Blood	92	100	83
	Heart	100	100	100
	Spleen	37	25	374
2¼ hours	Blood	84	75	36
	Heart	100	53	55
	Spleen	26	23	498
4 "	Blood	61	50	15
	Heart	135	71	49
	Spleen	56	43	769
5¼ "	Blood	44	33	8
	Heart	78	63	69
	Spleen	41	39	795
24 "	Blood	2	1	0

used. Counts of radioactivity were taken at the same time over the splenic area, and Table VII shows the results obtained. A concentration of radioactivity was found in this area, and in volunteer No. 3 it was remarkably high. We are not sure of the explanation of this, but it may be relevant that, although he was entirely symptomless, his serum bilirubin was 1.5 mg./100 ml. at that time. However, the spleen findings in general tend to support the view that coated cells are principally removed from the circulation by the spleen (see Jandl *et al.*, 1957 ; Mollison, 1959).

Discussion

The main findings in the experiments described were: (1) 10–20 ml. of plasma containing mainly complete anti-D failed to clear rapidly Rh-positive erythrocytes from the blood of Rh-negative male subjects and enhanced the immunization produced by these cells ; and (2) 35–50 ml. of plasma containing chiefly incomplete anti-D usually produced rapid clearing of Rh-positive red cells and considerably suppressed immunization by these cells in Rh-negative male subjects.

The relationship between the various factors may be considered under the following headings: (a) effectiveness of various anti-D antibodies in clearing injected Rh-positive cells from the circulation ; (b) relationship between the clearance rate of such cells and subsequent immunization ; and (c) relationship between differing amounts and types of anti-D antibody and subsequent immunization.

Antibody and Clearance.—Considering only the men treated with 35–50 ml. of plasma, it can be seen that in general when the plasma contained more than a trace of complete antibody only partial clearance was obtained in the first 24 hours. Rapid clearance was occasionally brought about by quite low-titre plasmas if they had no complete component—for example, L.V, first and second stimuli, and B.IV, first stimulus—but where there was more than a trace of saline activity a very high titre of incomplete antibody was needed to obtain satisfactory clearance—for example, B.III, first stimulus. Where the saline titre was more than 16, a good clearance was not found even if the incomplete titre was very high—for example, B.IV, third stimulus, and B.V, third and fourth stimuli.

Clearance of Injected Red Cells and Immunization.—Only those subjects in whom ^{51}Cr-labelled cells were followed for survival can give any information on this point. On examining the data in Tables IV, V, and VI it is obvious that immune antibody did not appear in most of the men in whom good clearance of the Rh-positive cells was obtained each time they were injected. Conversely, immunization occurred in many more of the men in whom only partial clearance was achieved than in those men in whom the cells were allowed to survive normally. This is shown in Table VIII. The data suggest that immunization is nearly always prevented in those volunteers in whom 95% of the injected cells have been cleared within 24 hours. One individual (B.II 2) developed antibodies in spite of good

TABLE VIII.—*Relationship Between Speed of Removal of 5 ml. of Injected Rh-positive Cells from Circulation and Whether or Not Immune Antibodies Developed*

R.B.C. Survival Score†	First Stimulus Only			Four Stimuli*		
	No. of Men	Developing Antibodies		No. of Men	Developing Antibodies	
		No.	%		No.	%
0–10	18	0	0	11	1	9·1
10–75	17	7	41·2	11	8	72·7
75–100	32	5	15·6	8	3	37·5

* An R.B.C. survival score has been calculated for each man in groups B.I.–B.V. by averaging the percentages of red cells remaining in the circulation 24 hours after each stimulus.
† Survival scores were grouped into the three categories after examination of the data had shown that the critical 24-hour level for protection might be 10%.

clearance rates on four successive occasions, but it might be important that 9% of the injected cells of the first stimulus survived 24 hours.

Immunization and Amount and Type of Antibody Used.—From a consideration of all the Tables it can be seen that when plasma containing a high titre of complete antibody was used several of the men became immunized (group L.I–III). When 10-ml. volumes were used, even though the anti-D was predominantly

incomplete but had some complete component, immunization often occurred (B.III–V). In the case of B.IV 1, who received at the third stimulus 50 ml. of plasma with a high titre of incomplete antibody but also showing considerable saline activity, the injection was followed by antibody formation. Only where the anti-D given had no activity in saline and was given in volumes of 35–50 ml. did most of the men obtain protection against immunization. As might be expected, the titre of such an antibody appeared to influence the result—for example, the use of 50 ml. of plasma with a weak incomplete anti-D in L.VI at the first stimulus was followed by the development of antibodies in one of the three men.

From the analysis of the data we interpret: (1) That any complete antibody in the plasma used is likely to enhance rather than prevent sensitization. (2) That plasma containing only incomplete antibody if given in volumes of 35–50 ml. will usually prevent immunization. Although there is not a clear relationship between the titre of such an antibody and immunization it would appear safer to use the highest titre antibody possible if immunization is regularly to be suppressed.

Some Immunological Problems

Red-cell Survival in Controls.—In most cases the first injection of Rh-positive cells into our controls was followed by normal survival of the cells with gradual clearance over a period of three months. Subsequent injections also had, in general, normal survival if no immune antibodies had developed. But in common with other workers (see Mollison, 1959) we occasionally found reduced survival time without demonstrable antibody. Two non-identical twins (B.V 5 and 6) had normal survival times with the first stimulus, and immune anti-D was subsequently detected in B.V 6 six weeks later. At the second stimulus both twins showed a marked and equal reduction in the survival time of the donor cells, but at the end of a further six weeks immune anti-D could not be detected in B.V 5 either by ourselves or by two other laboratories. A third stimulus was given and B.V 5 again had a reduced survival time, and on retesting six weeks later immune anti-D was detected for the first time. A similar situation occurred in B.II 4 and 6, in whom reduced survival times were demonstrated with their second, third, and fourth stimuli, again suggesting immunization. Immune antibody was finally demonstrated in B.II 6 five months after the fourth stimulus, but not in B.II 4. If this immunological state (reduced red-cell survival time without demonstrable antibody) had occurred in our " treated " series we should not have detected it, as their ^{51}Cr studies were always affected by the anti-D serum they had received. To safeguard against the late development of antibody (as in B.II 6) all subjects were retested about five months after their last stimulus.

Mechanisms of Protection and Enhancement.—The data presented are compatible with the hypothesis that incomplete anti-D prevents immunization by coating the red-cell surface and thus blocking the Rh antigen sites (Stern et al., 1961). The protection afforded by ABO incompatibility clearly cannot be due to the same mechanism, and Stern et al. (1961) have suggested that this may be due to a " clonal competition for antigen."

The enhancement of immunization by saline antibodies is more difficult to explain, although similar phenomena have been observed in other animal systems (see Cohen and Allton, 1962). We suggest as tentative hypotheses either that cells coated with saline antibody are dealt with at a different site in the reticulo-endothelial system at which, perhaps, immunization is more liable to occur ; or that the layer of complete antibody is more easily removed from the red-cell surface. In the latter case the saline anti-D would simply attract the Rh-positive cells to the reticulo-endothelial system, and then break off, leaving large numbers of partially coated cells in contact with immunologically competent cells.

Prevention of Rh Haemolytic Disease

Our previous studies (Finn *et al.*, 1961) suggested that Rh immunization was most likely to occur with " large " transplacental haemorrhages of foetal blood—that is, greater than 1 ml.—and bleeds of this size occur more commonly during delivery. On the other hand, we have observed occasional bleeds of the same order of magnitude to occur during pregnancy, and these probably account for a certain percentage of cases of primary immunization. There is also evidence (Kristoffersen *et al.*, 1962) that minute bleeds are not uncommon during the course of pregnancy, and it remains to be seen whether these are capable of inducing antibody formation in susceptible individuals or whether there is a critical size of bleed below which immunization is unlikely. On the whole we think that the evidence points to the fact that the majority of bleeds sufficient to cause immunization *do* occur during labour, and operative trauma at this time has been shown to increase their incidence (Wimhöfer *et al.*, 1962). If this be confirmed, then the present approach to the prevention of immunization by the use of incomplete Rh antibody could contribute considerably towards the prevention of Rh immunization, the antibody being given to an Rh-negative mother after the delivery of an Rh-positive child if foetal cells are demonstrated in her circulation.

Further Work Proposed

We are not entirely happy about giving whole plasma or serum, since it is not without risk of producing hepatitis. This difficulty can be overcome by using a concentrated gamma-globulin preparation containing only incomplete anti-D antibodies. We tested such a preparation and found that 5 ml. given intramuscularly was much more powerful in producing clearance than 50 ml. of high-titre antiserum given intravenously. As well as ease of administration and freedom from the risk of producing serum hepatitis, this technique has the advantage of reducing to negligible proportions the risk of enhancing immunization, because in the preparation of the gamma-globulin an adequate titre and lack of saline activity can be ensured.

Another aspect to be investigated is the delaying of the anti-D injection up to 48 hours after the Rh-positive blood, to see if immunization can still be prevented ; this is particularly important, since it is the situation which is apt to occur in hospital practice.

So far our experiments have only been in Rh-negative men using adult Rh-positive blood. We feel that it is essential now to find out if foetal blood can be cleared equally well and also to use sterile female volunteers, preferably pre-menopausal. If this is as successful as in the men we think that the evidence will be strong enough to try the technique on Rh-negative women who are having their first Rh-positive baby and in whom transplacental haemorrhage has occurred.

Summary

The results are described of experiments involving the injection of Rh-positive blood into 96 Rh-negative men

and designed to find out whether or not the production of immune anti-D can be prevented.

Giving 10–20 ml. of anti-D sera containing high titres of complete antibody half an hour after the Rh-positive blood, we found that only about 50% of the injected cells had been cleared within 48 hours and immune anti-D production was enhanced as compared with controls, who received only the Rh-positive blood.

Using 35–50 ml. of plasma containing predominantly incomplete antibodies, we found that only 3 out of 21 " treated " men developed immune antibodies after three or four stimuli as compared with 11 out of 21 control men, the difference being statistically significant ($P=0.02$).

Examination of these results and those of other experiments which are described suggests that about 95% of the injected cells have to be cleared from the circulation within 24 hours if immune antibody production is to be prevented. The anti-D antibody most likely to be effective in this should have no saline activity and as high an incomplete titre as possible.

Preliminary work with anti-D gamma-globulin given intramuscularly has shown that in appropriate dosage it is even more effective in rapidly clearing Rh-positive cells than the most powerful plasma we have used.

Before the stage is reached at which a clinical application of the technique in recently delivered Rh-negative women is justifiable, additional experiments are indicated and these are outlined. We are hopeful, however, that the technique will prevent most cases of Rh immunization and thus in time help to eliminate Rh haemolytic disease of the newborn.

We would first like to thank the Liverpool blood donors who volunteered for the experimental studies and who have so willingly attended for venesection on many occasions ; we are similarly grateful to the inmates of the Maryland State Penitentiary. We are indebted to Professor V. A. McKusick, Dr. R. R. Race, Dr. Ruth Sanger, Dr. A. E. Mourant, Dr. I. Dunsford, Dr. J. Shone, Dr. E. A. Murphy, and Miss Sarah Stallings for advice and help at various stages of this investigation. We are also grateful to Dr. W. Pollock, of the Ortho Research Foundation, and to Dr. J. Gorman and Dr. V. Freda, of Columbia University, for allowing us to test a sample of high-titre anti-D in the form of gamma-globulin. Our thanks are due to the medical and nursing staffs of the Maryland State Penitentiary, the Liverpool Regional Blood Transfusion Service, the Mersey Docks and Harbour Board, and the Dunlop Rubber Company Ltd., Liverpool, for much co-operation ; and to Mrs. Ruth Harris, Miss Maureen Shannon, and Miss Sheila Manning for great help with the field work and secretarial assistance. This work has been made possible by grants from the Research Committee of the United Liverpool Hospitals, under the chairmanship of Lord Cohen of Birkenhead, the Medical Research Council, the Nuffield Foundation, and the National Institutes of Health, U.S. Public Health Service.

REFERENCES

Cohen, C., and Allton, W. H. (1962). *Nature (Lond.)*, **193**, 990.
Finn, R., Clarke, C. A., Donohoe, W. T. A., McConnell, R. B., Sheppard, P. M., Lehane, D., and Kulke, W. (1961). *Brit. med. J.*, **1**, 1486.
—— McConnell, R. B., Woodrow, J. C., Kulke, W., Lehane, D., and Sheppard, P. M. (1962). *Nature (Lond.)*, **193**, 990.
Jandl, J. H., Jones, R. A., and Castle, W. B. (1957). *J. clin. Invest.*, **36**, 1428.
Kristoffersen, K., Jensen, K. G., and Felbo, M. (1962). *Dan. med. Bull.*, **9**, 203.
Levine, P. (1943). *J. Hered.*, **34**, 71.
Mollison, P. L. (1959). *Brit. med. J.*, **2**, 1035, 1123.
Race, R. R., and Sanger, R. (1950). *Blood Groups in Man*, 1st ed., p. 290. Blackwell, Oxford.
Stern, K., Goodman, H. S., and Berger, M. (1961). *J. Immunol.*, **87**, 189.
Wimhöfer, H. von, Schneider, J., and Leidenberger, F. (1962). *Geburtsh. u. Frauenheilk.*, **22**, 589.

From J. C. Woodrow et al. (1965). Brit. Med. J., 1, 279-283. Copyright (1965), by kind permission of the authors and the British Medical Association

30 January 1965

Prevention of Rh-Haemolytic Disease: A Third Report

J. C. WOODROW,* M.D., M.R.C.P.; C. A. CLARKE,* M.D., SC.D., F.R.C.P.; W. T. A. DONOHOE,* A.I.M.L.T.;
R. FINN,* M.D., M.R.C.P.; R. B. McCONNELL,* M.D., M.R.C.P.; P. M. SHEPPARD,† M.A., D.PHIL.;
D. LEHANE,‡ M.B., B.CH., F.C.PATH.; SHONA H. RUSSELL,§ M.B., B.CH., M.R.C.O.G.;
W. KULKE,‖ M.B., B.CH., D.M.R.T.; CATHERINE M. DURKIN,¶ M.B., B.CH., D.C.H.

Brit. med. J., 1965, 1, 279-283

In two papers (Finn *et al.*, 1961; Clarke *et al.*, 1963) we described experiments which were successful in preventing Rh immunization in Rh-negative male volunteers. The basis of the procedure was to remove rapidly from the circulation previously injected chromium-tagged Rh-positive red cells by giving high-titre incomplete anti-D either as an infusion of plasma or as gamma$_2$-globulin. In our second paper we stated that the next steps should be to find out whether foetal red cells could be cleared equally well as adult and whether female volunteers could be protected in the same way as men. The results of experiments to test these points form the first part (I) of the present paper. The second part (II) concerns two factors of great importance in the application of the technique to preventing Rh immunization due to pregnancy. These are the frequency with which transplacental haemorrhage from foetus to mother occurs during pregnancy as distinct from at delivery, and the relation of the production of immune antibodies to the size of transplacental haemorrhage assessed after delivery. In the third part of the paper (III) we discuss some of the details of the clinical trial, recently started in Liverpool, of anti-D gamma$_2$-globulin injection given to Rh-negative women after delivery.

I. Clearance of Rh-positive Foetal Cells in Women and its Relation to the Production of Immune Anti-D

Material and Methods.—Ten female Rh-negative blood-donor volunteers (all nulliparous and post-menopausal) took part in the experiment. Each was injected intravenously with 5 ml. of Rh-positive ABO-compatible foetal blood obtained from the umbilical veins of three babies. The actual Rh genotype of the injected blood varied on different occasions. Survival of the Rh-positive foetal cells was measured either by tagging them with ^{51}Cr or by using the Kleihauer acid-elution technique, which enables foetal cells to be demonstrated and counted among a population of adult red cells (Kleihauer and Betke, 1960). We counted the number of foetal cells in 50 low-power fields (diameter 940 μ) in each of two slides, and the average of the two counts was taken as the foetal-cell score. Where this resulted in a fraction the next higher digit was taken as the score. Half an hour after the injection of the Rh-positive red cells five of the volunteers received an intramuscular injection of 5 ml. of gamma$_2$-globulin prepared by the Blood Products Laboratory of the Lister Institute from the pooled sera of 11 hyperimmunized male volunteers. The anti-D titre of this gamma$_2$-globulin was 1 in 262,000 by the indirect Coombs test. The remaining five females acted as controls and received no antibody. The procedure was repeated three and six months later. Serum was obtained from the subjects at these times and again at least six months after the last stimulus, and was tested for the presence of complete and incomplete immune antibodies.

Results

The results are shown in Table I, from which it will be seen that in each of the treated volunteers the foetal cells were rapidly cleared from the circulation by the anti-D gamma$_2$-globulin. In the controls, on the other hand, the foetal scores generally remained much higher, though there are some results

* Nuffield Unit of Medical Genetics, Department of Medicine, University of Liverpool.
† Department of Genetics, University of Liverpool.
‡ Liverpool Regional Blood Transfusion Service.
§ Department of Obstetrics and Gynaecology, University of Liverpool.
‖ Radio-isotope Unit, Liverpool Radium Institute.
¶ Paediatric Registrar, Sefton General Hospital, Liverpool.

TABLE I.—*Clearance of Rh-positive ABO-compatible Foetal Blood by Incomplete Anti-D Gamma$_2$-globulin in Ten Rh-negative, Nulliparous, Post-menopausal, Female Volunteers (Two Series)*

	Treated			Controls			Treated		Controls		
Case No.:	1	2	3	4	5		6	7	8	9	10
Vol. anti-D gamma$_2$-globulin after each stimulus	5 ml.	5 ml.	5 ml.	0	0		5 ml.	5 ml.	0	0	0
First Stimulus : Percentage of Rh+ Cells Remaining (5 ml. = 100%)											
24/7/63: 5 ml. Rh+ foetal blood — ^{51}Cr (24 hr) / ^{51}Cr (48 hr)	3·1% / 0·1%	1·0% / 0·3%	3·8% / 0·0%	96·0% / 97·0%	N.T. / 67·0%	8/10/63: ^{51}Cr (48 hr) / ^{51}Cr (7 days)	0·8% / 0·2%	3·0% / 0·7%	84·4% / 76·0%	68·8% / 60·0%	79·5% / 64·5%
Immune-antibody formation (tested 19/11/63)	—	—	—	—	—	Tested (14/1/64)	—	—	—	—	—
Second Stimulus : Percentage of Rh+ Cells Remaining (5 ml. = 100%)											
19/11/63: 5 ml. Rh+ foetal blood	^{51}Cr results unreliable because of technical difficulties					14/1/64: ^{51}Cr (48 hr) / Kleihauer (48 hr.) / ^{51}Cr (8 days)	1·2% / 0·0%	2·8% / 0·0%	43·7% / 43·5%	N.T. / N.T. / 0·8%	89·1% / 86·7%
Immune-antibody formation (tested 3/3/64)	—	—	—	—	—	(Tested 7/4/64)	—	—	—	—	—
Third Stimulus : Percentage of Rh+ Cells Remaining (5 ml. = 100%)											
3/3/64: 5 ml. of Rh+ foetal blood — ^{51}Cr (48 hr.) / Kleihauer (48 hr.)	*	0·6% / 0·0%	0·8% / 0·0%	56·0% / 70·0%	1·8% / 0·0%	7/4/64: ^{51}Cr (48 hr.) / Kleihauer (48 hr.) / Kleihauer (9 days)	8·7% / 0·0%	0·1% / 0·0%	100·0% / 62·2%	4·0% / 37·1%	N.T. / N.T. / 85·7%
Immune-antibody formation (tested 10/11/64)	N.T.	—	—	—	—	(Tested 10/11/64)	—	—	—	†	—

* Left U.K. temporarily.   † Immune anti-D found.   N.T. = Not tested.

which are difficult to interpret. Thus in the controls there was, on occasion, a striking loss of foetal cells—for example, Case 5, third stimulus, and possibly Case 9, second and third stimuli. The reason for this finding is quite unknown, but it has been observed before, both by us and by other workers, and has sometimes been associated with the later production of antibody. In these two instances, however, no antibody has so far been produced. There are also two cases where the foetal-cell score was lower than expected—for example, Case 4, third stimulus, and Case 8, second stimulus. In the latter the third stimulus showed no similar drop, but the volunteer subsequently produced antibody. Again we have no explanation for this, but red-cell survival is a difficult subject and it is well known that many problems remain unsolved.

In both treated and control groups there was reasonable correspondence between the ^{51}Cr figures and those for the Kleihauer test, though there was one notable exception (control, Case 9, third stimulus) where we believe that the ^{51}Cr result may have been at fault because of the low initial dosage of the isotope.

It will be seen that in this experiment there was no suggestion of any enhancement of immune antibody production such as occurred in our earlier work when we used complete antibody in treatment (see Finn *et al.*, 1961). The only antibody produced was by one of the controls, and this is consistent with protection.

II. Frequency With Which Transplacental Haemorrhage Occurs During Pregnancy as Distinct From at Delivery, and the Relation of the Production of Immune Antibodies to the Size of Transplacental Haemorrhage Assessed After Delivery

The success or otherwise of preventing Rh-haemolytic disease by giving anti-D gamma$_2$-globulin after delivery depends on several factors, a crucial one being the time in pregnancy at which the transplacental haemorrhage occurs. Our view expressed in the earlier papers was that the majority of bleeds of sufficient size to cause immunization occur during labour, and we produced evidence in support of this. On the other hand, more recently, Cohen *et al.* (1964) and Cohen and Zuelzer (1964) expressed an entirely contrary opinion. The object of their first paper was to establish baseline data on transplacental haemorrhage in ABO-compatible pregnancies in unsensitized women. In 622 of such women foetal cells were demonstrated immediately post partum in about 50% of cases, and in about 10% of the series foetal losses, ranging from an estimated 0.5 ml. to 40 ml., were observed from examination of patients both before and after labour. Although the incidence of transplacental haemorrhage was higher after delivery than before, the authors did not think this indicated that delivery as such played an important part in producing transplacental haemorrhage. Furthermore, they were of the opinion that transplacental haemorrhage usually began well before the onset of labour.

In their second paper they investigated 127 Rh-negative mothers with respect to the production of antibody in relation to transplacental haemorrhage. Eight patients were found to have developed antibody, and four of these showed no foetal cells and four a transplacental haemorrhage at delivery of less than 1 ml. In 13 of their cases in which greater numbers of foetal cells were present at delivery no antibodies were found. However, they recorded the development of immune anti-D in two cases where massive transplacental haemorrhage had occurred but did not relate these to the study they were reporting. They conclude that their findings do not support " the current speculation that massive invasions of the maternal blood by fetal cells during labor is [*sic*] usually responsible for the sensitization of Rh-mothers, which concept has already led to efforts to suppress this hypothetical effect." An important criticism of their paper is that they do not state whether

the 127 mothers included multiparae as well as primiparae, and this is referred to again in the discussion.

We now have more data on the timing of transplacental haemorrhage and its relation to subsequent immunization.

(1) Timing of Transplacental Haemorrhage in Relation to Labour

We examined for foetal cells samples of blood from 200 mothers (random for blood group) before and after parturition, the " before " samples being taken anything from a few hours to a few days before the onset of labour and the " after " ones within 48 hours of it. Table II gives the results, and it will be

TABLE II.—*Timing of Transplacental Haemorrhage in Relation to Labour*

Time When Foetal Cells Found		Foetal-cell Score			
Before Delivery	After Delivery	<5	5–60	>60	Total
Present	Present	16	2	1	19
Absent	Present	26	10	4	40
Present	Absent	5	—	1*	6
Absent	Absent	—	—	—	135
Total		47	12	6	200

* In this case numerous foetal cells were seen, some in small clumps, in a sample six days before labour, but none were seen post partum.

seen that in 135 cases no foetal cells were observed either before or after delivery. In about two-thirds of the cases (40 out of 59) where foetal cells were detected after delivery they had not been present just before. In 19 out of the 59 cases, foetal cells were present both before and after delivery, but in four of these the number of cells was appreciably greater after parturition. In only six cases were foetal cells present before delivery and absent afterwards. Unfortunately we do not know the ABO blood group of the babies, but the data are still informative.

Bleeds which have occurred early in pregnancy may no longer be present in our pre-delivery sample if the baby is ABO-incompatible with the mother. On the other hand, if they have occurred at delivery, they may still be present in the after-delivery specimens, as some of these were taken very soon after the birth of the baby. This biases the data slightly by magnifying the importance of labour as a cause of transplacental haemorrhage. However, in the pre-delivery specimens there will be an accumulation of foetal cells deriving from the ABO-compatible cases, and this will argue in the opposite direction by minimizing the importance of labour as a cause of transplacental haemorrhage. Although we cannot allow for the two opposing biases we can say categorically that in the 59 samples of blood where foetal cells were present after delivery 40 of the haemorrhages had occurred during labour (or at any rate after the date of the pre-delivery sampling). In other words, the finding of foetal cells after delivery indicates in two-thirds of our cases that recent transplacental haemorrhage has occurred.

(2) Relation of Transplacental Haemorrhage to Subsequent Immunization

We next, in a new series, consider the relation of transplacental haemorrhage detected after delivery to the subsequent production of immune antibodies, and our work on this is still in progress. Using five Liverpool maternity units, blood samples are being taken from Rh-negative primiparae after delivery and foetal-cell scores made. Where the baby is Rh-positive, samples of serum are then obtained from the mother three and six months later (and wherever possible in a subsequent pregnancy) and tested for antibodies. The results for 216 ABO-compatible pregnancies followed up at three months, and for 126 of these for which information at six months is available, are set out in Table III, which shows that the incidence of immune-antibody formation increases with the number of foetal cells found. However, the subdivisions of the cell count in Table III are arbitrary, and we have therefore presented the data in a more absolute way (Table IV). Here only the presence or absence of foetal cells is considered in relation to antibody formation, and it will be seen that there is a highly

TABLE III.—*Relation of Transplacental Haemorrhage Detected After Delivery to Subsequent Immunization. The Cases are All Rh-negative Primiparae with Rh-positive ABO-compatible Babies*

		Foetal-Cell Count				Total
		0	1–4	5–60	60+	
(a) Tested at Three Months						
Antibody	..	3	4	3	3	13
No antibody	..	132	51	17	3	203
Total	..	135	55	20	6	216
(b) Tested at Six Months						
Antibody	..	4	4	1	2	11
No antibody	..	83	19	12	1	115
Total	..	87	23	13	3	126

(a) All 216 cases have been tested at three months.
(b) Of the 216 cases, 126 have been retested at six months. Although two new antibodies appeared, four cases which had antibodies at three months have not yet been retested at six months, and this is why the total count of antibodies recorded is two less at six months than at three months.

TABLE IV.—*Foetal Cells in Relation to Rh-immune-antibody Formation in 216 ABO-compatible Pregnancies. Tested at Three Months*

Immune Antibodies	Foetal Cells Present After Delivery	Foetal Cells Absent After Delivery	Total
Present	10	3	13
Absent	71	132	203
	81	135	216

P = 0·0053.
If a similar analysis is done for all cases based on the result of the latest test for antibodies carried out in each case—for example, three or six months—the result is even more highly significant (P = 0·0046).

significant relation between the presence of foetal cells in the post-delivery sample and the production of immune antibody ($P=0.0053$ using the test at three months, and $P=0.0046$ using the latest antibody test in each case). The basic data from which these tables are derived are given in the Appendix.

Our information also suggests that there is an increased probability of producing immune antibodies the greater the size of the haemorrhage, and the graph shows the weighted regression of antibody production on foetal-cell score. It will be seen that the y axis (percentage producing antibodies) has been transformed to angles and the x axis (foetal-cell score) to the square root of the cell score. This is because the direct relation between the two parameters was non-linear, but with the square-root transformation the relation became linear or almost linear over the range investigated. The weighted regression of antibody production on foetal-cell score is highly significant ($P<0.001$).

It will be seen from Table III that three patients developed immune antibodies even though we detected no foetal cells. We do not know (a) whether we failed to detect cells which were in fact present, (b) whether the cells had already disappeared after an ante-partum transplacental haemorrhage, or (c) whether immunization was due to some cause other than the trans-placental haemorrhage. We do not believe that the last-mentioned possibility is at all likely, and only further study of successive samples throughout pregnancy will decide how often foetal cells disappear during the ante-partum period.

Data on ABO incompatibility in relation to Rh-antibody formation are given in Table V. They show the incidence of antibody formation in our series when the pregnancies are divided according to whether or not the foetus is ABO-compatible with the mother. It will be seen that at three months no mother whose baby was incompatible on the ABO system has produced Rh antibodies. This finding is in agree-

ment with all previous work, demonstrating the protection afforded by ABO incompatibility as first noticed by Levine (1943).

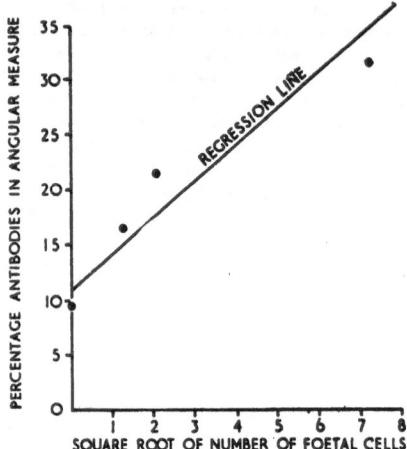

Weighted regression of the incidence of antibody formation on foetal-cell score. Regression coefficient b equals 3.24 and is highly significant ($P<0.001$). The y axis intercept a equals 10.83. (For the purposes of the regression calculation the data were grouped into four categories, each containing as nearly as possible the same number of individuals developing an antibody: This was because of the small number of individuals with a large foetal-cell score.)

TABLE V.—*ABO Incompatibility in Relation to Rh-antibody Formation Three Months After Delivery*

		Antibody	No Antibody	Total
ABO compatible	..	13	203	216
ABO incompatible	..	0	53	53
		13	256	269

The patients were all Rh-negative primiparae and the babies Rh-positive.

Discussion

We feel that our earlier studies demonstrated that it certainly is possible to prevent experimental Rh immunization, and similar results have been obtained by other workers. Thus Freda *et al.* (1964), who were the first to use gamma$_2$-globulin instead of whole plasma, showed that in a series of 38 volunteers (half of whom were used as controls) none of those "protected" developed immune antibody when followed up for a period of nine months, whereas 8 of the 19 controls did so. Again, Schneider and Preisler (personal communication, 1964), using much smaller volumes of Rh-positive cells and correspondingly smaller volumes of antiserum, obtained a rapid elimination of injected cells, and none of their 13 protected subjects developed an immune antibody, while 4 out of their 15 controls did so.

These experiments, however, represent an artificial situation, and the problem is whether the method is applicable in preventing Rh immunization due to pregnancy. The crux of the matter is the time at which the immunizing transplacental haemorrhage takes place, and the evidence provided by us on the one hand and that by Cohen and Zuelzer (1964) on the other is completely at variance. This may be because their series included multiparae as well as primiparae. If it did, one could not then be sure whether, in any particular case in which anti-D subsequently developed, it was due to primary immunization. Some of the multiparae may have been immunized by a previous pregnancy without the formation of detectable antibodies, and the pregnancy under study may simply have resulted in detectable anti-D, and in such cases very few or no foetal cells might be found. The fact that in their series two of the ABO-incompatible pregnancies were associated with the appearance of transient anti-D suggests that in these cases at least previous immunization had occurred. The interpretation is made more difficult because the authors do not make it clear whether foetal cells were found after delivery in these two mothers. If multiparae were indiscriminately included in Cohen and Zuelzer's series the data are not appropriate to determine the importance of the timing of transplacental haemorrhage in relation to primary sensitization.

Our investigation, using primiparae only, so strongly suggested that primary immunization was usually due to transplacental haemorrhage during labour that we felt a clinical trial of protection against Rh immunization was justified. This trial was begun in Liverpool in May 1964, and details of the organization are described. Unexpectedly, after only six months, some preliminary results also seem worth reporting.

III. Clinical Trial

The fact that we have found a correlation between the number of foetal cells in the maternal circulation after delivery and subsequent immunization has an important implication in the design of our trial. We believe that we are able to choose by the post-partum foetal-cell count those patients who are at greatest risk for Rh immunization. By using only these women in our treated and control groups we ought to be able to detect a significant difference between the two groups much sooner than if we took all Rh-negative mothers with Rh-positive babies regardless of the foetal-cell count. This is because the incidence of the appearance of anti-D following the first Rh-positive pregnancy is very low—in the order of only 5% in our series (see Table V). Thus if alternate cases, irrespective of the foetal-cell count, were treated with anti-D the series would have to be very large to produce significant evidence of protection by the gamma$_2$-globulin injection. Therefore, in our clinical trial we are including only those whom we consider " high-risk " primiparae.

Cases for the trial are chosen from the patients of five maternity units in Liverpool in co-operation with their medical staffs. The units are visited in the morning of each week-day, and a sample of blood is obtained from all Rh-negative women just delivered of their first babies. Films from these samples are immediately eluted and stained and counts of the number of foetal cells are made. Where the foetal-cell score is five or more and where the corresponding cord blood is Rh-positive and ABO-compatible with the mother, the case is included in the trial. Alternate cases are given, within 36 hours of delivery, 5 ml. of gamma$_2$-globulin containing high-titre (1:262,000 by indirect Coombs test) anti-D by intramuscular injection. The other cases are treated as controls and given no anti-D.

The patients are being followed up three and six months after delivery, when samples of blood are taken and tested for immune antibodies. Every effort is also being made to keep these women under observation when they become pregnant for a second time, since antibody formation sometimes becomes apparent only through the stimulus of a second pregnancy. We do not expect that significant results will be available until 1966, but after five months (November 1964) three out of eight of the controls have produced immune antibodies. Had the finding of an appreciable foetal-cell score after delivery made no difference to the probability of sensitization it is unlikely that there would have been any antibodies at all in such a small number of cases. In contrast, none of the six treated cases so far followed up has as yet presented any evidence of immune anti-D formation, although they all show a very weak indirect Coombs reaction consistent with the persistence of the administered anti-D, which we have previously been able to detect up to six months after injection. Further follow-up will be necessary to establish with certainty that these cases have not been immunized.

Clearly the bigger the clinical trial the sooner we shall have the answer to the problem of whether or not we can prevent the majority of cases of Rh-haemolytic disease. We are fortunate in having colleagues in Leeds, under Professor J. S. Scott; at Sheffield, under Dr. C. C. Bowley and Mr. Tom Smith; and at Baltimore, under Professor J. R. Krevans, who are collaborating with us and carrying out trials designed in the same way as our own. The results for the various centres will be the subject of other papers.

Appendix

1. A Note on the Kleihauer Technique

We find that the use of a sodium-phosphate-citric-acid buffer at pH 3.3 gives the best results. However, it still requires considerable experience to make accurate counts of foetal cells, particularly when the number is small. A subjective element is present in the assessment of any particular red cell, and small transplacental haemorrhages can be missed unless an experienced observer spends a considerable time reading the slides. The accurate estimation of the volume of foetal blood circulating in a mother requires measurement of the exact ratio of foetal to maternal red cells on the slide, and of the maternal red-cell mass. This has not been attempted in the present studies. The foetal-cell score used gives an approximate estimate of the size of the transplacental haemorrhage, a score of five representing approximately 0.25 ml. of foetal blood, and a score of 60 approximately 3 ml.

We have occasionally observed an appearance of blood films which makes the counting of foetal cells impossible. In these cases uneluted haemoglobin appears to be present in a considerable number of cells, but it varies greatly in amount from cell to cell. A graded appearance, from cells which are quite clearly adult to others which are indistinguishable from foetal cells, is seen, and it is impossible to assess if there has been a transplacental haemorrhage with these slides. The reason for this pattern of cells with uneluted haemoglobin is not known, and further studies are being carried out. There is evidence (Woodrow et al., in preparation) that they are of maternal and not of foetal origin, and they are therefore not being included in our clinical trial.

2. Details of Foetal-cell Scores in Relation to Subsequent Antibody Production

Results at Three Months After Delivery

No Antibody Found		Antibody Found	
Foetal-Cell Score	Frequency	Foetal-Cell Score	Frequency
0	× 132	0	× 3
1	× 11	2	× 2
2	× 24	3	× 2
3	× 8	6	× 2
4	× 8	13	× 1
5	× 4	64	× 1
6	× 3	70	× 1
8	× 3	200	× 1
12	× 1		
15	× 2		
18	× 1		
20	× 1		
25	× 1		
30	× 1		
67	× 1		
70	× 1		
400	× 1		

Results at Six Months After Delivery

No Antibody Found		Antibody Found	
Foetal-Cell Score	Frequency	Foetal-Cell Score	Frequency
0	× 83	0	× 4
1	× 4	2	× 2
2	× 11	3	× 2
3	× 3	6	× 1
4	× 1	70	× 1
5	× 4	200	× 1
6	× 2		
8	× 1		
12	× 1		
15	× 2		
20	× 1		
30	× 1		
400	× 1		

Summary

In previous papers we described experiments in which Rh immunization of Rh-negative male volunteers was successfully prevented by the intravenous injection of plasma containing a high titre of incomplete anti-D. In the present paper we describe experiments which show that Rh-positive foetal·cells can be cleared from the circulation of Rh-negative women as effectively as the Rh-positive adult cells were cleared from the Rh-negative men.

On three occasions we gave 10 Rh-negative post-menopausal nulliparae 5 ml. of Rh-positive foetal blood intravenously. In five of them each infusion was followed by an intramuscular injection of 5 ml. of anti-D gamma₂-globulin, and in each case this resulted in the foetal cells being rapidly cleared from the woman's circulation.

The other five women did not receive the anti-D gamma-globulin and served as controls. One of these controls and none of the treated women developed immune anti-D, a result which, though it does not demonstrate that protection was achieved, does rule out the possibility of this technique enhancing antibody production.

To find out if there is any relation between transplacental haemorrhage and labour, blood samples were taken from 200 women during the week preceding and the 48 hours following labour. Tests for foetal cells showed that in 135 patients none was present either before or after labour. Of the 65 where transplacental haemorrhage had occurred, in six this had taken place before labour and had disappeared after it. In 19 patients cells were present both before and after delivery, and in 40— that is, two-thirds—cells were not there before delivery but were present afterwards. We therefore consider that the majority of cases of transplacental haemorrhage occurred during labour or very shortly before it. Forty-seven haemorrhages were estimated to be less than 0.25 ml. of foetal blood in the maternal circulation, and of the 18 larger foetal haemorrhages 14 (78%) had occurred during or just before labour.

To find out if there is any relation between the presence of foetal cells in the maternal circulation after delivery and subsequent Rh immunization, a new series of Rh-negative primiparae is being examined for foetal cells in the maternal circulation after delivery, and if the baby is Rh-positive the serum of the women is being tested for antibodies three and six months later. Out of 216 women tested, no foetal cells were found in 135, and three of these developed anti-D ; of 81 women in whom foetal cells were found, 10 developed anti-D. There is thus a statistically significant relation between the detection of foetal cells and subsequent antibody production (P=0.005) ; moreover, the greater the number of foetal cells found the greater is the likelihood of immunization. A possible reason why Cohen and Zuelzer (1964) failed to find this relation is discussed.

Some details of the design and organization of a clinical trial of anti-D in selected women are given. For the trial the number of foetal cells after delivery is being used to detect Rh-negative primiparae " at risk " of Rh immunization, and alternate cases of such women are being given 5 ml. of intramuscular gamma₂-globulin with a high anti-D titre immediately after the birth of the baby. At the time of writing, this clinical trial has been in progress for only five months, but already the three-month follow-up shows that none of the six protected cases has any evidence of immune-antibody formation, while three out of eight untreated controls have produced immune anti-D. This preliminary result not only encourages the hope that a considerable proportion of Rh immunization can be prevented, but, in addition, it provides confirmatory evidence that women with a high risk of Rh immunization can be detected after delivery by examination of their blood for foetal cells.

In a note on the Kleihauer technique for the detection of foetal cells attention is drawn to the fact that certain women cannot be scored for the presence or absence of these because their blood contains not only large numbers of cells which look like foetal ones but also large numbers which are intermediate between adult and foetal cells in appearance. It seems probable that these cells with uneluted or partially eluted haemoglobin are of maternal origin.

We are grateful to the female blood donors who volunteered for the experimental studies and who attended on numerous occasions for injections and venesection. We would also like to thank those blood donors whose plasma has been the source of the gamma-globulin used in these studies and in the clinical trial. We are indebted to Dr. W. d'A. Maycock and his staff, of the Lister Institute of Preventive Medicine, who prepared the anti-D gamma-globulin. Our thanks are due to Lord Cohen of Birkenhead, Professor E. B. Ford, and Dr. R. R. Race for their helpful advice on various aspects of the work.

The survey and clinical trial could not have been carried out without the co-operation of Professor T. N. A. Jeffcoate and his consultant colleagues and the medical, nursing, and laboratory staffs of the Liverpool Maternity Hospital, Mill Road Hospital, Broadgreen Hospital, Sefton General Hospital, and Walton Hospital, and of the Liverpool Blood Transfusion Service.

We are grateful to Mrs. Ruth Harris, who has been responsible for the field work, both in the hospitals and in the follow-up of patients in their homes, and for the accurate record-keeping and secretarial work which these studies have entailed. We wish to thank Miss D. Townsend and Miss H. Millington for laboratory assistance, and Mrs. Doreen Macaulay for help in collecting the samples of blood.

This work has been made possible by grants from the Nuffield Foundation and the Research Committee of the United Liverpool Hospitals under the chairmanship of Lord Cohen of Birkenhead.

REFERENCES

Clarke, C. A., Donohoe, W. T. A., McConnell, R. B., Woodrow, J. C., Finn, R., Krevans, J. R., Kulke, W., Lehane, D., and Sheppard, P. M. (1963) *Brit. med. J.,* 1, 979.
Cohen, F., and Zuelzer, W. W. (1964). *Vox Sang. (Basel),* 9, 75.
—— —— Gustafson, D. C., and Evans, M. M. (1964). *Blood,* 23, 621.
Finn, R., Clarke, C. A., Donohoe, W. T. A., McConnell, R. B., Sheppard, P. M., Lehane, D., and Kulke, W. (1961). *Brit. med. J.,* 1, 1486.
Freda, V. J., Gorman, J. G., and Pollack, W. (1964). *Transfusion,* 4, 26.
Kleihauer, E., and Betke, K. (1960). *Internist (Berl.),* 1, 292.
Levine, P. (1943). *J. Hered.,* 34, 71.

Paper 34

34. Prevention of Rh-haemolytic disease: results of the clinical trial (1966). A combined study from centres in England and Baltimore. *Brit. Med. J., ii,* 907-914.

Commentary

Since four centres took part in this trial it has no authors and is usually referred to as 'A combined study, 1966'.

As was pointed out in the previous paper, this was a high risk trial designed on the assumption that the greater the number of fetal cells in the maternal circulation after delivery the greater the likelihood of immunisation, and the only women investigated were primiparae who had a fetal cell score of five or more in 50 low power fields. That in fact the supposition was correct was shown by the immunisation rate in the controls six months after delivery, for no less than 19 of these (22%) became immunised compared with no certain one in the treated. The figure for the controls is nearly three times that for all Rh-negative primiparae bearing Rh-positive ABO compatible babies if the fetal cell count is not considered.

The design of the trial had the additional advantage of eliminating primed cases, since the fetal cell score is unlikely to be high if there are occult antibodies. In other words, the results argued against Cohen and Zuelzer's view* that immunisation nearly always took place during pregnancy and that therefore giving anti-D after delivery would be ineffective.

The results given in the paper were those estimated six months after delivery. It was pointed out that the true protection rate would depend on the immunological state of the treated women after they had had a second Rh-positive baby. Preliminary data on this point both from the Combined Study trial and results in New York, Canada and Germany made all the teams optimistic that giving anti-D did protect against the disease in the next baby and not merely postpone the development of immunisation.

*Cohen, F. and Zuelzer, W. W. (1964). Identification of blood group antigens by immunofluorescence and its application to the detection of the transplacental passage of erythrocytes in mother and child. *Vox Sang. (Basel), 9,* 75.
Cohen, F., Zuelzer, W. W., Gustafson, D. C. and Evans M. M. (1964). Mechanisms of iso-immunisation. I. The transplacental passage of fetal erythrocytes in homo-specific pregnancies. *Blood, 23,* 621.

From Brit. Med. J., **ii,** *907-914. Copyright (1966), by kind permission of the British Medical Association*

15 October 1966

BRITISH
MEDICAL JOURNAL

Papers and Originals

Prevention of Rh-Haemolytic Disease: Results of the Clinical Trial
A Combined Study from Centres in England and Baltimore*†

Brit. med. J., 1966, **2,** 907–914

Finn (1960), in Liverpool, first put forward the idea that it might be possible to prevent immunization of Rh-negative mothers by giving them antibody to destroy Rh-positive foetal cells. The suggestion derived from our earlier work on ABO incompatibility in relation to Rh immunization (Clarke *et al.,* 1958), and the progress of the research since then has been described in four main papers. In the first two (Finn *et al.,* 1961 ; Clarke *et al.,* 1963) we described experiments which were successful in preventing Rh immunization in Rh-negative male volunteers. The basis of the procedure was to remove rapidly from the circulation previously injected chromium-tagged Rh-positive red cells by giving high-titre anti-D as an infusion of plasma. Later Gorman *et al.* (1963) (see also Freda and Gorman, 1962 ; Freda *et al.,* 1964) suggested the use of anti-D gamma-globulin instead of plasma, and since then we have used gamma-globulin.

In our third paper (Woodrow *et al.,* 1965) we showed that injected Rh-positive foetal cells could be cleared from the circulation of Rh-negative women volunteers as effectively as the Rh-positive adult cells were cleared from the Rh-negative men. We also produced evidence to show that the majority of cases of appreciable transplacental haemorrhage occurred during labour or very shortly before it, and, moreover, the greater the number of foetal cells found after delivery the greater was the likelihood of subsequent immunization. In this third paper we also stated that we had begun a clinical trial, in collaboration with colleagues working in Sheffield, Leeds, Bradford, and Baltimore, and the preliminary results of this were reported in August of last year (Clarke and Sheppard, 1965). Subsequently we described experiments which indicated that 1 ml. of gamma-globulin might be as effective in giving protection against the development of antibodies as the 5 ml. which we had used up to then (Clarke *et al.,* 1966).

In the present paper we describe the clinical trial, which has demonstrated that, anyhow up to six months after delivery, the technique which was successful in protecting against experimental Rh immunization has also protected women from Rh immunization by their Rh-positive foetuses.

Materials and Methods

Design of the Clinical Trial

The fact that we found a correlation between the number of foetal cells in the maternal circulation after delivery and subsequent immunization had an important bearing on the way we designed our trial.

We knew we were able to choose by the post-partum foetal-cell count a group of patients who were at considerable risk of developing Rh antibodies. By using only these women in our treated and control groups we thought we should be able to detect a significant difference (if one existed) between the two groups much sooner than if we took all Rh-negative mothers

with Rh-positive babies regardless of the foetal-cell count. Furthermore, we decided to limit the trial to primiparae in order to avoid any confusion due to possible effects of previous pregnancies, and thus we have included only those women whom we considered to be " high-risk " primiparae. In this way we made the best use of our limited supplies of gamma-globulin and kept this initial trial reasonably small so that in the event of any adverse effects the minimum number of people would have been treated.

The organization has been similar in all five centres, and the precise details of the Liverpool trial have been as follows. Five maternity units were visited in the morning of each week-day and a sample of blood was obtained from all Rh-negative women just delivered of their first baby. Films of these samples were eluted and stained and counts of the number of foetal cells in 50 low-power fields made (Kleihauer *et al.,* 1957 ; Woodrow *et al.,* 1965 ; Woodrow and Finn, 1966). Where the foetal-cell score was five or more, and where the corresponding cord blood was Rh-positive and ABO compatible with the mother, the case was included in the trial.

The aim was to treat alternate cases with 5 ml. of gamma-globulin containing high-titre anti-D (usually between 1 in 1,280 and 1 in 4,096 in albumin with R_2r cells) by intramuscular injection. However, for various reasons there has been considerable upset in the strict alternation of the cases. For instance, as we decided that the gamma-globulin should be given not later than 36 hours after delivery, all cases where the baby was born between Friday afternoon and Sunday morning have been used as controls and additional week-day deliveries treated to make the numbers equal. When gamma-globulin supplies have been short we have had runs of controls, and then compensated by treating several consecutive patients. Other difficulties encountered were delay in finding out the ABO group of the baby and the impossibility on occasion of reaching the patient within the time limit. Four patients refused treatment and were used as controls.

Nevertheless, despite these difficulties it will be seen that no large blocks of controls were unduly concentrated at any particular period of the trial. Even though a considerable proportion of the controls had to be chosen from the week-end deliveries, we are confident that there are no differences between

* The following took part in the study:
Liverpool Group : C. A. Clarke, M.D., Sc.D., F.R.C.P.; W. T. A. Donohoe, A.I.M.L.T.·; Catherine M. Durkin, M.B., Ch.B., D.C.H. ; R. Finn, M.D., M.R.C.P. ; D. Lehane, M.B., Ch.B., F.C.Path. ; R. B. McConnell, M.D., M.R.C.P. ; P. M. Sheppard, D.Phil., F.R.S. ; Shona H. Towers, M.B., Ch.B., M.R.C.O.G. ; J. C. Woodrow, M.D., M.R.C.P.
Sheffield Group : C. C. Bowley, M.B., B.S., M.R.C.O.G., F.C.Path.
Leeds and Bradford Group : Janet Shaw, M.B., Ch.B., M.R.C.O.G. ; R. B. Speight, F.I.M.L.T. ; L. A. D. Tovey, M.D.
Baltimore Group : Wilma B. Bias, Ph.D.; J. R. Krevans, M.D. ; Jeanette K. Light-Orr ; A. C. W. Montague, M.D.
† From the Nuffield Unit of Medical Genetics, Department of Medicine, University of Liverpool ; the Sheffield Regional Blood Transfusion Service ; the Department of Obstetrics and Gynaecology, the University of Leeds ; the Baltimore City Hospitals.

15 October 1966   Rh-Haemolytic Disease   BRITISH MEDICAL JOURNAL

the treated and control cases with regard to obstetric management. In fact, there is no significant difference between the mean foetal-cell scores for the combined control and the combined treated groups in the U.K. centres. (Mean square roots: 4.06 for controls and 4.511 for treated: S.E. of difference= 0.387, P>0.2). Similarly for the Baltimore data, where the results are expressed as volumes of foetal blood, the mean square roots are 0.802 for controls and 0.659 for treated, the S.E. of difference=0.112, P>0.2.

When the trial was started in May 1964 it was calculated on the basis of our previous work that 70 treated and 70 controls should be observed for six months after delivery, since this would be enough to give a statistically significant answer regarding the efficacy of the treatment (see Clarke and Sheppard, 1965). It was realized, however, that final proof of the complete prevention of immunization would only be obtained after the effects of second pregnancies had been observed.

Kleihauer–Betke Technique for Detecting Foetal Cells

This is an acid elution technique which enables foetal cells to be demonstrated and counted among a population of adult red cells (Kleihauer et al., 1957). The precise details of how we have used the test and the difficulties encountered with it have been described elsewhere (Woodrow et al., 1965 ; Woodrow and Finn, 1966). Thus in approximately 2% of post-delivery samples many intermediately staining cells are found due to an increase in maternal Hb F, and it is then impossible to obtain an accurate foetal-cell score. Before this was appreciated three such cases were treated, but the post-injection blood films showed no change. These cases, and subsequent similar ones, have been excluded from our trial. In general, however,

the technique has proved satisfactory and we had little difficulty in counting the foetal cells and selecting those cases with a count of 5 (or more), which we calculated was the equivalent of about 0.25 ml. of foetal blood. In the treated cases a foetal-cell count was usually carried out about 24 hours after the injection of the gamma-globulin, and in some patients this was repeated later to test further for the clearance of the foetal cells.

Tests for Antibody

In Liverpool, tests for Rh antibodies were made on samples of serum taken immediately after delivery and three and six months later. The sera were tested in the first instance against four different types of Rh-positive cells, and where a positive

TABLE I.—*Prevention of Rh-haemolytic Disease : Overall Results of Clinical Trial at Six Months or Later After Delivery*

Centre	Controls			Treated			
	No.	Immunized	Not Immunized	No.	Immunized	Not Immunized	Doubtful
Liverpool	40	10*	30	40	0	40	0†
Sheffield	15	5	10	14	0	12	2†
Leeds	5	0	5	6	0	5	1‡
Bradford	4	0	4	5	0	5	0
Baltimore	14	4	10	13	0	13	0
Total	78	19	59	78	0	75	3

* One of these had no antibody at delivery but had anti-D six months later, detectable only by papain technique (titre 1/4). Retested 18 months after delivery: findings similar.
† Three months after delivery reaction positive by papain technique, demonstrable only in neat serum. Negative Coombs test. Similar findings, though weaker, at six and eight months.
‡ Tests negative three months after delivery. Presence of anti-D queried at 10 months, but all tests negative 14 months after delivery (see Table IV for details).
Statistical analysis: Comparison of the combined control and treated groups for antibody production gives P=1·73×10⁻⁴ even if the three doubtful cases are regarded as immunized (one-tailed test).

TABLE II.—*Liverpool Series*

Controls

Serial No.	Date of Delivery	Foetal-cell Counts at Delivery	Cell Survival Where Known	Immune Antibody Production with Titres — 3 Months After Delivery	6 Months After Delivery
280	24/5/64	56, 78	—	Nil	Nil
292	29/5/64 r	13, 11; 5, 11; 8, 4; 5, 4	—	„	„
307	6/6/64 w	17, 19	—		„
362	2/7/64 r	7, 6; 5, 8	—	Anti-D present ICT 1/8 (ins.)	Anti-D present Alb. 1/16 Sal. nil ICT 1/16 Pap. 1/8
403	17/7/64 w	16, 18; 19, 17	—	Anti-D present Alb. 1/2 Sal. 1/2 ICT 1/2 Pap. 1/8	Anti-D present Alb. 1/16 Sal. 1/2 ICT 1/64 Pap. 1/4
446	8/8/64 w	74, 46; 81, 55	—	Anti-D present (ins.)	Anti-D present Alb. 1/2 Sal. 1/4 ICT nil Pap. 1/4
469	14/8/64 w	68, 71	5, 5 (20/10/64)	Nil	Nil
486	28/8/64 r	8, 7	4, 2 (20/10/64)	„	„
509	16/9/64	12. 14	7, 9 (20/10/64)	„	„
551	6/10/64 r	7. 7; 10, 6	8, 6 (22/10/64)	„	„
567	18/10/64 r	18, 8; 15	—	„	„
575	25/10/64 u	7, 8; 11, 8	5, 6 (11/11/64)	„	„
589	1/11/64 w	10, 8; 9, 7	12, 7 (10/11/64)	„	„
610	16/11/64 c	18, 14; 29, 30	—	„	„
617	21/11/64 w	17, 37; 36, 32	—	„	„
638	1/12/64 c	7, 7	—	„	Anti-D present Alb. 1/2 Sal. 1/2 ICT 1/4 Pap. 1/4
657	9/12/64 u	10, 15	—	?	Papain anti-D antibody Alb. nil Sal. nil ICT nil Pap. 1/4
659	10/12/64 u	10, 8	—	„	Nil
674	21/12/64	6, 4	—	Anti-D present (ins.)	Anti-D present Alb. 1/2 Sal. 1/2 ICT nil Pap. 1/4
698	8/1/65 g	18, 12	—	Anti-D present Alb. 1/4 Sal. 1/2 ICT 1/4 Pap. 1/2	Anti-D present Alb. 1/4 Sal. 1/2 ICT 1/8 Pap. 1/4
785	9/3/65	26, 32; 50, 41	—	Anti-D present Alb. 1/4 Sal. 1/2 ICT 1/2 Pap. 1/4	Anti-D present Alb. 1/2 Sal. 1/2 ICT 1/2 Pap. 1/2
798	13/3/65 w	27, 29; 30	0, 1 (4/5/65)	Nil	Nil
822	8/4/65	10, 11	0, 0 (25/5/65)	„	„
850	13/5/65	17, 17	—	„	„
868	27/5/65	5, 8; 11	—	„	„
869	29/5/65	6, 5; 6. 7	—	„	„
895	19/6/65	6, 3; 7, 8	1, 0 (2/8/65)	„	„
913	29/6/65 u	11, 8	3, 4; 6, 5 (5/8/65)	„	„
997	7/8/65	18, 20; 29, 26	1, 0 (1/10/65)	„	„
1042	6/9/65	23, 27; 25, 27	2, 0 (25/10/65)	Anti-D present Alb. 1/4 Sal. 1/4 ICT 1/8 Pap. 1/8	Anti-D present Alb. 1/4 Sal. Nil ICT 1/8 Pap. 1/8
1050	11/9/65 w	3, 7; 6, 5	1,0 (25/10/65)	Nil	Nil
1055	14/9/65 w	36, 38	4, 5; 7, 6 (19/10/65)	„	„
1061	17/9/65	16, 7	—	„	„
1068	18/9/65	9, 9	—	„	„
1080	26/9/65	8, 7; 8	—	Anti-D present Alb. 1/8 Sal. 1/8 ICT 1/4 Pap. 1/8	Anti-D present Alb. 1/8 Sal. 1/2 ICT 1/8 Pap. 1/8
1097	2/10/65	5, 6	—	Nil	Nil
1116	9/10/65 w	9. 14	1, 1 (15/12/65)	„	„
1140	23/10/65	27, 27	5, 5 (17/12/65)	„	„
1162	1/11/65	83, 44; 61	—	Anti Leᵇ	Anti Leᵇ
1221	8/12/65	72, 71; 69	27, 28 (10/1/66)	Nil	Nil

c = Cord blood group not available; baby grouped   u = Unable to   g = Gamma-globulin not available.   r = Refused treatment.   w = Week-end control.   ...pital to treat.   ins. = Insufficient serum for further tests.

result was obtained the sera were tested against a further panel of cells (R₁R₁, R₂R₂, R'r, R"r, R₁ʷr, and three different rr samples). This panel included all blood-group antigens apart from the extremely rare ones. Activity in saline and albumin, and by Coombs and papain techniques, was tested for routinely. Similar procedures were carried out in the other centres.

Results

Table I gives the overall findings together with the statistical analysis, and Tables II–VI the details for the five centres. Certain differences between the centres are dealt with below. Others, such as differences in the apparent length of survival of passive antibody in the treated cases and in the assessment of specificity of induced antibodies in the controls, probably reflect differences in technique in different laboratories.

Interpretation of Results of Clinical Trial

It is clear that the final results of this trial extend and confirm our preliminary report and there is no doubt that

anti-D gamma-globulin given soon after delivery is effective in preventing the development of immune Rh antibody in the subsequent six months. Taking the most favourable view—that is, when we compare the presence or absence of definite Rh immunization in the treated and controls—protection is complete (0 as against 19). However, it is possible that the two treated Sheffield women (Nos. 305 and 308) who still had antibodies eight months after delivery are in fact immunized, and, furthermore, the doubtful Leeds antibody (No. 13724/64) may indicate some unusual form of immunization rather than an error or the remains of the injected gamma-globulin. If these three cases are in fact failures, protection would still be of the order of 80% (3 as against 19). Nevertheless, passive antibodies can last longer than six months, and it is very unusual for immune antibodies, once formed, to disappear (though their titres may fluctuate), and we therefore feel that the three cases mentioned are in fact unlikely to be failures. However, we shall follow them up with great care and also the control whose antibodies were demonstrable only by the papain technique (Liverpool series, No. 657).

It can be seen that there is considerable variation between the five centres as regards the proportion of women in the controls who have developed antibodies, but statistical analysis shows that there is no significant heterogeneity between the centres.

It is encouraging that other clinical trials carried out in the U.S.A. (Freda et al., 1966 ; Gorman et al., 1966) and Germany (Preisler and Schneider, 1966) have produced similar findings to our own. The results of these, which are all based on tests for antibodies at six months or more after delivery, are shown in Table VII.

It is interesting to compare the proportion of immune antibodies found in the controls in the series of Pollack et al. (1966) (about 11%) with our own (about 24%). The explanation of this is that in the New York and California series all Rh-negative women delivered of Rh-positive ABO-compatible babies entered the trial, and the Kleihauer technique was not used. In our series, on the other hand, we treated high-risk cases only (foetal-cell count more than 5) and the higher immunization rate in our controls supports the view that the quantity of foetal cells detected after delivery is a guide to the degree of risk of immunization.

In the Freiburg series all Rh-negative women free of antibodies but regardless of parity and ABO group of the foetus, in whom one or more foetal cells were found in post-delivery blood films, were admitted to the trial. The inclusion of many low-risk cases as well as those with ABO incompatibility may account for the reduced incidence of antibodies among the controls. However, there may be other factors, and it will be interesting, when the full German data are published, to see the distribution of the foetal-cell scores, as it may well be that varying obstetrical procedures in different countries have a bearing on the frequency of Rh immunization.

From our earlier experiments with male volunteers and from a consideration of all the evidence on the timing of immunization we had anticipated that we ought to be able to protect about 75% of Rh-negative women, but we thought that our method might be too late for the remaining 25%. However, in the event the protection rate is probably very much higher. One reason for this may be that until the last few weeks of pregnancy transplacental haemorrhages large enough to cause immunization are much rarer than we had thought. In addition, we know (a) that Rh antibodies sometimes take six months or more to develop, and (b) that it is very unusual for a first Rh-positive baby to be affected. Yet another reason may be that, in contrast to the increase in titre of pre-existing antibodies which may occur in pregnancy, the primary immune response in the pregnant woman may be temporarily depressed as it is in some animals (Heslop et al., 1954 ; Medawar and Sparrow, 1956 ; Anderson and Benirschke, 1964 ; Anderson, 1965), and if this

TABLE II.—Contd.

Treated

Serial No.	Date of Delivery	Foetal-cell Counts at Delivery	Foetal-cell Counts after Treatment with 5 ml. Gamma-globulin Approx. 24 hr. Later	Subsequent Counts at Stated Times	Antibody Production 3 Months	6 Months
					After Delivery	
273	20/5/64	6, 7; 4, 3; 9, 13	2, 2	1, 0 (4 d.)	P	Nil
294	31/5/64	23, 28; 35, 24	N.T.	{ 5, 3 (42 hr.) 2, 1 (7 d.)	,,	,,
355	29/6/64	24, 26; 30, 33	0, 0	—	,,	,,
414	23/7/64	78, 86	18, 24	2, 2 (4 d.)	,,	,,
419	26/7/64	3, 6; 5, 6	6, 6	—	Nil	,,
436	3/8/64	24, 26; 21, 29	N.T.	1, 1 (46 hr.)	P	,,
453	10/8/64	16, 10; 8, 10	1, 0	—	,,	,,
504	13/9/64	5, 4; 6, 5	4, 4	1, 0 (3 d.)	Nil	,,
571	21/10/64	87, 96	5, 5	—	P	,,
583	29/10/64	3, 5 ; 8, 11	2, 1	—	Nil	,,
587	1/11/64	8, 5; 5, 4; 5, 5	0, 0	—	,,	,,
619	23/11/64	54, 58	4, 2	—	P	,,
656	8/12/64	16, 9; 10, 24; 24	4, 6	0, 0 (6 d.)	P	,,
665	13/12/64	4, 5; 6, 5	1, 0	—	,,	,,
668	15/12/64	34, 28	12, 12	—	Nil	,,
696	5/1/65	28, 30	0, 0	—	P	,,
767	24/2/65	67, 74	N.T.	2, 1 (36 hr.)	,,	,,
775	1/3/65	40, 38	3, 5	—	,,	,,
781	8/3/65	4, 9; 5, 10	2, 2	—	Nil	,,
782	8/3/65	7, 7	1, 1	—	P	,,
817	28/3/65	33, 30; 33	4, 10	2, 1 (3 d.)	,,	,,
820	31/3/65	7, 9	1, 2	—	,,	,,
840	26/4/65	20, 20	0, 1	—	,,	,,
844	3/5/65	31, 35	1, 2	—	,,	,,
884	10/6/65	13, 10; 13, 14	8, 7	0, 0 (48 hr.)	,,	,,
902	22/6/65	24, 15	0, 0	—	,,	,,
924	5/7/65	5, 8; 3, 4; 6, 5; 9	0, 1	—	,,	,,
979	28/7/65	82, 86; 81	N.T.	0, 1 (44 hr.)	,,	,,
992	4/8/65	123, 134; 116, 120	15, 12	1, 0 (48 hr.)	,,	,,
994*	6/8/65	5, 5	2, 2	0, 0 (48 hr.)	,,	,,
1013	20/8/65	15, 16	4, 6	0, 0 (48 hr.)	Nil	,,
1039	7/9/65	15, 16	2, 1	—	P	,,
1058	15/9/65	48, 55	2, 1	—	,,	,,
1120	12/10/65	4, 9; 6, 3; 6, 7	N.T.	0, 0 (48 hr.)	,,	,,
1143	26/10/65	6, 8	3, 4	—	,,	,,
1077	28/9/65	9, 8	0, 0	—	,,	,,
1166	4/11/65	52, 79	5, 6	—	,,	,,
1187	24/11/65	6, 8; 6, 10	0, 0	—	,,	,,
1191	26/11/65	6, 6	0, 0	—	,,	,,
1211	3/12/65	6, 4; 5, 3; 8, 3	0, 0	—	,,	,,
1224	9/12/65	29, 27	5, 5	—	,,	,,

N.T. = Not tested.
P = A weak reaction in albumin and by the Coombs and Papain techniques, demonstrable only with neat serum and presumably due to *passive* antibody.
* After submission of this paper it was discovered that this patient was not Rh-negative but Dᵘ-positive (R₁-r). She is therefore omitted from Table I and replaced by case 1224. It is of interest that patient 994 showed no adverse effects from the injection of anti-D and that the Rh-positive foetal cells were removed. However, since it has been shown that Dᵘ red cells take up only 7 to 25% as much antibody as ordinary D-positive cells, the foetal cells would preferentially absorb the injected anti-D and therefore be rapidly cleared.

Prevention of RH-haemolytic Disease: Clinical Trial. Liverpool Series
Each of the treated women was given 5 ml. of anti-D gamma-globulin intra-muscularly within 36 hours of delivery. In all but five of the treated women a sample of blood was obtained approximately 24 hours after treatment to determine clearance of foetal cells and in some cases samples taken later than this were also tested. In some of the controls samples of blood were obtained at varying times after delivery to determine cell survival.
To determine the foetal-cell score the routine practice was for one observer to count each of two slides. On occasion other observers repeated the counts, and these results are also included.

15 October 1966   Rh-Haemolytic Disease   Bartish MEDICAL JOURNAL

is so red cells crossing the placenta will not often evoke an antibody response until after delivery. If such suppression of antibody response really does take place the exact timing of a transplacental haemorrhage would be of academic importance only.

The above considerations have a bearing on the interesting work of Zipursky *et al.* (1965), who, because they thought it likely that about 25% of patients become immunized during pregnancy, set out to protect this group by giving anti-D to the mother during pregnancy. An initial dose of 1 ml. of anti-D gamma-globulin was given in the last trimester, followed at three-week intervals by 0.4 ml. This treatment was carried out on 45 women at the time of the report, and 30 of them had produced healthy Rh-positive infants, none of whom were anaemic though two had a weak-positive Coombs test on the red cells (*Medical World News,* 1965 ; Zipursky, 1965). We have as yet no information on how far the treatment prevents immunization, but it appears to be a safe procedure. However, it would not often be necessary if the initiation of Rh immunization is usually suppressed until after delivery.

Second Pregnancies

It has been suggested that by giving anti-D all we are doing is preventing immune-antibody production but that some of the women are in fact " sensibilized " (see Nevanlinna, 1953) and that in second pregnancies immune antibodies will become

TABLE IV.—*Leeds Series*

Controls

Serial No.	Date of Delivery	Foetal-cell Counts at Delivery	Immune Antibody 3 Months after Delivery	Immune Antibody 6 Months After Delivery or Later
12818/64	18/10/65	9, 6	Nil	Nil
13465/64	31/10/65	5, 8		,,
36228/64	25/11/64	5, 8	N.T.	,,
26709/64	4/3/65	11, 12	,,	,,
37991/64	3/4/65	100, 68	,,	,,

Treated

Serial No.	Date of Delivery	Foetal-cell Counts at Delivery	Score 24–48 hr. after Treatment with 5 ml. Gamma-globulin	Immune Antibody 3 Months after Delivery	Immune Antibody Six Months after Delivery or Later
18894/64	13/10/64	12, 6	2	Nil	Nil
13724/64	2/12/64	18, 20	6,6	,,	Doubtful*
28681/64	17/1/65	110, 100	20, 15	,,	Nil
6155/65	18/3/65	11, 8	0, 0	Anti-D present Alb. nil Enzyme positive (ficin and papain)	,,
4684/64	19/8/65	173, 117	75	Nil	,,
24286/65	1/9/65	26, 17	21, 20	,,	,,

N.T. Not tested.

* Although tests by the indirect antiglobulin technique suggested that a weak anti-D was present in this serum, further tests by Low's papain technique were negative and tests using ficinized cells gave inconclusive results. Unfortunately there was insufficient serum remaining of the specimen to confirm these results. Further samples at 14 months after delivery were tested both in Leeds and in Liverpool and found to be negative.

TABLE III.—*Sheffield Series*

Serial No.	Date of Delivery	Foetal-cell Score Delivery	24 hr	48 hr	3 mth	Antibody Production 3 Months After Delivery	Antibody Production 6 Months After Delivery	Serial No.	Date of Delivery	Foetal-cell Score Delivery	24 hr	48 hr	3 mth	Antibody Production 3 Months After Delivery	Antibody Production 6 Months After Delivery
				Controls								*Treated continued*			
27	13/1/65	17	19	—	0	Anti-D present Sal. 1/2 Alb. 1/4 ICT + Enzyme pp +	Anti-C + D present Sal. w Alb. + ICT + Enzyme pp +	143	21/5/65	9	2	1	0	Anti-D present Sal. nil Alb. nil ICT neg. Enzyme pp +	,,
51	15/2/65	254	234	161	0	Anti-D present Sal. 1/2 Alb. 1/4 ICT w Enzyme pp +	Anti-C + D present Sal. nil Alb. 1/2 ICT + Enzyme pp +	170	18/6/65	10	2	0	0	Anti-D present Sal. nil Alb. nil ICT neg. Enzyme pp w	,,
76	17/3/65	6	5	4	0	Nil	Nil	197	13/7/65	7	0	0	0	Anti-D present Sal. nil Alb. nil ICT neg. Enzyme pp +	,,
129	10/5/65	6	5	3	0	,,	,,								
167	13/6/65	15	15	15	0	,,	,,								
176	27/6/65	18	13	15	0	,,	,,	220	12/8/65	7	4	0	0	Anti-D present Sal. nil Alb. nil ICT neg. Enzyme pp +	,,
203	21/7/65	12	10	10	0	,,	,,								
230	28/8/65	5	6	6	0	,,	,,								
254	9/9/65	5	4	4	0	,,	,,	278	27/9/65	14	5	0	0	Anti-D present Sal. nil Alb. nil ICT neg. Enzyme pp w	Anti-D presen Sal. nil Alb. nil Enzyme pp w (absent at 8 months)
265	20/9/65	17	23	25	0	Anti-D present Sal. nil Alb. w ICT w Enzyme pp +	Anti-C + D present Sal. 1/1 Alb. 1/2 ICT + Enzyme pp +								
266	19/9/65	18	29	20	0	Nil	Nil	279	27/9/65	54	33	7	0	Anti-D present Sal. nil Alb. nil ICT neg. Enzyme pp w	Nil
303	9/10/65	20	18	16	0	Anti-D present Sal. nil Alb. nil ICT neg. Enzyme pp w	Anti-C + D present Sal. 1/1 Alb. 1/1 ICT + Enzyme pp +								
307	18/10/65	12	8	7	0	Anti-C + D present Sal. w Alb. w ICT w Enzyme pp +	Anti-C + D present Sal. 1/1 Alb. 1/1 ICT + Enzyme pp w	301	10/10/65	8	10	1	0	Anti-D present Sal. nil Alb. nil ICT neg. Enzyme pp +	,,
309	17/10/65	7	5	5	0	Nil	Nil	305	13/10/65	10	5	0	0	Anti-D present Sal. nil Alb. nil ICT neg. Enzyme pp +	Anti-D present Sal. nil Alb. nil ICT neg. Enzyme pp w (still present at 8 months)
331	9/11/65	9	13	12	0	,,	,,								
				Treated											
47	11/2/65	5	3	0	0	Anti-D present Sal. nil Alb. nil ICT neg. Enzyme pp w	Nil	308	18/10/65	8	5	0	0	Anti-D present Sal. nil Alb. nil ICT neg. Enzyme pp +	Anti-D present Sal. nil Alb. nil ICT neg. Enzyme pp w (still present at 8 months)
54	17/2/65	7	4	0	0	Nil	,,								
58	24/2/65	40	15	0	0	Anti-D present Sal. nil Alb. nil ICT neg. Enzyme pp w	,,								
118	22/4/65	5	2	2	0	Anti-D present Sal. nil Alb. nil ICT w Enzyme pp +	,,	315	20/10/65	22	7	0	0	Anti-D present Sal. nil Alb. nil ICT w Enzyme pp w	Nil

pp = Papainized panel. + = Present when tested with neat serum. w = Weakly present when tested with neat serum.

overt. It is likely that this state of affairs sometimes occurs naturally, the mothers being immunized by the first Rh-positive pregnancy even though no antibody can be detected in the post-partum period. Antibody may then appear late in the next Rh-positive pregnancy, probably as the result of a few foetal cells crossing the placenta.

We have studied six (untreated) primiparae who had a foetal-cell score of 5 or more after their first delivery, who were free of antibodies six months later, and who have produced an Rh-positive ABO-compatible second baby. Two of these six women developed antibody during the second pregnancy. If this small series is representative, then for every woman showing antibodies by six months after the first delivery approximately one other woman will develop them by the end of the second Rh-positive ABO-compatible pregnancy. This means that, untreated, about 50% of women in this category can be expected to have antibodies by the end of the second Rh-positive pregnancy. It is therefore important to note that six of the

treated women in our trial have been delivered of normal ABO-compatible Rh-positive second babies, and all are free of antibody. Furthermore, although it is likely that the risk of antibody developing during the second pregnancy is somewhat lower for the New York and the Freiburg series, the fact that six treated women in the former (Pollack, 1966) and six in the latter (Schneider, 1966) have reached the end of the second Rh-positive pregnancy without showing antibodies is very encouraging. (In the German series, the six women had had bleeds with the first baby of 0.16, 0.06, 0.12, 0.1, 0.17, and 0.05 ml. respectively—that is, " small " bleeds.)

There is also experimental evidence to support the view that we are not merely suppressing antibody formation. In a Baltimore study in 1963 (not previously reported) we gave 5 ml. of Rh-positive blood to 13 men who had earlier been protected by anti-D after four successive Rh-positive blood infusions. In 12 cases the injected blood survived normally, which makes it unlikely that the volunteers were in a state of " sensibilization." (The thirteenth case showed moderately reduced red-cell survival of both Rh-positive and Rh-negative cells.) Furthermore, Freda et al. (1966) gave 14 Rh-negative male volunteers three injections of Rh-positive blood, the first two stimuli being followed by injections of anti-D gamma-globulin and the third one not. This third injection of 1 ml. of blood was given 10 months after the second injection, and in no case was it followed by anti-D production. These workers were therefore mimicking a subsequent Rh-positive pregnancy, and they concluded that the protection afforded by the two gamma-globulin injections was complete. Taking all the available evidence into consideration, we feel that it argues strongly against the view that treatment with anti-D merely suppresses the appearance of immune antibody until the next pregnancy.

TABLE V.—Bradford Series

Serial No.	Date of Delivery	Foetal-cell Score at Delivery	Score 24 hr. after Treatment with 5 ml. Gamma-globulin	Immune Antibody 6 Months after Delivery
		Controls		
64/1627	1/12/64	10	—	Nil
65/124	1/3/65 (twins)*	14	—	,,
65/1406	7/8/65	8	—	,,
65/1402	20/9/65	19	—	,,
		Treated		
64/1780	26/12/65	17	8 (4 at 48 hr.)	Nil
65/143	8/3/65	10	2	,,
64/2318	26/3/65	6	2	,,
64/2254	21/4/65	16	6	,,
65/1230	16/9/65	65	16	,,

* One was Rh-positive; the other died soon after birth and was not grouped.

TABLE VI.—Baltimore Series

Date of Delivery	Estimated Volume of Foetal Bleed (ml.)	Immune Antibody 6 Months Post-delivery
	Controls	
7/1/65	1·4	Anti-D present
4/2/65	0·25	Nil
22/2/65	0·43	,,
7/3/65	3·0	,,
10/4/65	0·33	,,
20/4/65	0·25	Anti-D present
4/5/65	1·65	Nil
18/5/65	0·38	,,
22/5/65	1·0	Anti-D present
22/7/65	0·47	Nil
23/8/65	0·3	,,
13/10/65	0·26	,,
25/10/65	0·27	Anti-D present
7/12/65	0·84	Nil
	Treated	
25/1/65	0·58	Nil
23/2/65	1·65	,,
1/3/65	0·36	,,
7/4/65	0·36	,,
19/4/65	0·3	,,
19/4/65	0·48	,,
25/4/65	0·3	,,
25/4/65	0·25	,,
7/5/65	0·25	,,
22/5/65	0·26	,,
17/8/65	0·58	,,
20/8/65	0·5	,,
29/10/65	0·33	,,

TABLE VII

Centre	Controls			Treated		
	No.	Immune Antibody		No.	Immune Antibody	
		Present	Absent		Present	Absent
Trial begun April, 1964 — New York and California (Freda et al., 1966; Pollack, et al., 1966)	158	17	141	160	0	160
Trial begun October, 1963 — Freiburg (Schneider and Preisler, 1965; Preisler and Schneider, 1966)	47	2	45	55	0	55

Mechanism of Protection by Anti-D

The precise way in which the passively administered anti-D prevents active immunization is unknown, and more than one mechanism may be responsible.

1. Importance of Site to which Rh-positive Cells are Removed

An explanation of the protection conferred by maternofoetal ABO incompatibility is that in the presence of naturally occurring anti-A or anti-B, Rh-positive foetal red cells are either haemolysed intravascularly or are rapidly removed to the liver. In the latter case the paucity of immunologically competent cells results in a failure of the Rh antigen to stimulate antibody production. However, there is the anomaly that when a predominantly saline-active anti-D was used experimentally (Clarke et al., 1963) enhanced anti-D formation resulted. This may be because the red cells were not cleared from the circulation, or because of a difference in complement-binding, or because the lower titre of antibody may have resulted in the red cells being removed to the spleen (Mollison, 1961), where they would come into contact with numerous immunologically competent cells. On the other hand, we know that when incomplete anti-D is used removal is also to the spleen (Clarke et al., 1963), and yet in this case protection results and immune antibody is not formed. Thus the mechanism of protection by incomplete anti-D cannot depend on the site to which cells are removed.

2. Specific Inhibition of the Immune Response

It has been postulated that as part of a physiological homoeostatic mechanism regulating the production of antibody there is a " feed-back " effect by which passive antibody inhibits the further production of antibody (Uhr and Baumann, 1961). The great variety of antigenic systems in which suppression of primary immunization by the passive administration of antibody has been observed lends support to this view (see Neiders *et al.*, 1962). How the inhibition occurs is not known, but two possible modes of action have been suggested.

Blocking of Antigen Sites.—When the Rh-positive foetal cells encounter the injected incomplete anti-D coating of the cells occurs and the antigen sites are blocked by antibody. This blocking action may persist in the reticuloendothelial system of the spleen, and though there is no direct evidence to support this view the work of Stern *et al.* (1961) favours it. They demonstrated that if Rh-positive cells are coated with incomplete anti-D before injection into Rh-negative men the formation of antibodies is prevented. The cells were washed in saline before injection, and presumably there was no free antibody present. Finkelstein and Uhr (1964) suggest that the effect of such red-cell blocking might be that within the macrophage of the reticuloendothelial system there is a failure to "process" the antigen, and the lymphoid cells are thus not stimulated to produce antibody.

Inhibitory Effect on the Antibody-producing Cell.—Using sheep erythrocytes as antigen in rats, Rowley and Fitch (1964) showed in a series of experiments that passively administered antibody was apparently bound to potential antibody-forming lymphoid cells. This was associated with a failure of the cells to proliferate in response to administered antigen, and was interpreted as suggesting a direct inhibitory effect of the antibody on the potential antibody-producing cells.

It is uncertain how long the suppression of the immune response lasts after injection of the gamma-globulin, and Chown (1965) thinks that it may persist even after the passive antibody has disappeared. However, in our Baltimore study (see above), of the 13 men protected, four produced anti-D when challenged seven months later with 5 ml. of Rh-positive blood.

It is not known whether the giving of anti-D gamma-globulin will protect against the development of antibodies other than anti-D. This could be tested by giving a suitable dose of antibody directed against a red-cell antigen other than D and seeing whether or not anti-D was produced. An experiment based on this principle is in progress. Kell-negative Rh-negative volunteers have been injected with Kell-positive Rh-positive red cells, and then anti-Kell antibody administered. If protection is non-specific neither anti-Kell nor anti-D would be produced, but if the suppression of immunization is specific one would expect anti-D to be produced in some cases.

Design of our Further Clinical Trial

Earlier this year we showed that 0.5 ml. of gamma-globulin effectively clears 5 ml. of injected Rh-positive blood in 48 hours (Clarke *et al.*, 1966). Though, in a current experiment, we have not demonstrated protection with this dose—none of the controls and none of the treated has so far (nine weeks later) developed immune antibodies—yet we feel it is unlikely that we have caused enhancement, and therefore that we are justified in beginning a new clinical trial with a smaller dose of gamma-globulin than previously. This new trial began on 9 June 1966, and, as in the first clinical trial, only Rh-negative primiparae who have had Rh-positive ABO-compatible babies are being included. However, on this occasion we are treating, within 36 hours of delivery, alternate patients who have a Kleihauer score of from 0 to 4 inclusive, and these will be given 1 ml. of gamma-globulin. The original trial will be continued, and women with a foetal-cell score of five and over on the Kleihauer test will continue to be given 5 ml. of gamma-globulin.

ABO Incompatible Pregnancies

Although it is well recognized that ABO incompatibility between mother and foetus protects against Rh immunization, this is not invariably the case. In a six-month follow-up of 90 Rh-negative women who had Rh-positive ABO-incompatible first babies we found anti-D in one case. Since the incidence

of anti-D in a similar follow-up of ABO-compatible pregnancies is approximately 8%, and as compatible pregnancies are about four times as common as incompatible ones, it follows that of 32 antibodies developing after a first pregnancy approximately one will be the result of an ABO-incompatible pregnancy. In order to prevent these occasional cases of immunization it would be necessary to treat a considerable number of "low-risk" mothers, and perhaps this should be done only when supplies of gamma-globulin become freely available.

Supplies of Gamma-globulin

If the new clinical trial gives satisfactory results the reduced dosage will greatly ease the difficulty of providing gamma-globulin for the whole country, and the position can be further helped by the use of plasmapheresis. If all women "at risk" with Kleihauer scores of from 0 to 4 were given 1 ml. of gamma-globulin and the remainder 5 ml., it has been estimated that about 72,000 ml. of gamma-globulin a year would be needed. There are three possible sources from which this could be obtained, and they are listed in order of desirability:

1. Rh-negative women immunized by recent pregnancy who have high-titre incomplete antibodies in their serum. This source has the advantage that no booster doses are required, and therefore there is no risk to the donor.

2. Post-menopausal Rh-negative women sensitized by pregnancy or transfusion, and Rh-negative men sensitized by transfusion who would be prepared to agree to being hyperimmunized.

3. Post-menopausal Rh-negative women and Rh-negative men who would agree to being deliberately immunized.

Sources 2 and 3 carry the slight risk of homologous serum jaundice due to injection of donor blood, but this can be minimized by very careful selection of the donor.

By one or other of these methods, panels of donors could be established so that adequate sources of antibody would be available, and then by the use of plasmapheresis, whereby each donor provided 500 ml. of plasma at each attendance, ample supplies of gamma-globulin would be ensured. In order that excessive demands are not made on donors' time we feel that they should not be asked to attend more often than once a month.

Value of the Kleihauer Technique

In 1965 we published some information on the relation of foetal-cell score at delivery to production of Rh antibody six months later (Woodrow *et al.*, 1965), and we now have further results on this problem (see Table VIII).

It will be seen that there is an increasing likelihood of the mother developing antibodies as the foetal-cell count rises, and the Kleihauer technique is clearly of great value in assessing the risk of subsequent immunization. Because of this, and because of the uncertainty of how much gamma-globulin is needed to protect against large bleeds, we feel that at present it is wise to employ the Kleihauer technique wherever possible. It seems to us inadvisable simply to treat everyone with 1 ml., because this may not be enough to protect against a large transplacental haemorrhage—though this view may need revision in the light of further experience. Admittedly there are difficulties in learning the technique, and extra staff would be needed in the various regions if one were planning to use it

TABLE VIII.—*Relation of Foetal-cell Count After Delivery to Subsequent Rh Immunization as Measured Six Months After Delivery. Cases are All Rh-negative Primiparae with Rh-positive ABO-compatible Babies*

	0	1–4	5–60	60+	Total
Antibody (%) No antibody ..	5 (2·59) 188	11 (8·33) 121	9 (16·98) 44	3 (50) 3	28 (7·87) 356
Total ..	193	132	53	6	384

N.B.—The data do not represent a random sample of deliveries, as 37 women with a foetal-cell score of 5 or more (31 with a score of 5–60 and 6 with one of over 60) had been treated with anti-D gamma-globulin during this survey, and are not included.

Rh-Haemolytic Disease

on a national scale, the number depending on how often the ABO and Rh grouping of the baby is carried out at the hospital. Where it is, as few as two junior technicians (working under supervision) plus a full-time clerk might be able to do the work. In Liverpool two junior technicians carry out about 15 tests in one day, and this includes the time taken to prepare the buffer. If it were only a question of dividing big from small bleeds, very many more cases could be looked at. Where there was any doubt, the bleeds would be classed as "large" and those mothers with large bleeds and with "intermediate" or doubtful cells would be given 5 ml. of gamma-globulin, while 1 ml. should be sufficient to protect those with small or no bleeds.

Wider Applications of this Research

It is well known that in animals the giving of passive antibody has resulted in some prolongation of survival of grafts (Billingham *et al.*, 1956 ; Parkes, 1958 ; Brent and Medawar, 1961 ; Nelson, 1962), and it is possible that the immunological approach described here may have some practical application in the field of tissue transplantation in man. Furthermore, it might conceivably be of use in the prevention of some types of autoimmune disease. For example, it would be worth trying to protect NZB mice who are "at risk" for autoimmune nephritis (Russell *et al.*, 1966) by the injection of gamma-globulin from those animals which had already developed the disease.

Summary

A successful clinical trial of a method of preventing Rh immunization of Rh-negative mothers by their Rh-positive babies has been carried out. The technique has been developed over a period of six years, and was first shown to be successful in preventing Rh immunization of male volunteers.

Soon after the baby is delivered the woman is given an intramuscular injection of 5 ml. of gamma-globulin containing a very high titre of incomplete anti-D.

Included in this trial are 156 Rh-negative primiparae shown to be at considerable risk of Rh immunization because a number of foetal cells were detected in their blood after delivery of an Rh-positive baby. Half of the women were given 5 ml. of gamma-globulin and the other half served as controls.

Testing of the serum for antibodies at least six months after delivery has demonstrated no certain case of Rh immunization in the 78 treated women with 19 immunizations in the controls.

Three doubtful cases among the treated (two at Sheffield and one at Leeds) have occurred, and while reasons are given for thinking these women are not immunized the possibility remains that they may be ; but, even so, in these high-risk cases the order of protection would still be about 80%.

Workers in New York and California and Germany, using a similar type of approach, have also obtained very favourable results, though the design of their experiments differs slightly from our own.

Definite proof that Rh immunization can be prevented by this technique will rest on the immunological state of the treated women just after they have had a second Rh-positive baby. Results for this so far are encouraging, as no antibodies have developed in any of the 18 women who have had the treatment and who have had a subsequent Rh-positive ABO-compatible baby—six in our trial, six in Freiburg, and six in New York—and we can be very optimistic that the technique is not merely postponing the development of immune antibodies. The evidence to date seems to indicate that nearly all cases of maternal Rh immunization can be prevented by the injection after delivery of high-titre incomplete anti-D.

Experiments have been carried out which suggest that 5 ml. of gamma-globulin may be an unnecessarily large dose and that 1 ml. may be a safe dose for most women. A second clinical trial has been started in which alternate Rh-negative women whose blood after delivery contains no, or very few, foetal cells are being given 1 ml. of anti-D gamma-globulin.

The mechanism by which the injection of anti-D prevents Rh immunization, the problem of the supply of anti-D gamma-globulin, and the wider implications of this method of influencing immunological reactions are discussed.

We are grateful first of all to those mothers at the five centres who volunteered to enter the trial, and to the blood donors whose plasma has been the source of the gamma-globulin prepared in this country. The investigation here would not have been possible without the help of Dr. W. d'A. Maycock, Mr. L. Vallet, and the staff of the Lister Institute of Preventive Medicine, who prepared the gamma-globulin for us. Similarly, we acknowledge with thanks the Ortho Research Foundation, who provided it for the Baltimore trial.

The clinical trial in Liverpool could not have been carried out without the cooperation of Professor T. N. A. Jeffcoate, his consultant colleagues, and the medical, nursing, and laboratory staffs of the Liverpool Maternity Hospital and Mill Road, Broadgreen, Sefton General, and Walton Hospitals, and we are very grateful to them all. Similar acknowledgements are made to Professor J. S. Scott, who organized the starting of the trial in Leeds and Bradford, and to the obstetricians and staffs of the Maternity Hospital, Leeds, St. Luke's Maternity Hospital, Bradford, and the City General Hospital, Sheffield.

In Liverpool our thanks are due to Mrs. Rodney Harris, S.R.N., who was responsible for the field work in the hospitals and in the patients' homes, and to Miss D. Townsend, Miss H. Millington, and Miss C. Eunson for laboratory assistance with the Kleihauer technique ; also to Mrs. Carol Mortimer, A.I.M.L.T., and Mrs. Janthia Read, B.Sc., who carried out the laboratory work in Sheffield, and to Miss M. White, F.I.M.L.T., chief technician at St. Luke's Hospital, Bradford.

This research has been made possible by generous grants from the Nuffield Foundation and from the Research Committee of the United Liverpool Hospitals under the chairmanship of Lord Cohen of Birkenhead.

REFERENCES

Anderson, J. M. (1965). *Nature (Lond.)*, **206**, 786.
—— and Benirschke, K. (1964). *Brit. med. J.*, **1**, 1534.
Billingham, R. E., Brent, L., and Medawar, P. B. (1956). *Transplant. Bull.*, **3**, 84.
Brent, L., and Medawar, P. B. (1961). *Proc. roy. Soc. B*, **155**, 392.
Chown, B. (1965). Personal communication.
Clarke, C. A., Donohoe, W. T. A., McConnell, R. B., Woodrow, J. C., Finn, R., Krevans, J. R., Kulke, W., Lehane, D., and Sheppard, P. M. (1963). *Brit. med. J.*, **1**, 979.
—— Finn, R., Lehane, D., McConnell, R. B., Sheppard, P. M., and Woodrow, J. C. (1966). *Ibid.*, **1**, 213.
—— McConnell, R. B., and Sheppard, P. M. (1958). *Int. Arch. Allergy*, **13**, 380.
—— and Sheppard, P. M. (1965). *Lancet*, **2**, 343.
Finkelstein, M. S., and Uhr, J. W. (1964). *Science*, **146**, 67.
Finn, R. (1960). *Lancet*, **1**, 526.
—— Clarke, C. A., Donohoe, W. T. A., McConnell, R. B., Sheppard, P. M., Lehane, D., and Kulke, W. (1961). *Brit. med. J.*, **1**, 1486.
Freda, V. J., and Gorman, J. G. (1962). *Bull. Sloane Hosp. Wom. N.Y.*, **6**, 147
—— and Pollack, W. (1964). *Transfusion (Philad.)*, **4**, 26.
—— —— (1966). *Science*, **151**, 828.
Gorman, J. G., Freda, V. J., and Pollack, W. (1963). *Proc. 9th Congr. Int. Soc. Haematol.*, (Sept. 1962). Grune and Stratton, New York.
—— —— and Robertson, J. G. (1966). *Bull. N.Y. Acad. Med.*, **42**, 458.
Heslop, R. W., Krohn, P. L., and Sparrow, E. M. (1954). *J. Endocr.*, **10**, 325.
Kleihauer, E., Braun, H., and Betke, K. (1957). *Klin. Wschr.*, **35**, 637.
Medawar, P. B., and Sparrow, Elizabeth M. (1956). *J. Endocr.*, **14**, 240.
Med. Wld News, 1965, vol. 6, No. 36, p. 31.
Mollison, P. L. (1961). *Blood Transfusion in Clinical Medicine*, 3rd ed., p. 459. Blackwell, Oxford.
Neiders, M. E., Rowley, D. A., and Fitch, F. W. (1962). *J. Immunol.*, **88**, 718.
Nelson, D. S. (1962). *Brit. J. exp. Path.*, **43**, 1.
Nevanlinna, H. R. (1953). *Ann. Med. exp. Fenn.*, **31**, Supp. No. 2.
Parkes, A. S. (1958). *Transplant. Bull.*, **5**, 45.
Pollack, W. (1966). Personal communication.
—— Gorman, J. G., Freda, V. J., Jennings, E. R., and Sullivan, J. F. (1966). In press.
Preisler, O., and Schneider, J. (1966). *Bibl. gynaec. fasc.*, **37**, 1.
Schneider, J. (1966). Personal communication.
—— and Preisler, O. (1965). *Blut*, **12**, 4.
Rowley, D. A., and Fitch, F. W. (1964). *J. exp. Med.*, **120**, 987.
Russell, Pamela J., Hicks, J. D., and Burnet, F. M. (1966). *Lancet*, **1**, 1279.
Stern, K., Goodman, H. S., and Berger, M. (1961). *J. Immunol.*, **87**, 189.
Uhr, J. W., and Baumann, Joyce B. (1961). *J. exp. Med.*, **113**, 935.
Woodrow, J. C., Clarke, C. A., Donohoe, W. T. A., Finn, R., McConnell, R. B., Sheppard, P. M., Lehane, D., Russell, Shona H., Kulke, W., and Durkin, Catherine M. (1965). *Brit. med. J.*, **1**, 279.
—— and Finn, R. (1966). *Brit. J. Haematol.*, **12**, 297.
Zipursky, A. (1965). Personal communication.
—— Pollock, J., Chown, B., and Israels, L. G. (1965). *Birth Defects Original Article Series*, **1**, p. 84.

Paper 35

35. Pollack, W., Gorman, J. G., Freda, V. J., Ascari, W. Q., Allen, A. E. and Baker, W. J. (1968). Results of clinical trials of RhoGAM in women. *Transfusion, 8,* 151-3.

Commentary

This is the first USA paper with the results of a clinical trial and in it the anti-D was given as the proprietary preparation RhoGAM. Two dose levels were adopted (300 μg) and 1,000 μg) and in both the results were excellent (see Tables 2, 3, and 4).

At the time of writing the paper there had been a total of 145 patients from the treated and control groups of both series who had had a second Rh incompatible pregnancy and again the results were good. The conclusion was that a single dose of 300 μg or more of RhoGAM was an effective prophylaxis against Rh immunisation.

The names of those carrying out the trials are given in the paper but there are no references.

Results of Clinical Trials of RhoGAM* in Women

W. POLLACK,** J. G. GORMAN,† V. J. FREDA,† W. Q. ASCARI,** A. E. ALLEN** AND W. J. BAKER**

*From the Division of Diagnostic Clinical Pathology, Ortho Research Foundation, Raritan, New Jersey,** and the Departments of Obstetrics and Gynecology and Pathology, Columbia University, New York, New York†*

Intramuscularly administered RhoGAM, $Rh_o(D)$ Immune Globulin (Human) has been evaluated for its capacity to prevent the primary Rh immunization of Rh negative women giving birth to ABO compatible Rh positive infants. Since March 1964, over 3,000 women have been admitted to clinical studies in 43 centers ranging geographically from Argentina to Canada and from Australia to Scotland. RhoGAM prepared at the Ortho Research Foundation used throughout these studies is derived from plasma of persons previously immunized to the $Rh_o(D)$ antigen, and the antibody content of the final preparation is determined by a modification of the radioimmune assay of Hughes-Jones.[8]

Two studies, differing only in the dose of antibody administered, are presented separately and as a combined cumulative experience. In both studies, treated patients received a single intramuscular injection of RhoGAM containing either 5,000-6,000 μg of anti-$Rh_o(D)$ (5 ml study) or no less than 300 μg of anti-$Rh_o(D)$ (1 ml study) within 72 hours after delivery. For admission into either study patients met all of the criteria listed in Table 1.

Routine Rh typing and antibody screening were performed on a blood specimen of each candidate during the fourth to seventh month of her gestation. Screening

* Trademark of Ortho Diagnostics, Raritan, New Jersey.

Received for publication December 5, 1967; accepted March 25, 1968.

Transfusion
May-June 1968

TABLE 1. *Criteria for Admission to the RhoGAM Study*

The mother:	$Rh_o(D)$ negative Absence of serum anti-$Rh_o(D)$ prior to, and at the time of delivery.
The infant:	$Rh_o(D)$ positive ABO compatible Negative direct antiglobulin test of cord red blood cells.

tests to detect atypical antibodies were also performed at the time of delivery, five to ten days postpartum, and at one, three, and six months postpartum. After delivery of the infants, ABO and Rh typing and a direct antiglobulin test were performed on red cells of cord blood specimens. Mothers not meeting the criteria in Table 1 were excluded from the control as well as the treated groups. Patients were randomly allocated to control and treated groups so that both groups would have essentially the same characteristics with respect to socio-economic background, race, age, parity and gravidity. Prior to administration of RhoGAM, an indirect antiglobulin test

TABLE 2. *Results of Serologic Tests for Anti-$Rh_o(D)$ 5 ml Study [5,000 μg anti-$Rh_o(D)$]*

Patient Group	Positive	Negative	Total
Treated	0	300	300
Control	19	208	227
Total	19	508	527

$p < 0.001$.

Volume 8
Number 3

TABLE 3. *Results of Serologic Tests for Anti-Rh₀(D)*
1 ml Study [300 μg anti-Rh₀(D)]

Patient Group	Positive	Negative	Total
Treated	1	780	781
Control	32	467	499
Total	33	1,247	1,280

$p < 0.001$.

TABLE 5. *Results of Serologic Tests*
at Subsequent Delivery
1 ml and 5 ml Studies

Patient Group	Positive	Negative	Total
Treated	1	81	82
Control	7	56	63
Total	8	137	145

$p = 0.05$.

was performed using maternal erythrocytes and a 1:1,000 dilution of the RhoGAM to be used.

Results

Table 2 shows the results of the six month postpartum test of the sera of 527 patients admitted to the 5 ml study. Of the 300 treated patients, none was immunized, whereas 19 of the 227 control patients produced anti-Rh₀ (D).

Two thousand nine hundred twenty-nine patients were admitted to the 1 ml study. Of these, 1,901 were treated and 1,028 were followed as controls. Table 3 summarizes the serologic data related to patients who were followed for a minimum of six months postpartum. Of the 781 patients in the treated group, 1 (0.1%) became immunized, whereas in the control group 32 (6.4%) of the 499 produced anti-Rh₀ (D). The one failure had had a previously unprotected delivery of an Rh positive baby and, therefore, may have been actively immunized prior to this study. If so, her antibodies escaped detection by the methods employed.

Both dosage schedules appeared to offer

TABLE 4. *Results of Serologic Tests for Anti-Rh₀(D)*
5 ml and 1 ml Studies Combined

Patient Group	Positive	Negative	Total
Treated	1	1,080	1,081
Control	51	675	726
Total	52	1,755	1,807

$p < 0.001$.

significant protection. The combined results are shown in Table 4. A total of 1,081 patients have been treated and followed for a minimum of six months; only one of these developed anti-Rh₀ (D).

To date there have been a total of 145 patients from the treated and control groups of both series who have had a second Rh₀ (D) incompatible pregnancy. The criteria for including patients for the study of second pregnancies differ only in that patients are kept in the groups to which they were originally assigned and the ABO group of the infant was not considered. The results of antibody screening tests performed at the time of subsequent delivery are shown in Table 5. One of the 82 treated patients was found to be immunized, in contrast to 7 of the 63 control patients.

Conclusions

There is essentially no way of recognizing, *a priori,* which Rh negative women having Rh positive pregnancies will be immunized by fetal cells escaping into their circulation at the time of delivery. ABO incompatibility confers only incomplete protection.[2] The 11.1 per cent incidence of immunization in the control patients studied during subsequent pregnancies, when compared with the 7.0 per cent incidence of immunization in women in the combined studies of first pregnancies reflects the fact that immunization may escape detection unless there is another later exposure to the Rh antigen. This may account for the one apparent failure in the treated group.

It is concluded that a single dose of 300 μg or more of anti-Rh$_o$(D) immune globulin, RhoGAM, administered intramuscularly after each Rh incompatible pregnancy is an effective and antigenically specific prophylaxis against Rh$_o$(D) immunization. Since Rh immunization by pregnancy is the leading cause of clinically important hemolytic disease of the newborn, the use of this preparation should reduce, and may eliminate, this disease.

Acknowledgments

We would like to express our gratitude to the following investigators who contributed their time and energies to provide the clinical data summarized in this report.

A. A. Alter, M.D., Brooklyn, N. Y.

E. A. Banner, M.D., Rochester, Minn.

R. H. Barter, M.D., Washington, D. C.

R. S. Bayer, M.D., Syosset, Long Island, N. Y.

W. A. Bowes, M.D., J. J. Parks, M.D., Denver, Colo.

E. C. Bryant, M.D., Toronto, Ontario

L. R. Bryant, M.D., New Orleans, La.

L. P. Cawley, M.D., Wichita, Kansas

H. J. Chaplin, M.D., St. Louis, Mo.

S. H. Cherry, M.D., R. E. Rosenfield, M.D., New York, N. Y.

L. K. Diamond, M.D., I. Umansky, M.D., Boston, Mass.

W. D. Dolan, M.D., Arlington, Va.

S. R. Gambino, M.D., Englewood, N. J.

R. C. Goodlin, M.D., Palo Alto, Calif.

D. W. Huestis, M.D., Chicago, Ill.

G. R. Hewitt, M.D., N. Walsh, M.D., Ireland

J. L. Hutchison, M.D., Montreal, Canada

R. B. Jaffe, M.D., Ann Arbor, Mich.

E. R. Jennings, M.D., Long Beach, Calif.

W. L. Johnson, M.D., E. R. Giblett, M.D., Seattle, Wash.

J. R. Krevans, M.D., Baltimore, Md.

V. I. Krieger, M.D., Australia

R. L. Levin, M.D., Washington, D. C.

R. N. Levy, M.D., New Hyde Park, L. I., N. Y.

T. G. McElrath, M.D., Flemington, N. J.

H. G. McQuarrie, M.D., Salt Lake City, Utah

E. L. Macht, M.D., Abington, Pa.

A. J. Margolis, M.D., San Francisco, Calif.

M. Margulies, M.D., Buenos Aires, Argentina

S. P. Masouredis, M.D., Ph.D., Milwaukee, Wis.

N. G. Maxwell, M.D., Pittsburgh, Pa.

R. W. Preucel, M.D., Philadelphia, Pa.

J. T. Queenan, M.D., New York, N. Y.

J. G. Robertson, M.D., Edinburgh, Scotland

M. A. Stenchever, M.D., Cleveland, Ohio

L. Sussman, M.D., New York, N. Y.

L. L. deVeber, M.D., London, Ontario

M. E. Wade, M.D., New Haven, Conn.

H. Wallerstein, M.D., New York, N. Y.

V. E. Wendt, M.D., R. Visscher, M.D., Grand Rapids, Mich.

C. A. White, M.D., Iowa City, Iowa

S. J. Zwirek, M.D., J. W. Green, M.D., Lexington, Ky.

Paper 36

---

36. WHO Report (1967). The suppression of Rh immunisation by passively administered human immunoglobulin (IgG) anti-D (anti-Rh₀), *Bull. Wld. Hlth. Org., 36,* 467-474.

Commentary

By 1967 it was clear that suppression of Rh immunisation by the administration of anti-D was successful, and a meeting was called by WHO to discuss the policy to he adopted in providing the prophylaxis. The paper gives the conclusions that were arrived at by participants who represented the chief countries where early trials had been undertaken.*

Since the publication of the 1967 report H. H. Gunson, F. Stratton and P. K. Phillips (1971, *Brit. J. Haematol., 21,* 683-694) have pointed out that for immunisation of Rh-negative volunteers Rh-positve cells coated with complement enhance the frequency of the immune response, and this may be of importance when raising anti-D.

*See also World Health Organisation. (1971). Technical report series no 468.

From Bull. Wld. Hlth. Org., 36, 467-474. Copyright (1967), by kind permission of the World Health Organisation

THE SUPPRESSION OF Rh IMMUNIZATION BY PASSIVELY ADMINISTERED HUMAN IMMUNOGLOBULIN (IgG) ANTI-D (ANTI-Rh$_o$)*,†

Clinical trials carried out in several countries have established that primary immunization to the Rh antigen, which is liable to occur in certain Rh-negative women as a consequence of pregnancy, can be prevented by the injection of human immuno-globulin (IgG) anti-D (anti-Rh$_o$) shortly after delivery.

In this memorandum present knowledge of the subject is briefly reviewed and recommendations are made about methods of obtaining supplies of Rh antibody and of testing them for potency and about the selection of women to whom anti-D (anti-Rh$_o$) should be given while supplies remain inadequate for the treatment of all women at risk.

PROCUREMENT OF PLASMA CONTAINING ANTI-D (ANTI-Rh$_o$) ANTIBODY

In view of the anticipated demands for IgG anti-D (anti-Rh$_o$) there is an urgent need to mobilize all potential sources of human anti-D (anti-Rh$_o$) anti-bodies. There are two main sources of supply:

(*a*) persons already immunized by pregnancy or transfusion and having adequate anti-D (anti-Rh$_o$) antibody titres;

(*b*) deliberately immunized volunteers, who can be subdivided into two groups: (i) post-menopausal or sterilized women immunized by pregnancy or transfusion and men immunized by transfusion whose antibody titres require boosting; and (ii) men and post-menopausal or sterilized women who are not already immunized to the D (Rh$_o$) antigen.

Although, in those parts of Canada in which a prophylactic programme has been organized, enough plasma to meet all needs has been obtained by frequent plasmaphereses of already immunized women, it will be necessary, both there and in any other country planning a permanent programme of prevention, to supplement and eventually replace this source by deliberately immunized volunteers. The need to immunize volunteers may also arise if additional work shows that protection can be attained by the use of relatively small quantities of anti-D (anti-Rh$_o$) when this is " hyperimmune " (donors repeatedly restimulated). Deliberate immun-ization will also be required to replace the loss of naturally produced anti-Rh for blood-grouping sera.

Adequate supplies of IgG anti-D (anti-Rh$_o$) may be readily obtained by plasmapheresis (Janeway et al., 1963; Kliman et al., 1964; Kliman & Lesses, 1964). It should be pointed out, however, that, although healthy subjects have had 500 ml of plasma removed once a week for many months without suffering apparent ill-effects, nothing is known about any possible long-term or delayed effects. Detailed records of all plasma donors should be kept, includ-ing specification of antigen used, volume of plasma removed, physical examination, haemoglobin and plasma protein levels, leukocyte and platelet counts, liver function tests and such other data as may become indicated. It is desirable to recall all such donors at least annually for a complete health review. Some physicians consider that plasmapheresis should not be carried out more frequently than once a month.

* This statement, of which a French version will be published later, was drawn up by:

Dr B. Chown, Rh Laboratory, Winnipeg, Canada

Professor C. A. Clarke, Department of Medicine, The University of Liverpool, Liverpool England

Dr R. Finn, Nuffield Unit of Medical Genetics, The University of Liverpool, Liverpool, England

Dr K. L. G. Goldsmith, WHO International Blood Group Reference Laboratory, Medical Research Council, London, England

Dr H. C. Goodman, Chief, Immunology, World Health Organization, Geneva, Switzerland

Dr A. Hässig, Transfusion Service, Swiss Red Cross, Berne, Switzerland

Dr S. R. Hollán, Institute of Haematology, National Blood Centre, Budapest, Hungary

Dr N. C. Hughes-Jones, Experimental Haematology Re-search Unit, St Mary's Hospital Medical School, London, England

Professor J. J. van Loghem, Central Laboratory of the Netherlands Red Cross Blood Transfusion Service, Amsterdam, Netherlands

Dr W. D'A. Maycock, Lister Institute, Elstree, Herts, England

Dr S. P. Masouredis, School of Medicine, University of California, San Francisco, Calif., USA

Professor P. L. Mollison, Experimental Haematology Research Unit, St Mary's Hospital Medical School, London, England

Dr J. G. Robertson, Department of Obstetrics and Gynaecology, University of Edinburgh, Edinburgh, Scotland

Dr J. Schneider, University Clinic for Women, Freiburg im Breisgau, Germany

Dr V. Schönfeld, The Institute for Mother and Child, Prague, Czechoslovakia

Dr Z. Trnka, Immunology, World Health Organization, Geneva, Switzerland

Dr M. A. Umnova, Laboratory for the Study and Standardization of Blood Groups, Central Institute for Haematology and Blood Transfusion, Moscow, USSR

Dr C. van de Weerdt, Central Laboratory of the Nether-lands Red Cross Blood Transfusion Service, Amster-dam, Netherlands

† The dual nomenclature used in this memorandum has been adopted in conformity with the editorial policy of the *Bulletin of the World Health Organization*; it should not be taken necessarily to represent the preferences of the authors.

468

If it is assumed that for every million of a Caucasian population 1600 Rh-negative women will give birth each year to an Rh-positive ABO-compatible infant and that the suppressive dose is the amount of anti-D (anti-Rh_o) contained in 1.0 ml of an immunoglobulin solution containing 16 g per 100 ml, then about 90 litres of anti-D (anti-Rh_o) antibody-containing plasma will be needed annually. Using plasmapheresis and assuming that each donor gives 0.5 litre 12 times per year, 15 donors with acceptable antibody titre will be required for every million of population. If, as is probable, not all these donors will be available throughout the year, it may be necessary to have a group of 30 suitable donors available.

In the interim phase, when supplies of IgG anti-D (anti-Rh_o) are limited, the treatment of Rh-negative primiparae giving birth to ABO-compatible Rh-positive babies (about 550 per million in a Caucasian population) would require only about 30 litres of plasma per year.

Factors to be considered in a programme of active immunization of Rh-negative volunteers

1. A volunteer donor, whether of anti-D (anti-Rh_o) plasma or of Rh-positive blood for injection, must be in good health, meeting the same standards of health as those required for any blood donor.

2. An Rh-positive cell donor should be an R_2 blood donor who has given blood to at least 10 recipients, all of whom have been kept under supervision for a period of 6 months and have not developed jaundice. Ideally, the red-cell donor should lack antigens such as K and Fy^a which not infrequently stimulate the production of corresponding antibodies.

3. Before injection, the donor blood should be washed three times in the hope of reducing its white cell and platelet antigenicity and rendering it free of hepatitis virus (Haynes et al., 1960).

4. The dose should be 5 ml of red cells for the first injection of an unimmunized donor, and 2 ml for donors already immunized.

5. The interval between doses depends on the response of the recipient (Freda et al., 1966). If a volunteer has not developed antibodies by 6 months after the first dose of antigen, a second dose of 5 ml of cells should be given. The production of anti-Rh does not appear to be accelerated by giving repeated injections within the first 3 months. If the volunteer still has no antibodies at the end of the second 6 months, he should be rejected. There is evidence that a single injection of 5 ml of red cells will induce the formation of anti-Rh in about 50% of the recipients by the end of 6 months. At 3 months, approximately 25% of recipients have demonstrable antibodies (Freda et al., 1965). For a volunteer not

previously immunized, the second dose should be given as soon as antibodies first appear, and later doses at 6-month intervals.

For a volunteer who already has antibodies the interval should be 6 months.

6. The blood group of volunteers undergoing active immunization should be determined in order to exclude individuals lacking a high-frequency antigen such as k, Lu^b, against which they might become immunized.

Supervision and protection of deliberately immunized volunteers

Screening tests for liver function should be carried out on the volunteers before immunization and on several occasions during the 6 months' follow-up period.

Transfusion services or other organizations responsible for the deliberate immunization of volunteers should be in a financial position (possibly through insurance) to compensate donors for any accident, illness or other mishap attributable to their having been immunized. The risks being taken should be fully explained to the volunteers.

Volunteers who are actively immunized may be given a card to be carried at all times stating that their plasma contains anti-D (anti-Rh_o) antibody. They should be instructed that they must give this information should they themselves need transfusion.

PREPARATION OF IgG ANTI-D (ANTI-Rh_o)

Preparations of IgG anti-D (anti-Rh_o) should meet the Requirements for Human Immunoglobulins adopted by the WHO Expert Committee on Biological Standardization (1967). Such preparations can be expected to contain not less than about 90% of IgG; they may also contain traces of IgM.

It is preferable to use large pools of plasma, e.g., not less than 60 litres derived from not less than 10 donors (see page 471). Fractionation of large pools will tend to yield batches possessing more uniform potency and will allow a proportion of each batch to be set aside for possible future testing or as contributions to national reference preparations which might be used to establish an international reference preparation.

It is not yet possible to specify an acceptable minimum anti-D (anti-Rh_o) potency, expressed as μg anti-D (anti-Rh_o) antibody. (The minimum suppressive dose is discussed on page 471.)

There is at present little evidence about the stability of IgG anti-D (anti-Rh_o). Observations on changes in the potency of liquid and lyophilized preparations stored under different conditions are needed—liquid preparations stored frozen ($-30°C$ or less) and at $2°C–10°C$ and lyophilized preparations stored at $5°C$ and at $2°C–10°C$.

469

ASSESSMENT OF THE ACTIVITY OF IgG ANTI-D (ANTI-**Rh₀**) PREPARATIONS

The assessment of the biological activity of anti-D (anti-**Rh₀**) preparations in suppression of primary immunization could be carried out directly by clinical trials in which the effectiveness of graded doses of a particular preparation is determined. This method is, however, impracticable and reliance must be placed on estimates of other properties of the anti-D (anti-**Rh₀**) preparations, although these properties have not been shown to be directly related to that of immune suppression. Three methods can be considered: (1) determination of the antibody titre (anti-γ-globulin, enzyme or albumin); (2) estimation of both the concentration of anti-D (anti-**Rh₀**) antibody in μg/ml and the average value of the equilibrium constant; (3) determination of the ability to bring about destruction of Rh-positive red cells *in vivo*.

Determination of titre

The reaction between antibody and antigen is reversible ($Ab + Ag \rightleftharpoons AbAg$) and in any given system at equilibrium the relationship between the concentrations of the three components Ab, Ag and AbAg is given by the value of the equilibrium constant, K. The end-point of a titre is determined by the amount of antibody combined with the red cell (AbAg) and does not take account of the amount of free antibody (Ab) in the reaction mixture. However, it is probable that the activity of anti-D (anti-**Rh₀**) antibody in suppressing active immunization is dependent on the amount of antigen-antibody complex formed in the body. It is possible that there may be a correlation between the titre and the ability to suppress primary immunization.

The main disadvantage of the method is the great variability in the values obtained by different laboratories on the same sample (see, for example, Goldsmith, Mourant & Bangham, 1967). This variability would undoubtedly be considerably reduced if anti-D (anti-**Rh₀**) antibody titres were compared with that of a standard preparation of anti-D (anti-**Rh₀**) (see page 471).

Estimation of anti-D (anti-**Rh₀**) antibody content in μg protein/ml

This may be carried out using either (*a*) a quantitative ¹²⁵I-labelled anti-IgG technique, or (*b*) direct labelling of anti-D (anti-**Rh₀**) preparations.

¹²⁵*I-labelled anti-IgG.* The basis of this method is the calibration of ¹²⁵I-labelled anti-IgG, i.e., the determination of the number of molecules of ¹²⁵I-labelled anti-IgG that will combine with a ¹³¹I-labelled anti-D (anti-**Rh₀**) antibody molecule which is bound to the red cell surface. The estimation of the anti-D (anti-**Rh₀**) antibody content of a unknown sample of anti-D (anti-**Rh₀**) antibody is then carried out by absorbing the unknown anti-D (anti-**Rh₀**) on to Rh-positive red cells and estimating the amount absorbed using the previously-calibrated ¹²⁵I-labelled anti-IgG. The failure to absorb all the anti-D (anti-**Rh₀**) antibody on to red cells can be taken into account by using a graphical analysis of the results. This method also gives an estimate of the value of the equilibrium constant, which may be of importance in assessing potency. The details of this method are given elsewhere (Hughes-Jones, 1967).

The sensitivity of the method is high, the optimum concentration of antibody for estimation being 1-2 μg anti-D (anti-**Rh₀**) antibody/ml. Studies on several preparations of anti-D (anti-**Rh₀**) antibody suggest that an anti-IgG titre of 1 (indirect antiglobulin technique) is equivalent to an anti-D (anti-**Rh₀**) antibody content of 0.01–0.1 μg antibody protein/ml. The weakness of the method is the assumption that the calibration is applicable to all anti-D (anti-**Rh₀**) preparations. Inaccuracies involved in this assumption can be minimized by (i) calibrating against a pool of ¹³¹I-labelled anti-D (anti-**Rh₀**) antibody obtained from many donors, and (ii) using several ¹²⁵I-labelled anti-IgG preparations obtained from different animals.

*Direct labelling of IgG anti-D (anti-**Rh₀**) preparations.* This can be carried out with ¹²⁵I and the anti-D (anti-**Rh₀**) content determined by estimating the amount of radioactivity that can be specifically absorbed by Rh-positive cells. The disadvantage of this method is that the non-specific uptake of ¹²⁵I-labelled IgG by Rh-positive red cells is high compared with the specific uptake of anti-D (anti-**Rh₀**) antibody. Thus the method gives estimates in good agreement with the ¹²⁵I-labelled anti-IgG technique when the anti-D (anti-**Rh₀**) antibody content represents 0.3%-0.5% of the total IgG present, but less good agreement is obtained at lower concentrations.

Ability of anti-D (anti-**Rh₀**) preparations to bring about destruction of red cells in vivo

It seems desirable to obtain more information about the relation between the ability of a given batch of anti-D (anti-**Rh₀**) antibody to produce clearance of red cells from the circulation, and its ability to suppress primary immunization. Even though it may ultimately be shown that the suppression of immunization is not directly related to accelerated clearance, it seems quite likely that those properties of a particular anti-D (anti-**Rh₀**) preparation which make it relatively effective in producing clearance—for example, a high equilibrium constant—also make it relatively effective in suppressing immunization.

A subsidiary advantage of testing a particular batch of IgG anti-D (anti-**Rh₀**) in this way is that

470 / 471

red cell clearance may prove to be relatively reproducible between different subjects and may thus give an easily standardized measure of potency.

Nevertheless, it is by no means suggested that every batch of IgG anti-D (anti-Rh$_o$) should be tested in this way and it is thought that only a few centres will wish to carry out tests of clearance.

Selection of Rh-negative subjects as recipients

The requirements are the same as those for other volunteers receiving Rh-positive red cells (see page 468) with the additional requirement that the subjects must not have undergone splenectomy.

Selection of Rh-positive donor

See page 468.

Performance of the test

The IgG anti-D (anti-Rh$_o$) should be injected intramuscularly between 24 and 48 hours before injecting the Rh-positive cells. It is suggested that the amount injected should be of the order of 75 μg of antibody, as this gives a rate of clearance that can be conveniently measured. Tests should be carried out in not less than 2 subjects.

The volume of Rh-positive red cells injected should be approximately 0.5 ml (0.2 ml–2.0 ml). The cells should be labelled with ^{51}Cr (30 μCi should be a sufficient amount) and should be washed at least three times in saline before being injected intravenously.

An initial blood sample should be taken from the recipient at 10 minutes to provide an estimate of 100% survival; sufficient further samples should be taken to determine the maximal rate of destruction (see below); as a guide, if approximately 75 μg of anti-D (anti-Rh$_o$) are injected, further samples should be taken at approximately 8-12 hours, by which time a maximum of red cell destruction should have been established, and at 20-30 hours, when most of the red cells should have been eliminated; it is desirable to take one or two intermediate samples so as to define the slope of disappearance more precisely; the optimum time for taking samples will evidently vary with the dose of anti-D (anti-Rh$_o$).

The percentage survival of red cells (corrected for chromium elution) is then estimated for each sample and plotted on a logarithmic scale against time on a linear scale. The pattern of clearance observed is an initial lag phage, before the onset of destruction (due to the time taken for antibody to associate with the red cells), followed by disappearance of the cells which soon reaches a maximum rate. This maximum rate, expressed as a $T_{1/2}$ in hours, is taken as the rate of clearance. For further details, see Mollison & Hughes-Jones (1967).

THE NEED FOR STANDARD PREPARATIONS FOR INCOMPLETE ANTI-D (ANTI-Rh$_o$) ANTIBODY

Two types of standard preparation are required. On the one hand, whole-serum preparations are needed for comparison of the potency of anti-D (anti-Rh$_o$) antibody in the serum of those who are potential donors for the plasma pool, while, on the other hand, there is a need for standards of IgG anti-D (anti-Rh$_o$) to be used for assessing the relative potency of the IgG anti-D (anti-Rh$_o$) preparations used in the treatment of patients. Whole-serum preparations should be compared with national standard preparations of incomplete anti-D (anti-Rh$_o$), and these standards should themselves in turn have been tested in parallel with the International Standard for Anti-D (Anti-Rh$_o$) Incomplete Blood-Typing Serum. Ampoules of the International Standard, details of which have been published by Goldsmith, Mourant & Bangham (1967), may be obtained from the International Laboratory for Biological Standards, Statens Seruminstitut, Copenhagen. It should be pointed out that supplies of the International Standard are extremely limited and that it is to be used for comparison with national standards only.

The International Standard is not sterile and therefore cannot be used for *in vivo* studies, either to assess its protective effect or to determine its ability to clear Rh-positive cells.

Standard preparations of IgG anti-D (anti-Rh$_o$) will be required for assessing the relative potency of the IgG preparations of anti-D (anti-Rh$_o$) that are to be used therapeutically. These preparations must be tested for their potency by *in vitro* or *in vivo* methods and, in addition, they should have been used in clinical trials and shown to be effective.

THE OPTIMAL DOSE OF IGG ANTI-D (ANTI-Rh$_o$)

At the present time, there are no results available of a completed investigation in which the dose of IgG anti-D (anti-Rh$_o$) (measured in μg/ml) has been related to its effectiveness in suppression of the immune response.

In clinical trials carried out in Liverpool (Clarke et al., 1966), 5 ml of an anti-D (anti-Rh$_o$) preparation were used. The concentration of anti-D (anti-Rh$_o$) in this preparation is not known, but it is probably similar to the concentration found in later preparations which have been estimated. If this is so, then it is probable that a dose of approximately 750 μg was used and this was found to be completely effective. There is experimental evidence, however, that a smaller amount is also effective. Thus Freda and Gorman (unpublished observations) have found that 0.1 ml of an anti-D (anti-Rh$_o$) preparation protected 4 volunteers when given with 10 ml of blood on 6 occasions, and in the experiments of Zipursky.

472

and co-workers (presented in 1966 at the XIth Congress of the International Society of Blood Transfusion) both 5.0-ml and 1.0-ml doses of another anti-D (anti-Rh₀) preparation protected 12 volunteers when injected with 2 ml of blood. The anti-D (anti-Rh₀) concentrations of these preparations are also not known, but it is believed that they were of similar potency to later preparations from the same laboratories and thus the amount injected was probably of the order of 150 μg anti-D (anti-Rh₀) for Freda and Gorman and 60 μg–300 μg for Zipursky and co-workers.

Similarly, analysis of results obtained in Germany (Schneider & Preisler, 1966a) and by Freda and Gorman (unpublished observations) indicates that a dose of the order of 10 μg is insufficient to bring about suppression when 1ml–10 ml of Rh-positive blood are injected. It must be emphasized, however, that these values are only approximate and are suggested only as a tentative guide for further trials.

Until the mechanism of suppression of primary immunization is known, the possibility must also be considered that factors other than anti-D (anti-Rh₀) concentration are important. Thus, variation in the immunosuppressive activity of anti-D (anti-Rh₀) antibody obtained from different donors is possible, and it is for this reason that it has been recommended that IgG preparations are made from pools of at least 10 donors. Furthermore, it is recommended that clinical trials should be continued to compare the relative effectiveness of anti-D (anti-Rh₀) antibody obtained from mothers who have not been deliberately restimulated compared with that from donors who have been restimulated.

ENHANCEMENT OF IMMUNE RESPONSE TO D (Rh₀) ANTIGEN

There is experimental evidence in animals that under certain circumstances the passive injection of antibody enhances active antibody production. There is a report that this occurred in humans following the injection of serum containing anti-D (anti-Rh₀) saline agglutinins (Clarke et al., 1963) and it is now thought that enhancement was due to the presence of the IgM anti-D (anti-Rh₀). Experimental work carried out in New York (Freda et al., 1966) and London (Mollison, unpublished observations) suggests that there is no enhancement when IgG anti-D (anti-Rh₀) is injected in doses too low to bring about immune suppression, although this has yet to be established with certainty.

REPORTED CLINICAL TRIALS

Results 6 months post partum and later

Published results indicate that the administration of IgG anti-D (anti-Rh₀) within 72 hours of delivery is protective against the development of immune anti-D (anti-Rh₀) antibodies for 6 months or longer (Clarke et al., 1966; Schneider & Preisler, 1966b;

Freda et al., 1967). By March 1967, about 900 women had been studied for at least 6 months. Of these about half had received anti-D (anti-Rh₀) IgG and none of them had produced immune antibodies, whereas 60 of the controls had done so. Although the protocols of these studies differed in terms of the selection of patients, the sources of the immunoglobulin and the doses employed for prevention, the results indicate that the anti-D (anti-Rh₀) immunoglobulin was uniformly protective.

Results from subsequent pregnancies

The references already quoted also give the latest information on subsequent pregnancies in women given anti-D (anti-Rh₀) immunoglobulin following their earlier delivery. In such treated women, no Rh antibodies have yet been detected during or immediately after the following pregnancy, suggesting that primary immunization had been entirely prevented, although, since the number of cases is still small (40 at March 1967), the results cannot yet be considered to be conclusive.

RECOMMENDATIONS REGARDING PRIORITIES

At the present time, the amount of IgG anti-D (anti-Rh₀) available is limited and it is recommended that steps be taken to accumulate stocks of this material as quickly as possible. In the transition period, trials should be continued to obtain further information about the treatment; for example: (*a*) two dose levels could be compared since the minimum suppressive dose is not yet known (see " The optimal dose of IgG anti-D (anti-Rh₀)," page 471; (*b*) the effectiveness of small doses of anti-D (anti-Rh₀) in bringing about immunosuppression could be studied in those women who have relatively high foetal cell counts. During this interim period, if no trials are carried out, an alternative would be to treat only those women shown to have a high foetal cell count following delivery.

As supplies of IgG anti-D (anti-Rh₀) increase, the order in which groups of women at risk qualify for protection will depend on local factors, including obstetrical, geographical and legal considerations; but it is recommended that all Rh-negative primiparae with ABO-compatible Rh-positive infants, regardless of the foetal cell count in the maternal circulation, be given first priority.

473

Below is an example of the groups and numbers involved using a country with a population of approximately 5 million (Scotland) where the frequency of Rh-negative persons is 15%:

	No. per million of total population
Total births per annum	20 000
Total births from primiparous women	6 500
Number of abortions (estimated)	2 000
Rh-negative primiparae with ABO-compatible Rh-positive infants (8%)	550
Rh-negative primiparae regardless of blood grouping of infants (15%)	1 000
All births to Rh-negative women with ABO-compatible Rh-positive infants (8%)	1 600
All births to Rh-negative women regardless of blood grouping of infants (15%)	3 000
All pregnancies of Rh-negative women with ABO-compatible Rh-positive infants (8%) + 15% of abortions	2 000
All pregnancies of Rh-negative women regardless of blood grouping of infants (15%) + 15% of abortions	3 300

The estimated number of patients requiring treatment per annum ranges from 550 per million to 3300 per million of population.

Suggested routine tests when using IgG anti-D (anti-Rh₀)

It is considered very valuable that all sera obtained from patients should be kept for reference purposes for one year.

Tests following delivery :

(a) Determination of the ABO and Rh groups of the mother, if not previously determined.

(b) Examination for anti-Rh antibodies by indirect antiglobulin and enzyme tests.

(c) Foetal cell counts, where possible.

(d) Cord blood testing of the infant for ABO and Rh groups and direct antiglobulin test.

(e) A compatibility test between the IgG anti-D (anti-Rh₀) and the mother's red cells is carried out at some centres, but is not considered essential except for those using large doses of very potent preparations.

Cord blood may be obtained before or after delivery of the placenta, but maternal blood should be obtained after delivery of the placenta if foetal cell studies are being carried out.

Subsequent tests in mothers :

(a) After a pregnancy in which IgG anti-D (anti-Rh₀) is given: test for antibodies by antiglobulin and enzyme techniques at 6 months post partum.

(b) In the next following pregnancy: test for antibodies by antiglobulin and enzyme techniques during the pregnancy and immediately and 3 and 6 months after delivery.

PROBLEMS REQUIRING SOLUTION

The need to define more precisely the optimum effective dose for immunosuppression has already been discussed. Other problems which require consideration are as follows:

1. The latest time after delivery at which an injection of IgG anti-D (anti-Rh₀) is effective requires further elucidation.

2. The effect of medical termination of pregnancy on the frequency of the subsequent anti-D (anti-Rh₀) isoimmunization should be determined.

THE ESTIMATION OF FOETAL CELLS IN THE MATERNAL CIRCULATION

Several methods exist for the demonstration of foetal cells in the maternal circulation, but the acid elution technique (Kleihauer et al., 1957) has been most widely used. It should be emphasized, however, that the experimental conditions are critical (Cohen et al., 1964). Fresh buffer should always be used and a pH of 3.2–3.3 is recommended. Various methods of scoring the foetal cells have been described (Schneider & Ludwig, 1965; Woodrow & Finn, 1966). The conversion of foetal cells scores into absolute volumes of foetal blood is inaccurate, and the expression of results as a ratio of foetal to adult cells is to be preferred.

It should be emphasized that this technique requires experience and cannot successfully be performed as an occasional test. There are several inherent difficulties in the interpretation of the slides, because the acid elution technique does not distinguish between maternal and foetal HbF. Maternal HbF levels are increased in thalassaemia and in some other haematological disorders, and there may also be an increase in maternal HbF during pregnancy. False positive results may also occur in association with a marked reticulocytosis. With experience, it is usually, although not invariably, possible to identify those conditions with a high maternal HbF, because the HbF is usually unevenly distributed among many cells rather than concentrated in a few cells, as in a true transplacental haemorrhage (Woodrow & Finn, 1966). In a few cases, this distinction is not possible with the acid elution technique.

The acid elution technique has proved of great value in elucidating the natural history of Rh sensitization and has emphasized the importance of delivery in the sensitization process. It has further been possible to divide cases into high-risk and low-risk groups. The risk of sensitization is related to the number of foetal cells found in the maternal circulation following delivery (Woodrow & Finn, 1966; Schneider & Preisler, 1966b). In about half the cases where sensitization occurs, less than 0.2 ml of foetal blood is detected following delivery.

474

Although the acid elution technique is very valuable as a research method, the difficulties in obtaining reproducible results with the technique make it unlikely that it will come into use as a method of deciding whether or not to give prophylactic treatment. When sufficient supplies of IgG anti-D (anti-Rh_o) become available, it is envisaged that all women at risk will be treated regardless of whether a transplacental haemorrhage has been demonstrated or not. In the interim phase, when supplies of IgG anti-D (anti-Rh_o) are limited, the acid elution technique may be used to select a high-risk group and thus allow the available supplies of IgG anti-D (anti-Rh_o) to be used to the best advantage.

The acid elution technique has shown that there is an increased risk of transplacental haemorrhage following various obstetrical procedures, such as manual separation of the placenta (Finn et al., 1963) and it is therefore recommended that such procedures should be performed with extreme care in Rh-negative women. Transplacental haemorrhages have also been described following abortion (Hollán et al., 1967), and eventually protection may also have to be provided in these cases.

REFERENCES

Clarke, C. A. et al. (1963) *Brit. med. J.*, 1, 979

Clarke, C. A. et al. (1966) *Brit. med. J.*, 2, 907

Cohen, F., Zuelzer, W. W., Gustafson, D. C. & Evans, M. M. (1964) *Blood*, 23, 621

Finn, R., Harper, D. T., Stallings, S. A. & Krevans, J. R. (1963) *Transfusion (Philad.)*, 3, 114

Freda, V. J., Gorman, J. G. & Pollack, W. (1966) *Science*, 151, 828

Freda, V. J., Robertson, J. G. & Gorman, J. G. (1965) *Ann. N.Y. Acad. Sci.*, 127, 909

Freda, V. J. et al. (1967) *J. Amer. med. Ass.*, 199, 390

Goldsmith, K. L. G., Mourant, A. E. & Bangham, D. R. (1967) *Bull. Wld Hlth Org.*, 36, 435

Haynes, L. L. et al. (1960) *J. Amer. med. Ass.*, 173, 1657

Hollán, S. R., Szelenyi, J. G. & Sötér, V. (1967) *Acta med. Acad. Sci. hung.*, 24 (in press)

Hughes-Jones, N. C. (1967) *Immunology*, 12, 565

Janeway, C. A. et al. (1963) *Vox. Sang. (Basel)*, 8, 93 (Panel discussion)

Kleihauer, E., Braun, H. & Betke, K. (1957) *Klin. Wschr.*, 35, 637

Kliman, A., Carbone, P. P., Gaydos, L. A. & Friedrich, E. J. (1964) *Blood*, 23, 647

Kliman, A. & Lesses, M. F. (1964) *Transfusion (Philad.)*, 4, 469

Mollison, P. L. & Hughes-Jones, N. C. (1967) *Immunology*, 12, 63

Schneider, J. & Ludwig, G. A. (1963) *Klin. Wschr.*, 41, 563

Schneider, J. & Preisler, O. (1966a) *Blut*, 12, 1

Schneider, J. & Preisler, O. (1966b) *Obstet. and Gynec.*, 28, 615

WHO Expert Committee on Biological Standardization (1967) *Wld Hlth Org. techn. Rep. Ser.*, 361

Woodrow, J. C. & Finn, R. (1966) *Brit. J. Haemat.*, 12, 297

Paper 37

37.   Hughes-Jones, N. C. (1967). The estimation of the concentration and equilibrium constant of anti-D. *Immunology*, *12*, 565-571.

Commentary

This is not an easy paper to understand, but it is important because it describes a method which gives more accurate information about the efficiency of an anti-D antibody than does titre.[*]

It must be appreciated that the antigen-antibody reaction on the red cell is not a once-for-all static event, but a dynamic situation in which some antibody molecules are attaching themselves to the red cells while others are leaving them to enter the plasma. Where the affinity is great most of the antibody is on the red cells at equilibrium, and the value of the equilibrium (binding) constant is then high.

It is possible, however, to have a high average equilibrium constant (K) and yet a weak antibody (i.e. one with low concentration) and Table 1 shows that the two are independent of each other—but both are important. So too is the heterogeneity index (a) of the values of K for different anti-D molecules within a particular sample of anti-D serum. A wide spread of the values of K within a sample means that a large number of anti-D molecules will have a high value for the equilibrium constant, and hence the biological efficiency (i.e. destruction of red cells) will be high, since more anti-D molecules will be bound to the cell surface.

The object of Hughes-Jones' test is to determine the concentration in μg/ml and the value of the equilibrium constant of any particular anti-D, and he does this by means of an indirect method, which can be called a 'quantitative antiglobulin test'. The quantitative aspect lies in the use of ^{125}I-labelled antiglobulin. This reagent is initially calibrated to find out its combining ratio with anti-D on the surface of the red cells on a weight for weight basis. The calibration is carried out by incubating ^{125}I-labelled antiglobulin with red cells which are coated with ^{131}I-labelled anti-D. Since the two isotopes of iodine are readily distinguished, the amount of antiglobulin which can combine with 1μg of anti-D under the conditions of the assay is easily determined.

The estimation of the anti-D content of an unknown sample of anti-D is then carried out by first absorbing it on to Rh-positive red cells and then estimating the *amount* absorbed by using the previously calibrated ^{125}I-labelled anti-IgG. Since the reaction between anti-D and red cells is reversible and obeys the law of mass action, some anti-D is always left free in solution and is not absorbed by the Rh-positive red cells. In measuring total anti-D concentration, it is clearly necessary to take this unbound anti-D into account. This has been done by absorbing several aliquots of anti-D with different volumes of Rh-positive cells and measuring the amount of anti-D absorbed on to the cells in each case. The total amount of anti-D in the solution can then be derived by a graphical representation of the data (the Scatchard plot).

The same graph can also be used to obtain the value of the equilibrium constant, which is the reciprocal of the free D-antigen concentration when half the anti-D is bound to red cells at equilibrium.

It will be seen from Table 2 of this paper how the equilibrium constant influences the amount of antibody which is required in the plasma to give a similar concentration of anti-D bound to the red cells. Thus with 1 ml of red cells present in the circulation, 21 times as much of a weakly binding antibody was required compared to the strongly binding antibody. When there are 400 ml of cells in the circulation, only 3 times as much weakly binding antibody is required as of the strongly binding one.

[*]The titre of a serum is expressed as the reciprocal of the greatest dilution of the serum
   which will produce a detectable reaction with selected red cells.

37. Commentary cont.

reciprocal of moles/litre. (A mole is the molecular weight in grammes dissolved in a litre of water, and the molecular weight of gamma-G-globulin is about 160,000). This unit can be derived from the equation for the law of mass action at equilibrium, $[AbAg]/[Ab_{free}] \times [Ag_{free}] = K$ (where Ab = anti-D and Ag = D-antigen), if all concentrations are expressed as moles/litre. In order to derive the unit for K, moles/litre is substituted in the mass action equation thus:

$$\frac{\text{moles/litre}}{\text{moles/litre} \times \text{moles/litre}} = \frac{1}{\text{moles/litre}} = \text{litres/mole}$$

Definition of the Unit used for the value of K (litres per mole).
The unit used for the value of the equilibrium constant is litres/mole, which is the

From N. C. Hughes-Jones (1967). Immunology, 12, 565-571. Copyright (1967), by kind permission of the author and Blackwell Scientific Publications

Immunology, 1967, **12**, 565.

The Estimation of the Concentration and Equilibrium Constant of Anti-D

N. C. HUGHES-JONES

Experimental Haematology Research Unit, Wright-Fleming Institute of Microbiology, London, W.2

(*Received* 16th *September* 1966)

Summary. A method is described for estimating the concentration and equilibrium constant of the blood group antibody, anti-D. The principle of the method is based on the fact that the reaction between anti-D and red cells is reversible and obeys the law of mass action. D-positive red cells at five different concentrations were added to aliquots of antisera containing anti-D and the reaction allowed to come into equilibrium. The amount of anti-D bound to the red cells in each case was estimated using ^{125}I-labelled anti-γ-globulin. The results of these estimates were then analysed according to two derivations of the law of mass action. Twenty-one examples of antisera containing anti-D were examined and the estimated range of values was as follows: concentration, $0 \cdot 3$–$7 \cdot 2$ μg/ml; equilibrium constant, $1 \cdot 4 \times 10^7$ to $1 \cdot 2 \times 10^9$ l/mole; index of heterogeneity, $a = 0 \cdot 6$–$0 \cdot 9$.

INTRODUCTION

The reaction between anti-D and red cells is reversible and when equilibrium is reached antibody is present free in solution as well as bound to red cells. The extent of the agglutination produced by the addition of antiglobulin serum is dependent only on the amount of anti-D bound to the cells and an estimate of the titre of the antibody does not take into account the amount of antibody remaining free in solution. In any given mixture of D-positive red cells and anti-D, the amount of free antibody depends on the initial concentration of antibody, its equilibrium constant, and on the amount of red cells present. Similar considerations apply to the amount of anti-D which will combine with D-positive red cells in the circulation. Elucidation of the action of anti-D *in vivo* is thus dependent on a knowledge of the concentration and equilibrium constant in each particular case. This report presents a method of measuring these two factors.

The number of molecules of the Rh antibody, anti-D, bound to red cells can be estimated using iodinated anti-γ-globulin (Costea, Schwartz, Constantoulakis and Dameshek, 1962; Rochna and Hughes-Jones, 1965); this technique can be adapted to measure the anti-D content of serum. The principle of the method depends on the fact that the reaction between anti-D and red cells is reversible so that, at equilibrium, the amounts of bound and free anti-D are given by the law of mass action. Red cells at several different concentrations are added to aliquots of the serum containing anti-D and allowed to come into equilibrium. The amount of anti-D bound to the red cells in each case is estimated using ^{125}I-labelled anti-γ-globulin ([^{125}I]anti-γ-globulin) and the total antibody content of the serum can be calculated by an analysis of the results according to a derivation of the law of mass action.

MATERIALS AND METHODS

Serum containing anti-D

Twenty-one sera, obtained from women at the time of delivery of a child suffering from haemolytic disease of the newborn, were kindly supplied by Dr W. Walker of Newcastle.

Red cells

Red cells (from a single CCDee donor) were used in all experiments for adsorption of the anti-D. The concentration of D antigen sites was estimated to be 313 p-moles/ml red cells by the method of Rochna and Hughes-Jones, 1965. The cells were washed three times before use, and white cells and platelets were removed.

[^{125}I]Anti-γ-globulin

Anti-human γ-globulin was obtained from a sheep and purified by absorption and elution from CM-cellulose to which human γ-globulin had been attached (Weliky, Weetall, Gilden and Campbell, 1964). This antibody was labelled with ^{125}I by the method of McFarlane (1958) and the combining ratio between this anti-γ-globulin and anti-D adsorbed onto red cells was estimated using an [^{131}I]anti-D. The anti-D used for calibration was obtained from a single donor. Details of these procedures and those used for determining specific activity and purity of the anti-γ-globulin are given elsewhere (Rochna and Hughes-Jones, 1965).

Procedure for estimating anti-D content of sera

The estimation of the anti-D content of sera is most accurate when there is approximately 0·2–2·0 μg of anti-D/ml of solution. It was found that antisera diluted 1:5 with 0·17 M NaCl, pH 7·0, usually gave a suitable concentration. If the initial estimate of antibody showed the concentration to be outside the optimal range, the procedure was repeated at the correct dilution.

Five 1-ml aliquots of the diluted antiserum were obtained and the R_1R_1 red cells were added in the following amounts, 2, 10, 50, 100 and 200 μl. The suspensions were then incubated at 37° for 2 hours with frequent mixing. This is sufficient time to bring the reactants into equilibrium. The suspensions were then centrifuged at 4° and the cells washed three times with 2 ml of ice-cold saline. One millilitre of [^{125}I]anti-γ-globulin (15 μg antibody/ml) was then added and after rapid mixing with a pipette, the suspensions were placed at 37° for 10 minutes without further disturbance. The suspensions were centrifuged and the supernatant saved for estimates of the free anti-γ-globulin concentration. The cells were transferred to another container with 2 ml of ice-cold saline, centrifuged, the supernatant removed and the ^{125}I content of the cells estimated. The amount of anti-D bound to the cells was then calculated using the previously determined combining-ratio between anti-D and anti-γ-globulin at the particular free anti-γ-globulin concentration present at the end of the 10-minute incubation period (see Rochna and Hughes-Jones, 1965).

Analysis of results

The results were analysed according to the derivation of the law of mass action derived by Scatchard (1949). The derivation is as follows: $r/[Ag]_{(free)} = Kn - Kr$ where r = the equilibrium concentration of antigen–antibody complex, n = the maximum amount of antigen–antibody complex that is formed when all the antibody is bound to antigen, K = the equilibrium constant and [Ag] = the free antigen concentration at equilibrium (derived as $[Ag]_{(total)} - [AgAb]_{(eq)} = [Ag]_{(free)}$). The value of n, which is equivalent to the total antibody concentration of the diluted antiserum, can be obtained by plotting $r/[Ag]$ against r and extrapolating to the abscissa, for, when $r/[Ag] = 0$, then $n = r$. In order to obtain the equilibrium constant, the data were analysed according to the derivation of Karush (1962) as follows: $\log r/n - r = a \log [Ag]_{(free)} + a \log K$. If $\log r/n - r$ is plotted against $\log [Ag]_{(free)}$, then the value of K is equal to $1/[Ag]_{(free)}$ when $\log r/n - r = 0$; the slope of the line gives the heterogeneity index, a. The molar concentration of antibody was calculated assuming a molecular weight of 160,000 for γG-globulin.

Antiglobulin titres on all twenty-one sera were estimated at the same time by a standard technique, using cells at a final concentration of 4 per cent and reading the results on a semi-opaque tile.

RESULTS

An example of the analysis of the results obtained in a typical case is shown in Figs. 1 and 2. The estimated concentrations, the values of the equilibrium constants and indices of heterogeneity are given in Table 1 and are shown graphically in Fig. 3. The relationship between titre and antibody concentration is shown in Fig. 4.

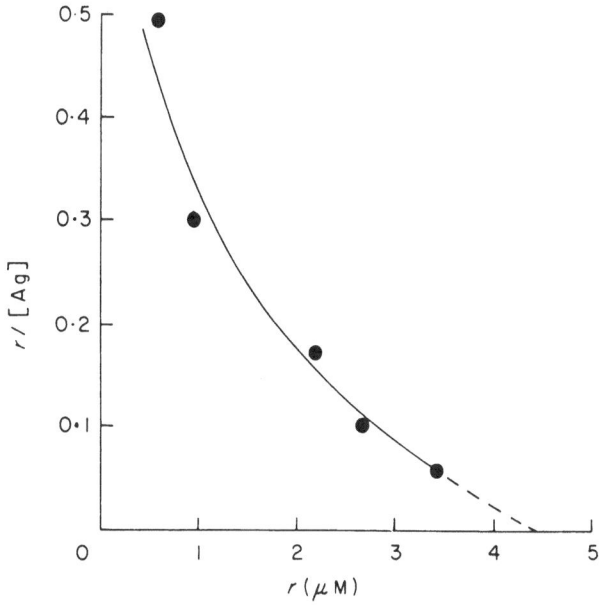

FIG. 1. An example of the plot of $r/[Ag]$ against r. The extrapolation to the abscissa gives the concentration of antibody in the diluted antiserum.

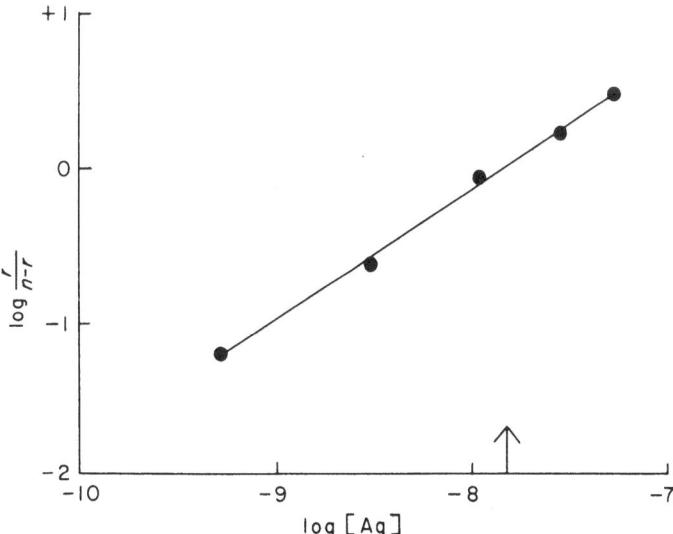

FIG. 2. An example of the plot of $\log r/n-r$ against $\log[Ag]$. The slope of the curve gives the heterogeneity index. The reciprocal of the molar concentration of [Ag] at the point when $\log r/n-r = 0$ gives the value of the equilibrium constant K in l/mole.

TABLE 1

THE ESTIMATED VALUES OF THE CONCENTRA-
TION, EQUILIBRIUM CONSTANT (K) AND
HETEROGENEITY INDEX (a) OF ANTI-D PRESENT
IN TWENTY-ONE SERA OBTAINED FROM WOMEN
AT THE TIME OF DELIVERY OF A CHILD
SUFFERING FROM HAEMOLYTIC DISEASE OF THE
NEWBORN

Serum	Concentration (μg/ml)	$K \times 10^{-7}$ l/mole	a
1	2·2	7	0·85
2	1·3	16	0·6
3	7·2	10	0·7
4	3·2	18	0·9
5	3·2	120	0·61
6	6·0	62	0·8
7	4·2	12	0·75
8	0·6	5	0·8
9	3·6	7	0·81
10	4·2	1·4	0·86
11	1·2	100	0·65
12	3·7	14	0·89
13	0·3	20	0·75
14	1·4	11·2	0·82
15	1·6	18	0·68
16	2·4	31	0·86
17	2·0	12	0·65
18	5·0	14	0·74
19	2·9	28	0·76
20	0·3	20	0·9
21	3·4	3·5	0·85

DISCUSSION

There are two main sources of error in this technique of measuring anti-D concentration. (1) The concentration must be estimated by extrapolation of a curved line, which could introduce an error of 10–20 per cent. (2) A more serious source of error derives from the assumption that the [^{125}I]anti-γ-globulin combined to the same extent with unknown examples of anti-D as it did with the [^{131}I]anti-D with which it was calibrated. An experiment was carried out to investigate the error introduced by this assumption. Ten examples of anti-D were purified and labelled with ^{131}I and their combining ratio with the [^{125}I]anti-γ-globulin determined. It was found that there was a variation in the combining ratios of these ten examples compared with the original anti-D used for the calibration. Eight of the ten examples gave combining ratios within 25 per cent of that of the 'calibrating' anti-D, the other two gave ratios 40 per cent lower. The estimates of the anti-D concentration are thus probably within a factor of 0·6–1·5 of the true anti-D concentration.

Although the average values of the equilibrium constant vary widely, there being approximately a 100-fold difference between the lowest and highest values, twelve out of the twenty-one values fall within the narrow range $1·0$–$3·0 \times 10^8$ l/mole.

The heterogeneity index used here is that initially suggested by Nisonoff and Pressman (1958) and is based on the surmise that the distribution of equilibrium constants is normal or Gaussian around the mean. If this is so, then the plot of $\log r/n - r$ against $\log[\text{Ag}]_{(\text{free})}$ should·be linear. Within experimental error, the data obtained in this investigation fit linear curves, and this provides evidence that the distribution does approximate to a normal curve. A heterogeneity index of $a = 1·0$ indicates homogeneity, and values below indicate heterogeneity, the lower the value, the greater the heterogeneity. To give an

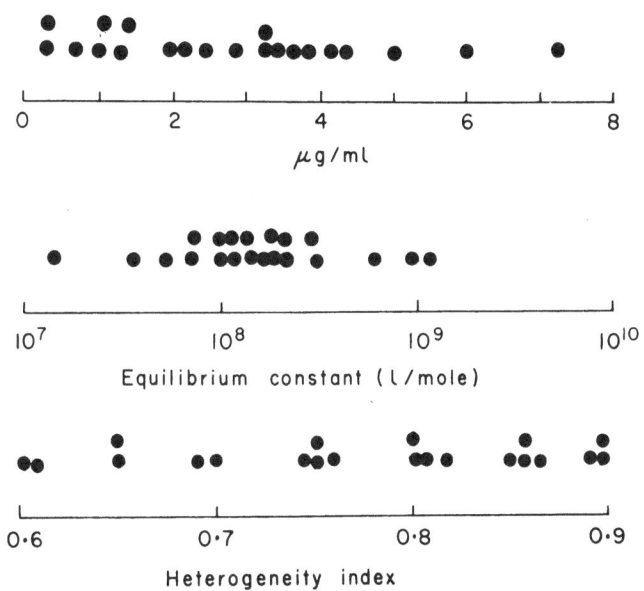

Fig. 3. Graphical representation of the estimates of antibody concentration, equilibrium constant and index of heterogeneity of twenty-one examples of anti-D.

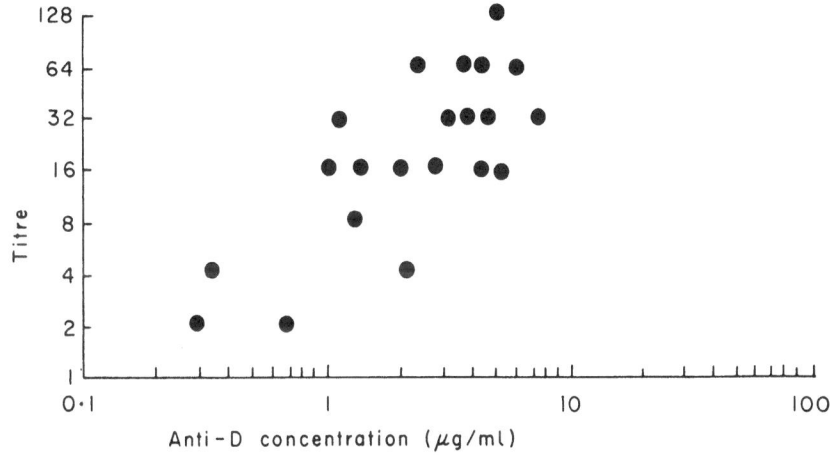

Fig. 4. The relationship between the anti-globulin titre and the anti-D concentration.

indication of the range, it can be calculated (Fujio and Karush, 1966) that an antibody with a mean equilibrium constant of 1×10^8 l/mole and heterogeneity index $a = 0.6$ will have two-thirds of all the molecules with constants within a range 1×10^7 to 1×10^9 l/mole and 95 per cent will be inside the range 1×10^6 to 1×10^{10} l/mole.

The relationship between titre and concentration of anti-D given in Fig. 4 shows that the correlation is poor, e.g. a titre of 32 being given by examples of anti-D in the range 1·2–7·2 μg/ml. There are two reasons for this poor correlation. (1) The error involved in the estimation of titre is recognized to be large; duplicate estimates frequently show a two-fold and sometimes a four-fold difference in strength. (2) The titre of an antibody not only depends on its concentration but also on the values of the equilibrium constant, the degree of heterogeneity and on the concentration of red cells. It has been found (unpublished observations) that at the end-point of the titration (standard anti-globulin test) there is approximately 1 μg anti-D/ml of red cells or 350 molecules/red cell. This is of the same order as that given by Dupuy, Elliot and Masouredis (1964). The titre gives no indication of the amount of antibody free in solution at the end-point, an amount which is dependent on the values of K and a. Thus, it can be calculated that two antibodies

TABLE 2

TOTAL AMOUNT OF ANTIBODY (μg/3000 ml) WITH TWO DIFFERENT VALUES OF K WHICH ARE REQUIRED IN THE PLASMA TO GIVE A CONCENTRATION OF ANTI-D BOUND TO RED CELLS OF 0·03 μg/ml RED CELLS

D-positive red cells in circulation (ml)	Antibody	
	$K = 1 \times 10^7$ l/mole	$K = 1 \times 10^9$ l/mole
1	4·2 μg	0·2 μg
400	39 μg	13 μg

The heterogeneity index is taken to be $a = 0·7$ in both cases.

present at a concentration of 1 μg/ml but which have values of K equal to 1×10^7 and 1×10^9 l/mole would give titres of 2 and 22 respectively, provided that there was no heterogeneity of the equilibrium constant in each example. Antibodies are, however, always heterogeneous and if a value of $a = 0·7$ is taken for each, then the titres become 4 and 20 respectively, provided that the final concentration of R_1R_1 cells used for the titre is 4 per cent. Thus equal concentrations of anti-D whose equilibrium constants fall at either end of the range found in this investigation would have a five-fold difference in titre.

The rate of red cell destruction *in vivo* caused by antibodies depends on the number of antibody molecules attached to red cells (Mollison and Hughes-Jones, 1967). The rate of destruction brought about by a particular antibody is thus dependent on its concentration and on the average value and the extent of heterogeneity of the equilibrium constant, that is, the same factors which affect the titre of an antibody. The titre and the biological activity of an antibody however are not necessarily related.

This results from the fact that the titre is usually estimated using a fixed quantity of red cells (4 per cent) whereas the number of red cells to be destroyed in any individual obviously varies from case to case. This can be illustrated as follows. Assuming that the minimal amount of anti-D on the red cells must be 0·03 μg/ml for destruction to take place (Mollison and Hughes-Jones, 1967) the total amount required in the plasma of an adult can be calculated for the two situations where there is either 1 ml or 400 ml of R_1R_1 cells in the circulation of an Rh negative individual. The values are shown in Table 2; it can be seen that with 1 ml of cells present in the circulation, 21 times as much of the weakly-binding antibody ($K = 1 \times 10^7$ l/mole) is required compared to the stronger binding antibody. When there are 400 ml of cells in the circulation only 3 times as much weakly-binding antibody is required as stronger binding antibody. These two antibodies give a five-fold difference in their titres. Titre and biological effectiveness would be related if the titre were estimated using the same concentration of D-positive cells as would be found in the circulation in any particular case *in vivo*.

REFERENCES

COSTEA, N., SCHWARTZ, R., CONSTANTOULAKIS, M. and DAMESHEK, W. (1962). 'The use of radioactive antiglobulin in the detection of erythrocyte sensitization.' *Blood*, **20**, 214.

DUPUY, M. E., ELLIOT, M. and MASOUREDIS, S. P. (1964). 'Relationship between red cell bound antibody and agglutination in the antiglobulin reaction.' *Vox Sang. (Basel)*, **9**, 40.

FUJIO, H. and KARUSH, F. (1966). 'Antibody affinity. II. Effect of immunization interval on antihapten antibody in rabbit.' *Biochemistry*, **5**, 1856.

KARUSH, F. (1962). 'Immunological specificity and molecular structure.' *Advanc. Immunol.*, **2**, 1.

MCFARLANE, A. S. (1958) 'Efficient trace-labelling of proteins with iodine.' *Nature (Lond.)*, **182**, 53.

MOLLISON, P. L. and HUGHES-JONES, N. C. (1967). 'The clearance of Rh-positive cells by low concentrations of Rh antibody.' *Immunology*, **12**, 63.

NISONOFF, A. and PRESSMAN, D. (1958). 'Heterogeneity and average combining constants of antibodies from individual rabbits.' *J. Immunol.*, **80**, 417.

ROCHNA, E. and HUGHES-JONES, N. C. (1965). 'The use of purified ^{125}I-labelled anti-γ-globulin in the determination of the number of D antigen sites on red cells of different phenotypes.' *Vox Sang. (Basel)*, **10**, 675.

SCATCHARD, D. (1949). 'The attractions of proteins for small molecules and ions.' *Ann. N.Y. Acad. Sci.*, **51**, 660.

WELIKY, N., WEETAL, H. H., GILDEN, R. V. and CAMPBELL, D. H. (1964). 'The synthesis and use of some insoluble immunologically specific adsorbents.' *Immunochemistry*, **1**, 219.

Paper 38

38. Mollison, P. I., Hughes-Jones, N. C., Lindsay, M. and Wessely, J. (1969). Suppression of primary Rh immunisation by passively-administered antibody: Experiments in volunteers. *Vox Sang., 16*, 421-439.

Commentary

Two important concepts in immunology are 'priming' and 'augmentation'.

'Priming' indicates that immunisation has taken place but that antibodies cannot be detected by routine laboratory tests. They can be detected, however, by red cell survival studies, since red cells do not live their normal 100 days when there are occult antibodies present. Rh-negative women who have been primed by a *previous* Rh-positive pregnancy will routinely be classed as having 'no demonstrable antibodies' and may therefore be given anti-D after their next Rh-positive pregnancy. This will of course be too late. Previous priming is the most important cause of the small anti-D failure rate.

'Augmentation', in the connexion of prophylaxis of HDN by the giving of anti-D, means that anti-Rh antibodies are formed more readily than if anti-D had not been given. This possibility has worried anti-D research workers ever since the first Liverpool experiments when it appeared to have taken place. Subsequent follow up, however, made it much more likely that the complete (19S) anti-D just had no effect, i.e. it neither protected nor augmented.

In the paper under discussion, Mollison *et al.* show convincingly, by studies on cell survival in Rh-negative male volunteers given Rh-positive cells, that when the conventional antibodies (i.e. those detected by routine tests) had been excluded from the controls (2 cases) it was still possible to show priming in six out of thirteen other controls. This was demonstrated by giving Rh-positive cells tagged with ^{51}Cr six months after the original stimulus—a proportion of these cells was eliminated by the hidden antibody. By contrast, none of those treated with 75 μg of anti-D after the first stimulus had abnormal cell survival after the second injection, and only two out of eight had slightly subnormal curves at that time, even those to whom a very small dose (15 μg) of anti-D had been given. Thus they were much better off than most of the controls in spite of the smallness of their protective dose. This shows that augmentation had not occurred in this experiment.

The paper strikingly anticipates the findings that a much smaller dose of anti-D than had at first been thought is effective in preventing immunisation (Paper 46).

The reason for the additional discussion after this paper is that it formed part of a conference on Recent Advances in Immunopathology and Blood Transfusion.

From P. L. Mollison et al. (1969). Vox Sang., 16, 421-439. Copyright (1969), by kind permission of the authors and S. Karger

Vox Sang. *16:* 421–439 (1969)

Suppression of Primary Rh Immunization by Passively-Administered Antibody. Experiments in Volunteers

P. L. Mollison, N. C. Hughes-Jones, Margaret Lindsay and Jane Wessely

MRC Experimental Haematology Research Unit, St. Mary's Hospital
Medical School, London

Summary. Rh-negative volunteers were given an injection of 1 ml of Rh-positive red cells, either alone or with 15 μg or 75 μg anti-D. Six months later anti-Rh was detected in 2 out of 14 subjects who had originally received Rh-positive red cells alone but in none out of 8 subjects who had also received 15 μg anti-D and in none out of 15 subjects who had also received 75 μg anti-D.

Six months after the start of the experiment, thirty-four of the subjects were injected with 1 ml of ^{51}Cr labelled red cells without anti-D. At 7–11 days after injection, survival was normal in all of 13 subjects who had received 75 μg anti-D with their first injection of red cells. By contrast, survival was subnormal in seven out of 13 cases who had received no anti-D with their first injection of red cells. This difference is significant (p $=$ 0.027) and is taken to indicate that primary immunization occurred when 1 ml of Rh-positive red cells was given alone but was prevented when 1 ml of red cells was given with 75 μg anti-D. Survival at 7 days was slightly subnormal in 2 out of 8 subjects who had received 15 μg anti-D with their first injection of red cells; this is taken as evidence that no augmentation of primary immunization was produced with this dose.

In a follow-up study of another series of Rh-negative volunteers, who had been injected with 0.3 ml of Rh-positive red cells at a time when they had between 0.6 and 4 μg anti-D in their circulation, 3 to 8 months later the survival of injected Rh-positive red cells was normal in 5 out of 6 cases, suggesting that there had been no augmentation of primary immunization.

There is abundant evidence that when 'excess' antibody is administered passively with antigen, primary immunization is inhibited, and it has been shown that the higher the binding constant of the passively administered antibody, the smaller is the amount required for inhibition [7]. Nevertheless, for any given antigen-antibody system the minimum amount of antibody required for suppressing primary immunization by a given amount of soluble antigen cannot yet be predicted precisely, and an added complication is introduced when the antigen is not soluble but is cell-borne. Accordingly, at the present time, the precise amount of passively-administered antibody required to inhibit primary immunization by a given amount of cells must be determined by experiment.

The object of the present work was to define more closely the minimum amount of IgG anti-D required to inhibit primary Rh immunization by 1 ml of Rh-positive red cells.

Methods

Subjects. Rh-negative blood donors were interviewed in groups and told of the object of the work; the risks of becoming isoimmunized and of developing hepatitis were explained. The donors were given forms and asked to return these, after reflection, to indicate whether or not they were prepared to take part.

Fifty-nine subjects received injections of Rh-positive red cells: of these, 52 were men and 7 were post-menopausal women; three of the women had never been pregnant; the four remaining women had each had two or more pregnancies and, as mentioned below, were excluded from some of the analyses; results in one non-parous woman were also excluded when, on further questioning, it was discovered that she had received a transfusion of Rh-positive blood many years previously. No other subjects had been transfused with Rh-positive blood.

Three experiments were carried out:

Experiment I. Thirty-six subjects were enrolled and were divided at random into three groups of 12; in March 1967 all 36 subjects received an intravenous injection of 1 ml of red cells from an Rh-positive donor (MES; further details are given below). The first group (A) received only red cells; the second and third groups (B and C) received an intramuscular injection of 15 μg and 75 μg, respectively, of anti-D (immunoglobulin batch N49G; see below) given at the same time as the red cells.

Six months later, the subjects were re-injected with 1 ml of Rh-positive red cells from the same donor but on this occasion the red cells were labelled with 30–50 μc ^{51}Cr, after being washed in citrate pH 6.9 [2, p. 724]. Samples were taken at 10 min, 24 h, 7 days (11 days in 2 cases) and 28 days. The radioactivity of all samples was determined at the end of 28 days, after lysing the samples with saponin. The haemoglobin concentration of all the samples was determined in duplicate by the cyanmethaemoglobin method and results were then expressed as counts per min of haemoglobin in the samples. Then, taking the counts per min haemoglobin in the 10 min sample as 100%, the percentage survival at 24 h, 7 days and 28 days was determined.

Samples of serum were examined for anti-Rh immediately before the second injection (six months after the first) and one month and four to five months after the second injection.

In a preliminary experiment, the effect of intramuscular injections of 15 μg, 45 μg and 75 μg of anti-D (batch N49G) in clearing Rh-positive red cells from the circulation was tested in three additional subjects. In these cases the injections of immunoglobulin were given 24 h before an injection of 1 ml of ^{51}Cr labelled red cells from donor MES. Supplementary observations were made in two of the subjects taking part in series C but in these cases, as in the rest of series B and C, the injections of gamma globulin were given at the same time as the red cells.

Experiment II. The second experiment, conducted at the same time as the first, differed only in the following ways: first, only 8 subjects were enrolled and these were divided into two series: X, in which the subjects received an intravenous injection of 1 ml of red cells alone and Y, in which they received the same amount of red cells but also received an intramuscular injection of 75 μg antibody (N49G); second, a different donor, selected because he was Bu(a+) as well as Rh-positive, was used (all the recipients were Bu(a–)); third, following the second injection of red cells (given 6 months after the first) samples were taken at 10 min, 11 days and 28 days. In this experiment, as in experiment I, the red cells of the second injection were labelled with ^{51}Cr and their survival estimated.

Experiment III. This experiment was a continuation of one previously reported in which the main object was to determine the effect of small amounts of Rh antibody, passively-administered, on the survival of a small volume of Rh-positive red cells in previously unimmunized Rh-negative subjects. As reported previously [3], 10 male subjects, who had not previously been transfused, were given an intravenous injection of 0.29–0.43 ml of red cells (average 0.34 ml) from donor MES; 7 of the subjects received an intramuscular injection of anti-D immunoglobulin (from a single donor 'Av') at the same time as the red cells and 3 received an injection of anti-D 24–48 h before the cells; the amount of anti-D injected ranged from 1 to 1000 μg. Between 6 and 22 weeks later, 5 subjects were given a second injection of ^{51}Cr labelled red cells; by comparing the rate of clearance with that observed following the first injections, which had been given within 24 h of injecting the anti-D, the amount of anti-D remaining in the body at the time of the second injections could be calculated. It was concluded that the amount of anti-D remaining in the 5 cases was between 0.6 and 4 μg and it was further concluded that the anti-D had been disappearing from the circulation with a T$\frac{1}{2}$ of 16 days.

In the present work 9 of the 10 subjects were given further injections of ^{51}Cr-labelled red cells between 250 and 295 days after the first injections. Assuming that the anti-D had continued to disappear from the body with a T$\frac{1}{2}$ of 16 days, the amount remaining at the time of the final injections of red cells was calculated to be less than one ten thousandth of the amount originally injected. Thus, in the subject who had originally received 1000 μg, the amount remaining at 295 days was 0.1 μg and in the other cases was very much less.

Donors. All the injections of red cells given in experiments I and III came from a particular group O R$_1$r donor (MES) whose blood had been given to a number of recipients on previous occasions and had not been known to induce hepatitis in any of them. The number of D antigen sites on the red cells of this donor, estimated by the method of Rochna and Hughes-Jones [6], was 18,000.

The injections given in experiment II were from a group O R$_2$r donor who had given 16 donations for therapeutic transfusions without known ill effects to the recipients; as already mentioned, this donor was Bu(a+).

Serological tests. All serum samples were tested by the indirect antiglobulin method and were also tested against enzyme-treated cells. In both cases, 1000 volumes of serum were incubated with one volume of red cells; in the antiglobulin test the period of incubation was 3 h and the red cells, after being washed as usual, were tested with a specific anti-IgG serum. In the enzyme test, red cells were first treated with papain for 7 min and then, after being washed, were incubated with serum for 1$\frac{1}{2}$ h before being examined microscopically for agglutination.

Results

Rate of clearance produced by anti-D immunoglobulin, batch N49G. Figure 1 shows the results of the preliminary experiments in which different amounts of anti-D (N49G) were injected into 3 subjects and in which, 24 h later, the survival of 1 ml of ^{51}Cr-labelled Rh-positive red cells was estimated. In the subject injected with 15 μg there was a delay ('lag') of approximately 25 h and the cells were then cleared with a T$\frac{1}{2}$ of 24 h; in the subject who received 45 μg of antibody the lag was 15 h and the subsequent T$\frac{1}{2}$ 12 h; and in the subject who received 75 μg the lag was approximately 5 h and the subsequent T$\frac{1}{2}$ of 9 h.

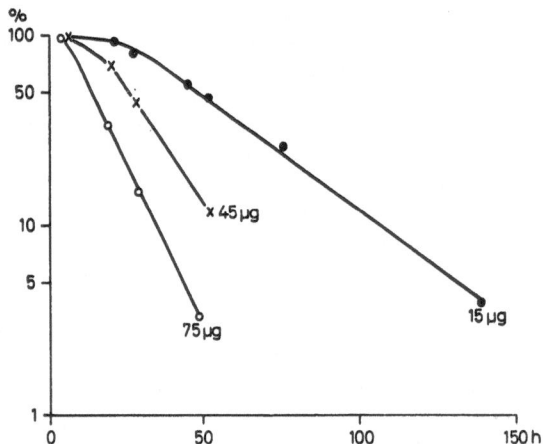

Fig. 1. Rate of clearance of 1 ml ^{51}Cr-labelled Rh-positive red cells (donor M.E.S.) in three Rh-negative subjects, injected 24 h previously with 15, 45 and 75 μg anti-D (Batch N49G), respectively.

In two of the subjects from group C who received 75 μg anti-D (N49G) at the same time as the initial injection of 1 ml of red cells, ^{51}Cr survival was as follows: in one case, lag 5 h, T$\frac{1}{2}$ 6 h; in the second, lag 15 h, T$\frac{1}{2}$ 12 h. These differences presumably reflect varying rates of absorption of anti-D immunoglobulin from the site of injection.

Experiments I and II

Series A (subjects receiving only red cells). Amongst the 12 subjects originally enrolled in this series there was one parous woman. One of the remaining 11 subjects developed hepatitis 187 days after the

Table I. ^{51}Cr red cell survival results (second injections of red cells) in experiments I and II

Amount of anti-D with first injection of red cells	Series	Subject	^{51}Cr Survival 24 h	7 (or 11) days	28 days	Anti-Rh at 4–5 months
Nil	A	Old	99.5	89.5	60	0
		Mor	96.5	86.5	58.5	0
		San	96	87.5	56	0
		Byr	97	(78.0)[1]	52.5	0
		Slo	91	78.5	42	0
		Bol	93.5	75.5	0	0
		Den	95.5	75	33	+
		Gra	92.5	(67.5)[1]	3	+
		Wal	89.5	66.5	0	+
		Ben[2]	32	0	0	+
		(PW)Mil	73.5	23.5	0	+
	X	Ric	....	(80.5)[1]	58	0
		Mis	....	(68)[1]	3	+
		Buc[2]	....	(0)[1]	0	+
15 μg	B	Fre	103	88	57.5	0
		Pit	94.5	85.5	3	0
		Cun	....	84	58	+
		Mah	93.5	83.5	55.5	0
		Hig	96	82	58	0
		Edw	92.5	81	0	0
		Ash	93.5	76	0	0
		Woo	91	75.5	0	0
		(PW)Str	93	75.5	0	0
		(PW)And	85	61.5	0	+
		(PW)McK	58.5	0	0	+
75 μg	C	O'Br	99	87	45	+
		Roc	98	86.5	51	0
		Rev	93.5	86.5	50.5	+
		Chi	96	84	5	0
		MacT	97	82.5	25	0
		McK	96	83	43.5	0
		Tay	91.5	82	20	0
		All	94	80.5	38.5	0
		Mof	93	80	49.5	0
		Bes	89.5	77.5	43.3	0
	Y	Bro	....	(76.5)[1]	48	0
		Lar	....	(76)[1]	1	0
		Wel	....	(75.5)[1]	54	0

PW = parous woman
[1] ^{51}Cr survival at 11 days [2] Anti-D present before 2nd injection .... Not estimated

initial injection of red cells and received no further injections. [51]Cr survival results following the second injection in 11 subjects (including the one parous woman) are shown in table I.

Series B (subjects receiving red cells and 15 µg antibody). This series included 3 parous women and one other woman who was withdrawn from the experiment after it was discovered that she had previously been transfused with Rh-positive blood. [51]Cr survival results following the second injection of red cells are shown in table I.

Series C (subjects receiving red cells and 75 µg antibody). One subject withdrew from the experiment shortly after receiving the first injection and one other subject attended 6 months after the initial injection to give a blood sample but then withdrew from the experiment. [51]Cr survival results following the second injection of red cells in the remaining 10 subjects are shown in table I.

Series X (subjects receiving red cells alone). Of the 4 subjects enrolled, only 3 completed the experiment.

Series Y (subjects receiving red cells and 75 µg antibody). Of the 4 subjects enrolled in this series all were tested 6 months after the initial injection but only 3 subjects received a second injection of red cells (table I).

Formation of detectable anti-Rh following the initial injection of red cells. Six months after the first injection of red cells, the results were as follows (excluding the parous women): in series A, one out of 11 subjects formed anti-Rh; in series B none out of 8 and in series C none out of 11 formed anti-Rh. In series X one out of 3 and in series Y none out of 4 formed anti-Rh. Thus, if experiments I and II are pooled the results are as follows: subjects receiving red cells alone initially, anti-Rh formed in two out of 14 cases; subjects receiving cells with 75 µg of antibody initially, anti-Rh formed in none out of 15 cases.

[51]Cr red cell survival results (table I, II and fig. 2). In series A, B and C all the subjects except one were tested at 24 h; excluding the parous women, there was only one subject (Ben) who had a grossly reduced red cell survival at this time and this was the only one whose serum contained detectable anti-Rh before the injection was given. Amongst the four parous women survival at 24 h was obviously reduced in two cases and probably reduced in a third case.

At 7–11 days, ^{51}Cr survival was estimated in all except one subject (Cun, series B) either at 7 days or (in subjects Byr and Gra, Series A) at 11 days. Taking 77% as the lower limit of normal survival (see below), in series A, 4 were normal and 4 abnormal; in series B, 5 were normal and 2 abnormal and in series C all 10 results were normal.

Taking 70.5% survival as the lower limit of normal at 11 days (see below) one out of two results in series A and two out of three results from series X were abnormal but all of the three results in series Y were normal.

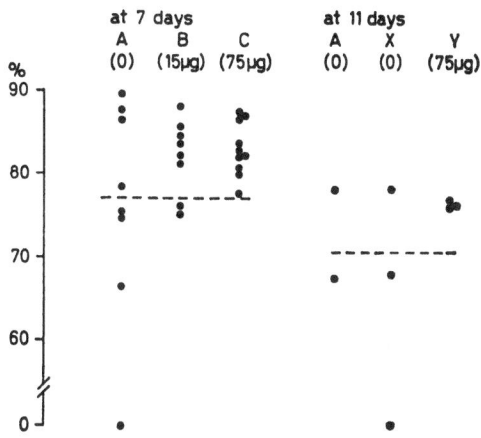

Fig. 2. ^{51}Cr survival at 7 or 11 days, following the injection of 1 ml of ^{51}Cr-labelled Rh-positive red cells (donor M.E.S.) in experiments I (A,B,C) and II (X, Y). All subjects had received an injection of 1 ml of Rh-positive red cells six months previously; the amount of anti-D given with the first injection is shown in brackets. The dotted line shows the levels taken as the lower limit of normal ^{51}Cr survival (see text).

Table II. ^{51}Cr survival, at 7–11 days, of a second injection of red cells given six months after the first injection

Series	No. of subjects	First injection 1 ml red cells with	Second injection ^{51}Cr survival (%) at 7–11 days	
			normal	subnormal
A + X	13	no anti-D	6	7
B	8	15 μg anti-D	6	2
C + Y	13	75 μg anti-D	13	0

(A + X) vs. (C + Y); p = 0.027

Table III. Relation between ^{51}Cr red cell survival results (second injection of red cells) at 7–11 days[1]

No. of donors	Survival at 7–11 days	Survival at 28 days			
		Normal (47–60%)	Slightly subnormal (38–45%)	Definitely subnormal (20–33%)`	Nil (0–5%)
25	Normal (77% at 7 d. or 70% at 11 d.)	14(1)	5(1)	2	4
7	Slightly subnormal (75–76% at 7 d. or 67–68% at 11 d.)	0	0	1(1)	6(3)
3	Definitely subnormal (23.5–66.5% at 7 d.)	0	0	0	3(3)
3	Nil (0.5% at 7–11 d.)	0	0	0	3(3)

The figures in brackets indicate the number of subjects developing anti-Rh within 4–5 months of the injections.

[1] Four parous women are included in this table.

Of the 4 parous women, all had subnormal ^{51}Cr survival at 7 days.

The lower limit of normal survival at 7 days, referred to above, is simply the mean -2 S.D. of series C (i.e. 82.95 $-2 \times 2.9 = 77.05$). Since mean normal ^{51}Cr survival at 11 days is approximately 6.5% lower than at 7 days [2, p. 24, method b] the lower limit of survival at 11 days may be taken as 77–6.5 or 70.5%.

Table II summarizes the ^{51}Cr survival results at 7–11 days; when the pooled results of series A and X (no anti-D with first injection) are compared with the pooled results of series C and Y (75 μg anti-D with first injection) there is a significant difference (p = 0.027).

Table III, which includes the results in the 4 parous women, shows the relationship between ^{51}Cr survival at 7–11 days and at 28 days. When survival was normal at 7–11 days it was 5% or less at 28 days in only 4 out of 25 cases. However, when it was slightly subnormal at 7–11 days it was 5% or less at 28 days in 6 out of 7 cases. When it was definitely subnormal at 7 days it was always nil at 28 days.

Formation of anti-Rh, detectable in vitro, *four to five months after the second injection of red cells.* As table I shows, excluding parous women, the incidence of detectable anti-Rh was as follows: Series A + X (red cells only) 6 out of 13; Series B (red cells + 15 μg anti-D) 1 out of 8; Series C + Y (red cells + 75 μg anti-D) 2 out of 13.

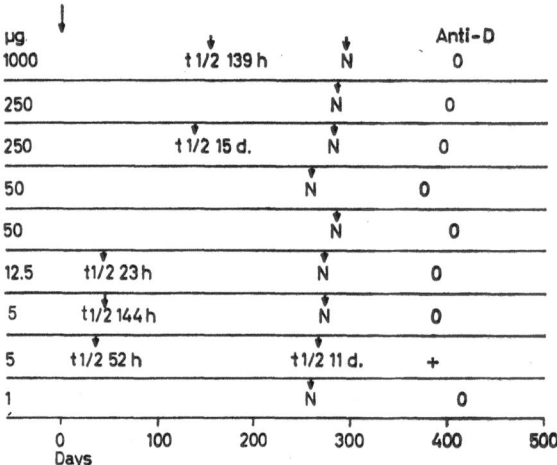

Fig. 3. Experiment III. At zero time, all subjects received an injection of 0.3 ml Rh-positive red cells together with 1–1000 μg anti-D. Within the following six months five subjects received a second injection of red cells; the T½ ^{51}Cr is shown. At 260–295 days all subjects received a further injection of 0.3 ml of ^{51}Cr-labelled Rh-positive red cells and at about 400 days the serum of all subjects was tested for anti-D. Only one subject had a diminished red cell survival and he was the only one who formed detectable anti-D. $N =$ normal ^{51}Cr survival. *Anti-D =* an indirect antiglobulin test for anti-D; antibody (titre 1) was detected in only one case (marked +).

As table III shows, diminished ^{51}Cr survival at 7–11 days was clearly correlated with the subsequent formation of detectable antibody. Thus, of 25 subjects in whom survival at 7–11 days was normal, two developed antibody. Of seven subjects with a slightly subnormal survival at 7–11 days, four developed antibody and all of six subjects with definitely subnormal survival at 7–11 days developed antibody (2 had already developed antibody before the second injection of red cells). Similarly, in 12 subjects who developed anti-Rh, ^{51}Cr survival had been normal at 28 days in only one case and had been less than 5% in 9 cases.

In several cases, anti-Rh was first detected using enzyme-treated cells at a time when the indirect antiglobulin test was negative, but in all these cases the indirect antiglobulin test later became positive.

In many cases the antibodies were very weak and could not be detected by a 'standard' antiglobulin test in which 20 volumes of serum were incubated with 1 volume of red cells.

Anti-Bu^a could not be detected in the serum of any of the six subjects (series X and Y) who had been injected with Bu(a+) cells.

Experiment III

In the present work, between 260 and 295 days after the beginning of the experiment, nine out of ten subjects received another injection of 0.3 ml of red cells from MES. In eight cases ^{51}Cr survival was normal (47–59.5%) at 28 days; testing of these subjects 101–120 days later did not reveal anti-Rh in any of them. In the ninth subject ^{51}Cr red cell survival was definitely diminished (T$\frac{1}{2}$ 11 days) and very weak anti-Rh was detected in the serum when retested 100 days later, although no antibody could be found at the time of the ^{51}Cr red cell survival test (fig. 3).

Discussion

FREDA et al. [1] found that a single injection of 10 ml of Rh-positive (R$_2$r) blood (approximately 4 ml of red cells) induced the formation of anti-Rh in 6 out of 13 subjects within the following 6 to 9 months. When experiments I and II of the present work were planned it was hoped that 1 ml of Rh-positive blood (R$_1$r) would be an equally effective stimulus but in fact, it induced the formation of detectable anti-Rh in only 2 out of 14 subjects. Evidently then, in deciding whether primary immunization had occurred in a significant number of cases in this group, compared with the control series, analysis of the ^{51}Cr red cell survival results is all important.

In using the ^{51}Cr red cell survival results as an index of the presence of a very low concentration of antibody it seems clear that survival at 7–11 days is more important than survival at 28 days, since by 28 days primary immunization might have occurred as a result of the second injection. As described in Results, if the criterion of normal survival at 7 days is taken as the mean −2.S.D. of the results in series C, and normal survival at 11 days is taken as a level of 6.5% below the lower limit for 7 days, then it is possible to show a significant difference between series A and X (red cells alone) on the one hand, and series C and Y (red cells and 75 μg anti-D) on the other. Some justification for regarding these criteria of normal survival as valid is supplied by the observation that of the cases showing slightly subnormal survival at 7–11 days as many as 6 out of 7 had nil survival at 28 days, contrasted with only 4 out of 24 in cases with normal survival at 7–11 days.

It would have been less biassed to have taken, for the lower limit of normal ^{51}Cr red cell survival, figures obtained in normal subjects injected with their own red cells. However, although figures have been given [2, p. 25], they were obtained using various slightly different methods of red cell labelling and they show a distinctly wider scatter than observed in series C in the present experiments. Thus, the figure for the lower limit of normal at 7 days is 73.5% and for 11 days 68%. Using these criteria, only 4 out of 13 cases in series A and X would be abnormal (and of course none in series C or Y).

The conclusion that 75 μg of anti-D inhibits primary immunization by 1 ml of Rh-positive red cells does not disagree with previous observations. POLLACK et al. [4] obtained evidence of complete suppression when 300 μg anti-D was given with approximately 4 ml of Rh-positive red cells and they later [5] found that 40 μg anti-D given with 2 ml of red cells was ineffective or only partially effective.

POLLACK et al. [5] concluded that primary immunization was probably augmented when 10 μg anti-D was given with 2 ml of R_2r red cells. In the present work no evidence of augmentation was obtained.

In series B the proportion of abnormal survival results at 7 days (2 slightly subnormal out of 8) is evidently not greater than in series A. Thus, no evidence was obtained that primary immunization was augmented by giving 15 μg anti-D with 1 ml of red cells. In experiment III, there were 6 subjects who had been injected with 0.3 ml Rh-positive red cells at a time when they were calculated to have between 0.6 and 4.0 μg of anti-D in their circulation. When these subjects were subsequently challenged with a further injection of Rh-positive red cells, ^{51}Cr survival was diminished in only one case. This incidence of primary immunization is lower than that observed in series A in which 1 ml of red cells from the same donor was given without anti-D, but the difference may be due either to chance or possibly to the fact that only 0.3 ml of red cells was used in experiment III. In any case, it seems safe to conclude that primary immunization was not augmented by giving 0.3 ml red cells to subjects with between 0.6 and 4.0 μg of anti-D in their circulation.

References

1. FREDA, V. J.; GORMAN, J. G. and POLLACK, W.: Rh factor: Prevention of iso-immunization and clinical trials on mothers. Science *151:* 828 (1966).
2. MOLLISON, P. L.: Blood transfusion in clinical medicine; 4th ed. (Blackwell, Oxford 1967).
3. MOLLISON P. L. and HUGHES-JONES, N. C.: Clearance of Rh-positive red cells by low concentrations of Rh antibody. Immunology, Lond. *12:* 63 (1967).

4. POLLACK, W.; SINGHER, H. O.; GORMAN, J. G. and FREDA, V. J.: The prevention of isoimmunisation to the Rh factor by passive immunisation with Rh₀(D) immune globulin (human). American Association of Blood Banks, New York, October 1967. Scientific exhibit.

5. POLLACK, W.; GORMAN, J. G.; HAGER, H. J.; FREDA, V. J. and TRIPODI, D.: Antibody – mediated immune suppression to the Rh factor: Two mechanisms by which this can occur. Transfusion, Philad. *8:* 151 (1968).

6. ROCHNA, E. and HUGHES-JONES, N. C.: The use of purified ^{125}I-labelled anti-γ globulin in the determination of the number of antigen sites on red cells of different phenotypes. Vox Sang. *10:* 675 (1965).

7. WALKER, J. G. and SISKIND, G. W.: Studies on the control of antibody synthesis. Effect of antibody affinity upon its ability to suppress antibody formation. Immunology, Lond. *14:* 21 (1968).

Authors' address: Prof. Dr. P. L. MOLLISON, Dr. N. C. HUGHES-JONES, Dr. MARGARET LINDSAY and Dr. JANE WESSELY, MRC Experimental Haematology Research Unit, St. Mary's Hospital Medical School, *London W.2* (England).

Discussion

E. REYNIERSE. I want to present some evidence that the *in vitro* properties of anti-D preparations may not give too much information about the *in vivo* activity, especially in the suppression of Rhesus immunization.

Table I

C.L.B. I		C.L.B. I		C.L.B. II–III	C.L.B. II–III	
μg/ml	250 μg	250 μg	3 h 50′	210 μg	210 μg	10 h 05′
K (l/mole)	1.6×10^8		3 h 20′	1.8×10^8		6 h 40′
a	0.79	500 μg	3 h	0.65	420 μg	6 h 30′
titer	1/4000		3 h	1/6000–1/8000		7 h
T½ Cr^{51}		1250 μg	1 h 30′		840 μg	4 h 30′
125 μg .	8 h 50′		0 h 55′			3 h 50′
	7 h					

The two preparations anti-D prepared at our laboratory did not differ very much as far as their properties *in vitro* are concerned, as could be expected.

Preparation I contained about 250 μg of anti-D per ml, preparation II contained 210 μg.

The mean affinity constant was practically the same in the two preparations, perhaps slightly higher in the second, whereas the heterogeneity index was lower in the second preparation.

This would mean, that the titer of the second preparation ought to be higher than that of the first, which is indeed the case. We tested the two preparations *in vivo*.

Rh negative volunteers were given intramuscularly from 125 μg to 1250 μg anti-D. About 48 h later they were given intravenously about 2 ml of packed ^{51}Cr labelled Rh positive red cells. It can be seen that, although we would expect that there are more antibody molecules per cell with preparation II, the survival *in vivo* is much longer with the second preparation than with the first one. About 850 μg of preparation II fall into the same range as 250 μg of the first preparation, so that we think that there are other properties which cannot be determined yet, that are important for the *in vivo* effect of anti-D.

E. BORST. In 1966 a controlled clinical trial was started in ten obstetrical departments simultaneously. This trial differed in two respects from those carried out elsewhere. In the first place a comparatively low dose of anti-D immunoglobulin was used, i.e. 250 μg, and in the second place the trial comprised all non-immunized Rhesus negative women with a Rhesus positive child, irrespective of parity or ABO compatibility.

The women were randomized by treating those with odd-numbered birthdays. Tests for antibodies were carried out immediately after delivery and four to six months later.

Blood samples taken after delivery were also examined for the presence of foetal red cells, according to the method of KLEIHAUER, BRAUN and BETKE. The results are shown in table II.

Table II. Results of a controlled clinical trial with 250 μg of anti-D immunoglobulin

Approximate amount of foetal blood in the maternal circulation after delivery	Control No.	Imm.	Treated No.	Imm.
none found	163	2	163	0
<0.1 ml	123	8	105	0
0.1– 1 ml	27	2	37	0
1– 10 ml	2	1	2	0
10–100 ml	0	0	4	0
≥ 100 ml	0	0	2	2
total	315	13 (4%)	313	2 (0.6%)

$\chi_0^2 = 6.91$ $P < 0.01$

In the treated group, only 2 out of 313 women showed active immunization. In both these cases an exceptionally large transplacental haemorrhage had taken place.

In the control group 13 out of 315 women formed Rhesus antibodies. In four of these cases the baby's ABO group was incompatible with that of the mother. It should further be noted that two women showed active Rhesus immunization despite the fact that immediately after delivery no foetal red cells had been found in their circulation.

It is concluded that a dose of 250 μg of anti-D immunoglobulin probably suppresses Rhesus immunization in all cases with transplacental bleeds up to 25 ml and that this form of treatment should be extended as soon as possible to all Rhesus negative women with a Rhesus positive child, irrespective of ABO compatibility or outcome of Kleihauer technique after delivery.

N. C. HUGHES-JONES. I think the results of Dr. REYNIERSE are interesting because they are unexpected. One would expect the biological activity of pools made from large numbers of donors would be similar and that the same number of micrograms would have given the same rate of removal *in vivo*. We have evidence that different examples of anti-D from different donors will give different rates of destruction *in vivo*. But it was certainly our belief that if you pooled sera from a large number of donors, the differences between donors would average out. This opens questions that are in a field that we know nothing about, and these interesting results must be followed up.

CH. M. VAN DER WEERDT. I should like to stress that the second pool was larger than the first one. The second pool was 175 l, the first one was only 20 l. So perhaps that might be of some importance.

N. C. HUGHES-JONES. Yes, perhaps the 20 l pool was too small. Did it contain more than 20 donors?

CH. M. VAN DER WEERDT. Yes, 35 donors.

R. E. ROSENFIELD. There are two possibilities to explain the observed difference in these two immunoglobulin preparations: (1) that other factors have to be taken into account and (2) that the assay in its present form does not give quite the information that it is alleged to. I favour the second. I think, however, that Dr. HUGHES-JONES is to be congratulated, even if he was at least partly wrong. I think

Table III

1. MDH

	before	1st Injection	1	14	2nd and 3rd injections	5	14	21	60 days
Group 1	177		—	117		83	89	97	106
Number n	10		—	10		9	9	9	8
Group 2	199		89	139		65	111	82	97
n	10		10	10		10	10	9	9
Group 3	225		125	161		115	141	95	125
n	10		10	6		9	9	10	10
Group 4	244		123	158		135	104	103	86
n	10		10	10		10	9	10	10

2. LDH

	before	1st injection	1	14	2nd and 3rd injections	5	14	21	60 days
Group 1	212		—	218		126	124	133	59
Number n	10		—	10		10	9	9	8
Group 2	202		158	146		130	107	107	104
n	10		10	10		10	10	9	8
Group 3	204		146	150		117	97	100	75
n	10		10	10		10	10	10	10
Group 4	202		161	143		116	94	97	87
n	10		10	10		10	9	10	10

3. GPT

	before	1st injection	1	14	2nd and 3rd injections	5	14	21	60 days
Group 1	9.6		—	9.0		8.2	8.1	8.2	10.4
Number n	10		—	10		9	8	9	9
Group 2	9.2		9.9	7.9		7.0	8.4	7.4	8.7
n	10		10	10		10	10	10	8
Group 3	10.6		10.9	5.0		5.6	8.2	8.7	8.5
n	8		8	8		8	9	10	10
Group 4	8.3		10.7	5.4		7.9	4.4	6.7	8.1
n	10		10	10		10	9	10	10

1. Malatdehydrogenase (MDH)
2. Lactatdehydrogenase (LDH)
3. Glutamat-Pyruvat-Transaminase (GPT) before and after i.v. injection of 3×10 ml Rh + blood.

Group 1 received no anti-Rh$_0$-immunoglobulin, group 2 – 1200 μg, group 3 – 600 μg and group 4 – 300 μg anti-Rh$_0$-immunoglobulin 24 h later. (Enzyme units in international units).

10 ml O DCe/DCe blood i.v. by O dce/dce male persons

300 μg anti-Rh$_0$(D) immunoglobulin, e.g. 1200, 600, 300 μg for each male person

Table IV.

Group 1 Untreated control group. (no anti-Rh₀(D) immunoglobulin)	6 persons (60%) formed Rh-antibodies 4 an anti D + C (titre up to 1:2000 anti-D[1] 1:16 anti-C) 2 an anti-D[1] (titre 1:16)	5 persons (50%) had formed already after the second injection Rhesus-antibodies
Group 2 24 h after i.v. blood injection 1200 μg (min. 1100 μg)[3] anti-Rh₀(D) immunoglobulin (1 ml 16 or 16.5%)	None of the 30 persons formed antibodies against the donorerythrocytes. Continued controls were made over 9 months (6 months after last blood injection)	According to the half-life ($T\frac{1}{2}$) of the passive immunised anti-Rh₀(D) antibodies, these could still be tested. Up to 2 months after the intramuscular injection (indirect anti-Rh₀(D) Coombs test, with the donor blood positive up to 1:4 in one case 1:8)[2]
Group 3 24 h after i.v. blood injection 600 μg (min. 550 μg)[3] anti-Rh₀(D) immunoglobulin (0.5 ml 16 or 16.5%)		
Group 4 24 h after i.v. blood injection 300 μg (min. 275 μg)[3] anti-Rh₀(D) immunoglobulin (0.25 ml 16 or 16.5%)		

[1] All titres were done with the same Coombs serum (same charge No.) under the same laboratory conditions The 800 tests (2×800 tests $= 1 \times$ immediately, $1 \times$ at the end of the series after 9 months with frozen serum) were done.

With a special Coombs serum we got titre values up to 1:4096 anti-D. The test erythrocytes were the same donor blood corpuscles as we used for passive immunization.

[2] The same as above. We got titre values up to 1:32 anti-D with a special Coombs serum.

[3] Tolerance rate of the used one-way injection syringes.

Each group consists of 10 male persons with the blood formula O dce/dce. Each person received 10 ml whole blood of the formula O DCe/DCe intravenously for three times in time intervals of 28 days. 24 h after each injection group 2 got 1200 μg, group 3 600 μg and group 4 300 μg anti-Rh₀ immunoglobulin.

he has opened up a subject that is difficult but of extreme importance. There is absolutely no question that 2 different sources of anti-D can differ tremendously in their biological activity. The measurement of the average constant of binding, to my mind, is the absolute essential beginning.

A. E. G. Kr. von dem Borne. May I ask Dr. Hughes-Jones if he finds any correlation between immunization time, the number of immunizations and the value of K, the equilibrium constant?

N. C. Hughes-Jones. We have looked into this and in the cases that we have done, the value of the equilibrium constant seems to be unchanged over many months and once at a certain level, it remains at that level. We thought it might increase, as happens in animals, but I think that if the increase does occur, it probably takes place during the first few months, or even the first few weeks. Those donors whom we examined received their original primary immunization many years ago.

Ch. M. van der Weerdt. I would like to ask Dr. Hughes-Jones a question. Have you any data about the extent of loss of specific activity during the fractionation of the plasma pool to obtain IgG preparations? Is there much loss of anti-D activity during the procedure.

N. C. Hughes-Jones. The recovery of both anti-D and γ-globulin are approximately 70%.

G. A. GATHOF. We tested an anti-D immunoglobulin to find out:

1. The activity of the red blood cell enzymes MDH + LDH after immunization and after injection of anti-D immunoglobulin. GPT was estimated as a control (table III).

2. The minimal dosage (table IV).

3. How long after injection of anti-Rh₀(D) immunoglobulin can passive anti-D antibody be demonstrated with serological tests? (fig. 1).

4. Immunization rate in Rh negative persons after injection of Rh positive blood (fig. 2).

The test procedure was as follows: 4 groups of 10 male Rh negative volunteers, got three intravenous injections of 10 ml Rh positive (R_1R_2) blood with a time interval of twenty-eight days. Twenty four hours later we injected intramuscularly anti-D immunoglobulin: group 2 1200 (min. 1100)μg, group 3 600 (min. 550)μg, group 4 300 (min. 275)μg.

The most interesting fact we found in these experiments was an unexpected decrease of enzyme activity of red blood cells (the enzyme control GPT stayed at the same level).

C. VERMYLEN. I like to comment briefly on the results in Belgium. Until now 1280 patients are treated with anti-Rh₀(D) immunoglobulin, but only the results of 300 patients are yet available, because the 700 remaining cases are not controlled

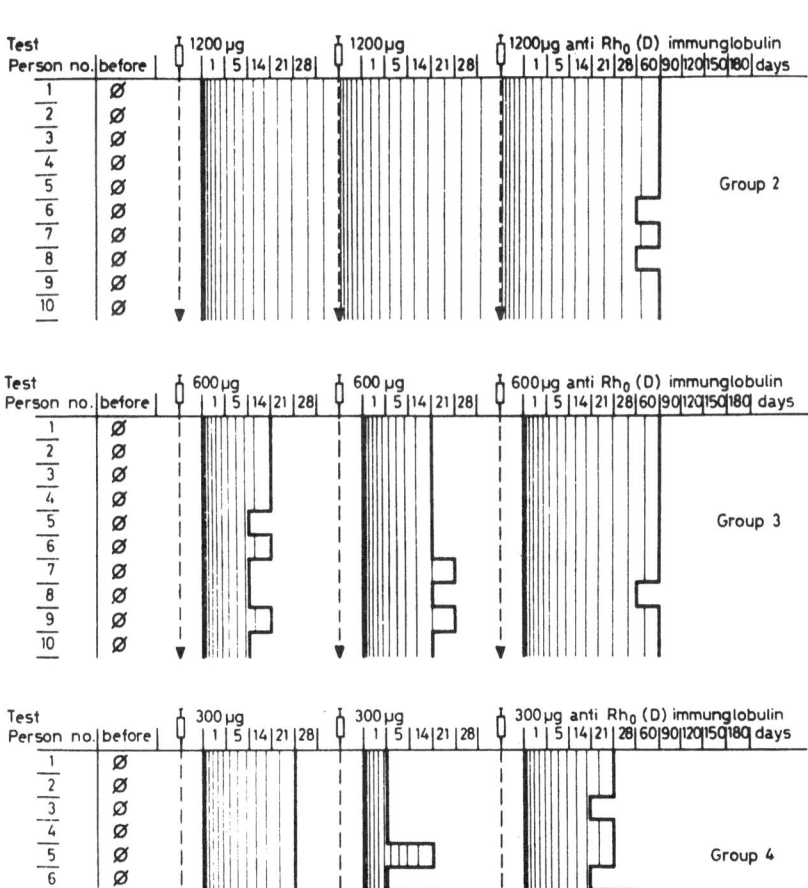

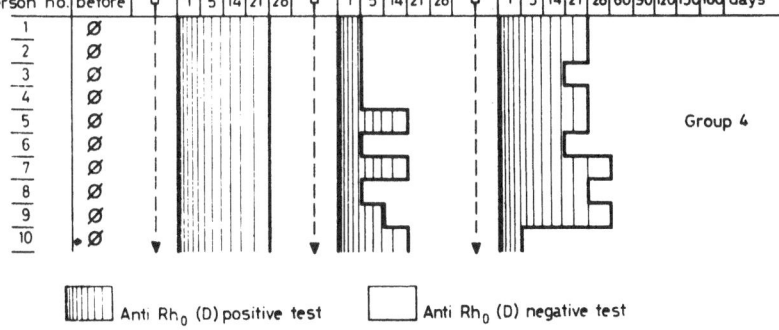

Fig. 1. Serological test proof of passively immunisation with Rh-antibodies (anti-Rh₀[D] immunoglobulin) by intramuscular injection.

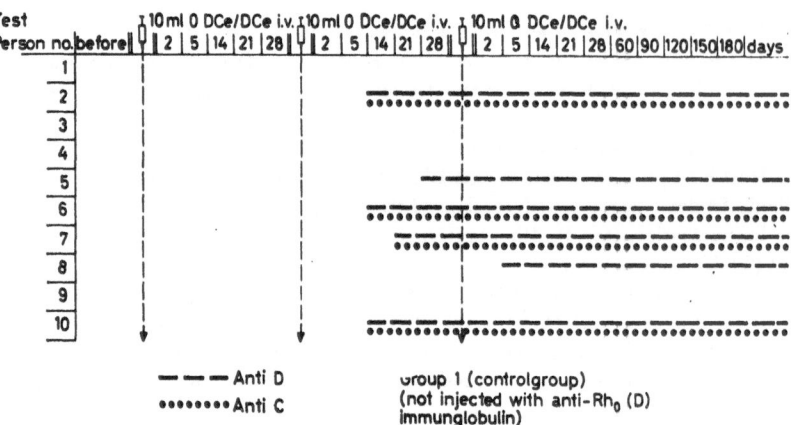

Fig. 2. Rh-antibodies appearing in O dce/dce kk-persons after 2 or 3 intravenous injections with 10 ml O DCe/DCe kk blood.

six months after therapy. In this group of 300 treated patients, 3 immunizations occurred. One of the immunized women was a primipara. The group contained 120 primiparae. In the immunized woman a large fetal maternal bleeding of 180 ml was demonstrated. The other two immunized women were multiparous and no antibodies could be demonstrated at the moment of delivery.

We still think that these two cases are cases of indistinct immunization, existing at delivery but not detectable by our serological tests. The selection of patients in the whole study is based on an ABO-compatible pregnancy and the demonstration of a negative indirect Coombs test at the moment of delivery between the serum of the mother and the red cells of the newborn.

A. M. JOSEPHSON. Two questions: (1) instead of using the word pool size, I am wondering how many donors there were in the two different pools, which might make a lot of difference. (2) Have any of the groups, in Europe at least, worried about concentration of other antibodies in this hyper immune-anti-D and are you cross matching the material with mothers cells?

CH. M. VAN DER WEERDT. I cannot give the exact number of donors in each group. In the first group there were about 35 different donors and I guess there were about 200 different donors in the second pool, but I might be wrong for some 25 donors.

We only exclude donors giving plasma for the production of anti-D immunoglobulin, when they have very high titers of contaminating antibodies, and yet in the end product, the IgG preparation, only a very low titer of contaminating antibodies is present. With large pools you dilute out most of the antibodies that are present in some of them.

H. W. KRIJNEN. May I ask whether somebody in the audience has perhaps experience concerning the stability of these anti-D immunoglobulin preparations.

C. VERMYLEN. We made several preparations on a small scale of anti-Rh$_0$(D) immunoglobulin and we had very bad experience with the stability of the anti-D titer. After 4–5 months at least 25–30% of the original activity was lost, and that is the reason why we try lyophilization at present.

H. W. KRIJNEN. May I ask you, Dr. VERMYLEN, what the preparation method was in which you saw this decrease in anti-D titer?

C. VERMYLEN. Electrodecantation followed by an ethanol precipitation. You can use the electrodecanted preparation but we include ethanol precipitation as a final step to eliminate the danger of hepatic virus contamination. We perform this final step to be in accordance with the W.H.O. recommendations.

H. W. KRIJNEN. And this final preparation, was this a 16% solution and was the solvent 0.3 Molar glycine?

C. VERMYLEN. The solvent is 0.3 Molar glycine and the concentration of the proteins varies between 12 and 16 g%.

N. C. HUGHES-JONES. We had one example from the Lister Institute. Two vials of the same preparation were kept for 2 years; one vial was kept at –40°C and another at +4°C. After storage there was no difference in the anti-D activity between the vials. The preparation was a 10% solution of γ-globulin produced by Cohn fractionation.

H. W. KRIJNEN. Also dissolved in 0.3 Molar glycine?

N. C. HUGHES-JONES. There was no glycine present, only thiomersal.

R. E. ROSENFIELD. In our experience, whole serum is variable and often highly unstable. We are, however, extremely pleased with the stability of ORTHO concentrated material. This is quite stable at 4°C. If frozen, however, it loses about 30% of its activity.

Perhaps Dr. PENNELL would comment on the general problem of instability of fraction II preparations.

R. B. PENNEL. I think I have rather little to say in general and although the proof is not perfect, the instability seems to parallel the contamination with plasminogen. Perhaps some of the methods used here, are more heavily contaminated with plasminogen than our usual standard fractionation products. That would be my guess to account for the variability.

C. VERMYLEN. Yes, we think we can completely agree with Dr. PENNELL. I am not quite sure if the agent is plasminogen. What we know is that an esterase is present in the gamma globulin preparations, which is easily demonstrated by TAME hydrolysis. Changing the solvent from 0.3 Molar glycine to 3% epsilon aminocaproic acid, we get a preparation which is much more stable regarding anti-D activity.

C. P. ENGELFRIET. I would like to ask Dr. MOLLISON if the protective mechanism for 2 different antigens on the cell surface would be as antigen specific as for 2 different soluble antigens. Would not one expect to have found, e.g., some anti-C in a number of the protected women, for anti-C is formed quite frequently in pregnancy and no anti-C has ever been found so far I think.

P. L. MOLLISON. The experiments of POLLACK et al. [Transfusion, Philad. 8: 151, 1968], in animals suggest that for red cell antigens, as for soluble antigens, suppression by passively-administered antibody is highly specific: rabbits of group Hg (A–F–) injected with Hg(A+F+) red cells and with anti-HgA formed anti-Hg^F but not anti-Hg^A.

On the other hand, as you say, it does appear that anti-C formation is inhibited by passively-administered anti-D. Possibly, the discrepancy is due to the fact that C does not normally act as a separate antigen but acts in collaboration with D so that the antibody formed is anti-CD (G) rather than anti-C + anti-D. However, this explanation does not seem entirely convincing.

Paper 39

39. Chown, B. (1967). Prevention of Rh hemolytic disease. *Canad. Med. Ass. J., 97,* 1294-1296.

Commentary

It is no secret that Dr Bruce Chown, who in 1967 was the Director of the Rh laboratory in Winnipeg, wrote the editorial reprinted as Paper 39. The Liverpool and New York experiments mentioned at the beginning of his second paragraph have already been described and the Canadian work on prophylaxis during pregnancy is given in Paper 40.

From B. Chown (1967). J., 97, 1294-6, Copyright (1967), by the kind permission of the author and
Canadian Medical Association

1294 EDITORIALS AND ANNOTATIONS

Canad. Med. Ass. J.
Nov. 18, 1967, vol. 97

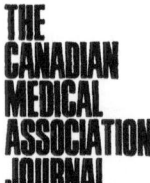

THE CANADIAN MEDICAL ASSOCIATION JOURNAL

LE JOURNAL DE L'ASSOCIATION MÉDICALE CANADIENNE

November 18, 1967

PREVENTION OF Rh HEMOLYTIC DISEASE

IN LESS than 30 years our understanding of rhesus hemolytic disease of the newborn has run full cycle from hypothesis to prevention. Recent studies, such as the one by Zipursky and Israels, published in this week's issue (p. 1245), encourage the belief that the disease can be practically eradicated.

In the years around 1960 three groups—one in Liverpool, one in New York and one in Winnipeg—set out independently to investigate the possibility of preventing Rh hemolytic disease, all having in mind the use of anti-Rh antibodies as the protective agent. While the Winnipeg group, supported by a grant from the United States Public Health Service, was attempting to define in precise terms the mode and condition of primary immunization,[1] both the Liverpool and New York groups were making a direct frontal attack on the problem: they injected Rh-negative volunteers with Rh-positive red cells and then with anti-Rh antibodies. The Liverpudlians at first used whole serum[2] but later anti-Rh gamma globulin. From the beginning, the New Yorkers used gamma globulin G extracted from whole anti-Rh plasma by a modification of the Cohn cold ethanol process.[3] Although the Liverpudlians were left with some fascinating problems[4] which have not yet been solved, both groups obtained a clear answer to the question they had asked: "Will passively given anti-Rh antibodies prevent Rh-negative volunteers, injected with Rh-positive blood, from becoming actively immunized?" The answer was "Yes, if the antibodies belong to the incomplete or immunoglobulin G class." Both groups then moved boldly forward and set up experimental programs for the prevention of Rh-antibody formation in women. Their boldness has been more than justified.

Both groups (and they were shortly joined by a group in Freiburg, Germany)[6] used anti-Rh immune globulin in a dose of 5 ml. and gave this to Rh-negative women who had no Rh antibodies at the time they gave birth to an Rh-positive ABO-compatible baby. (A mother and baby are said to be ABO compatible if the mother is of such an ABO group that she does not have an A or B antibody which will react with the baby's cells, e.g. mother O, baby O; mother A, baby A or O and so on. In the presence of ABO incompatibility Rh immunization is very rare.) In detail the two studies differed.

The number of fetal erythrocytes present in the maternal circulation increases as pregnancy progresses and is greatest immediately after delivery.[9] Although Zipursky and Israels comment on the comparatively "crude methods" of estimating circulating erythrocytes, the Liverpool group, early in their study, observed[5] that there was a direct relationship between the number of fetal cells present in a woman's blood immediately after delivery and the probability of her developing antibodies: if no fetal cells were found, the chance that the woman would develop antibodies was 1 in 30; if very few were found, the chance was 1 in 15; if a moderate number were found, the chance was 1 in 7; if many were found, the chance was 1 in 2. The last two categories, which together had about a 1 in 4 chance of antibody formation, were classed as a "high-risk" group; that is, there was a high risk of antibody formation. As Zipursky and Israels point out, this view is not supported by Cohen and Zuelzer,[10] who reported that only one of eight women developing Rh antibodies after pregnancy had a "large" number of fetal erythrocytes in her circulation post partum. Furthermore, the data presented by Zipursky and Israels concerning 573 women with Rh-positive babies showed that more of those who had a postpartum cell scan of four erythrocytes or less (they include their definition of a cell scan) developed Rh isoimmunization following pregnancy than those who had more fetal erythrocytes. Their series also showed that only three who had less than four fetal erythrocytes on a cell scan developed Rh isoimmunization and only five women who had had "large" numbers of these fetal cells in their circulation developed Rh antibodies, whereas 13 who had no fetal cells at all in their circulation post partum developed Rh isoimmunization. They suggest an explanation for this lack of "fetal erythrocytes" in the maternal circulation immediately after delivery (p. 1248).

For three reasons, only the high-risk group was chosen for treatment by the Liverpudlians: the amount of anti-Rh gamma globulin was limited; if the method of prevention was effective, this group would most likely quickly prove that this was so; if by any chance the treatment proved to be harmful and increased the chances of

Canad. Med. Ass. J.
Nov. 18, 1967, vol. 97

TABLE I.—RESULTS OF TRIALS USING ANTI-RH GAMMA GLOBULIN FOR THE PREVENTION OF RH-ANTIBODY FORMATION IN WOMEN

Study centre	Type of women in the study	Dose of anti-Rh antibody	TREATED SUBJECTS			UNTREATED CONTROLS			
			Total	Antibodies formed	Antibodies not formed	Total	Antibodies formed	Antibodies not formed	Antibodies formed %
Liverpool (and associates)	"high-risk" primiparas	5 ml.	123	1	122	130	26	104	20.0
Liverpool (and associates)	"low-risk" primiparas	1 ml.	97	0	97	103	3	100	2.9
Freiburg	"high-risk" women	5 ml.	52	0	52	74	4	70	5.4
New York (and associates)	any woman "at risk"	5 ml.	160	0	160	158	17	141	10.8
New York (and associates)	any woman "at risk"	1 ml.	716	1	715	561	42	519	8.1

The British preparation of anti-Rh gamma globulin contained about 200 μg. of anti-Rh antibody per ml. The New York 5-ml. preparation contained about 1500 μg. of anti-Rh antibody per ml. but their 1-ml. preparation only 300 μg. The current Connaught product contains about 290 μg. of anti-Rh antibody per ml. and is being used experimentally in 1.5- and 0.5-ml. doses. In all cases the conclusion as to whether a woman had or had not developed antibodies was based on tests for antibodies carried out at least six months after delivery.

immunization, few women who would otherwise not have been immunized would be exposed to the risk. The women treated were all primiparas, so that the issue could not be confused by sensitization resulting from an earlier pregnancy. The selection of women to be treated or to be left as untreated controls was made on a random basis. The treated subjects received treatment within 36 hours after delivery. The Freiburg group followed the same plan as the Liverpudlians.

The New York group, more accurately called the New York and associated groups, because the anti-Rh gamma globulin was distributed for experimental use in a number of cities, used all women at risk in their study, either for treatment or as controls without reference to the presence or absence of fetal cells and without regard to parity. Treatment was given up to 72 hours after delivery. After an extended trial in New York and in Long Beach, California, with a prophylactic dose of 5 ml. of anti-Rh gamma globulin, this group reduced the dose to 1 ml. and distributed the gamma globulin to 42 hospitals for trial.

The latest results[7] from the British, German and American groups are presented in Table I.

One conclusion is clear: this method of prophylaxis is highly successful; it appears to give almost 100% protection. In addition, data are now available (see table below) on 122 women from the Liverpool and New York series who had no antibodies six months after delivery and

	Treated	Antibodies present after subsequent delivery	Untreated	Antibodies present after subsequent delivery
Liverpool (and associates)	14 (primiparas only)	0	25 (primiparas only)	2
New York (and associates)	44 (any parity)	0	39 (any parity)	12

who have gone through another pregnancy and been delivered of another ABO-compatible Rh-positive baby.

Whatever else may be deduced from the figures, it is clear that the injection of anti-Rh gamma globulin after one pregnancy has not, under the conditions of the experiment, increased the probability of antibody formation in the succeeding pregnancy.

The results reported from the various centres are in agreement in principle, though they differ in detail. For example, the difference in frequency of antibody formation by the controls in the Liverpool and associates series as compared with the Freiburg series is statistically significant, as is the difference in the frequency of antibody formation in the "second" pregnancy of the untreated controls of the Liverpool group as compared with the New York group. There is obviously room for investigation of these disparities. The Winnipeg authors point out that the incidence of transplacental hemorrhages at the time of delivery may vary in different centres, and that these variations may explain the differences in different geographical areas.

Nor is it known how the anti-Rh gamma globulin brings about the results that are so much to be desired: this presents an intriguing problem in immunology that will require for its solution research work both in human volunteers and with animals. Since the number of suitable and willing volunteers is limited, it would be desirable if the experimental work with them in Canada could be co-ordinated across the country. It may well be that the present method of prevention is not the ideal method.

1296 EDITORIALS AND ANNOTATIONS

Canad. Med. Ass. J.
Nov. 18, 1967, vol. 97

There remains also the practical problem of the provision of adequate supplies of potent anti-Rh gamma globulin. Last year the Winnipeg group invited the western medical schools and the University of Western Ontario, the Department of National Health and Welfare, and the Connaught Medical Research Laboratories to take part in a planning conference. It was decided that the represented medical schools (Manitoba, Saskatchewan, Alberta, British Columbia and Western Ontario), with the co-operation of the local Red Cross Blood Transfusion Depots in Edmonton, Calgary and Vancouver, would collect plasma from selected Rh-negative women who already had anti-Rh antibodies; that this would be pooled, processed to gamma globulin by the Connaught Medical Research Laboratories, and then used by the contributing centres in a planned and co-ordinated study of the prevention of primary Rh immunization. The Department of National Health and Welfare made research grants to the Winnipeg, Saskatoon and Vancouver groups, while the Department of Health of Alberta made grants to Edmonton and Calgary. In the course of six months more than 200 litres of plasma was collected in the Red Cross Depots of Winnipeg, Edmonton, Calgary and Vancouver. It then took three months to process this to anti-Rh gamma globulin: the co-ordinated study in the four cities began on March 1; the Winnipeg group had already been carrying out experimental studies with earlier lots of anti-Rh gamma globulin.

It can be estimated that about 7% of all newly delivered women are at risk; that is to say, about 7% of newly delivered women will be Rh-negative and have given birth to an Rh-positive, ABO-compatible baby. With regional variation, about 20,000 women per million of population are delivered of a live baby each year, or 400,000 women a year in Canada.

Seven per cent or 28,000 are at risk, so that at present 28,000 doses of anti-Rh gamma globulin a year are needed. Connaught Laboratories recovered a maximum of 14 "prophylactically adequate" doses of gamma globulin per litre of plasma. On this basis, 2000 litres of plasma a year would be required. While this amount is easily within the capabilities of the already immunized women, it is not desirable to collect more plasma than is necessary. Studies are already under way to determine whether prophylaxis can be attained with smaller doses; whether whole plasma from selected donors will produce more than 14 doses per litre; and whether such material will be as effective as gamma globulin and at the same time safe. A preliminary report on the use of whole plasma in prophylaxis was made from St. Mary's Hospital, St. Louis, Mo., at the recent meeting of the American Association of Blood Banks.[8]

Indeed, if the program of prevention is successful, women who might act as plasma donors will become increasingly uncommon, and one will have to turn to intentionally immunized men (Zipursky and Israels, p. 1250) or postmenopausal or sterile women.

The Red Cross Transfusion Service has accepted responsibility for collecting the necessary plasma, but to be a success this program will require the active support of practising physicians and co-ordination with research conducted by the university groups.

REFERENCES

1. ZIPURSKY, A. et al.: Lancet, 2: 489, 1963.
2. FINN, R. et al.: Brit. Med. J., 1: 1486, 1961.
3. FREDA, V. J., GORMAN, J. G. AND POLLACK, W.: Transfusion, 4: 26, 1964.
4. CLARKE, C. A. et al.: Brit. Med. J., 1: 979, 1963.
5. WOODROW, J. C. et al.: Ibid., 1: 279, 1965.
6. SCHNEIDER, J. AND PREISLER, O.: Blut, 12: 4, 1965.
7. FINN, R. AND SCHNEIDER, J.: Papers presented at the American Association of Blood Banks, New York, October 24, 1967.
8. Paper presented at the 20th annual meeting of the American Association of Blood Banks, New York, October 24, 1967.
9. COHEN, F. et al.: Blood, 23: 621, 1964.
10. COHEN, F. AND ZUELZER, W. W.: Vox Sang., 9: 75, 1964.

Paper 40

40. Zipursky, A. and Israels, L. G. (1967). The pathogenesis and prevention of Rh immunisation. *Canad. Med. Ass. J.*, *97*, 1245-57.

Commentary

The early part of this paper deals with the relation between transplacental hae-morrhage and the development of immunisation, but we are concerned here only with the section on prophylaxis given during pregnancy. The Canadian group were very early in experimenting with ante-partum anti-D, and Zipursky and Israels report here the results of two series treated in this way.

To begin with, in order to obtain evidence about possible damage to a fetus, two Rh-positive babies (one aged two months and one aged eighteen months) were given 5.0 ml of ^{51}Cr tagged autologous blood. Forty-eight hours later each received 0·5 ml of Rh-immune globulin, and the older child received a second dose of 0·5 ml one week later. After these injections the calculated half-life for red cell survival was found to be 21 days in one child and 31 days in the other (a half-life of 21 days is normal for the erythrocytes of an infant of two months). It was considered therefore that if these quantities of antibody (which were far greater than a fetus could receive if its mother were given the usual protective dose of anti-D) did not shorten eryth-rocyte life span, treatment during pregnancy would be safe.

The authors describe the results of giving anti-D gammaglobulin in two series of Rh-negative pregnant women.

Series A

A single dose of 0·4 ml was given one week before delivery in the first cases, but this was later altered to a single dose of 1 ml given at this time. Finally, it was decided that the programme should be 1 ml given at what was judged to be the 28th week, followed by two 0·4 ml doses four weeks apart. Forty-seven Rh-negative women were treated and 35 of the babies were Rh-positive. The direct Coombs test was weakly positive in five of these, and two of the five were ABO incompatible, which the authors think may explain the positive test. In one of them (born one day after the mother received 0·4 ml of anti-D gammaglobulin) the bilirubin rose to 14·0 mg per cent by day 3 (this was considered to represent a case of ABO haemolytic disease). All infants were otherwise well. Of the women followed up at the time of writing (20 for six months and 5 for four months) none had developed antibodies.

Series B

This comprised three groups, one of 20 women who received 1.5 ml of anti-D at the 36th week, another of 20 women who received 1 ml immediately postpartum, and one of 21 women acting as controls. Of the controls one, and of the treated none, had developed anti-D when tested 6 months or later post-partum. ABO incompat-ibility between mother and fetus was found in 2 of the 21 controls, in 4 of the women who received anti-D post-partum and in 5 of the 20 injected at 36 weeks. All the babies were normal and with one exception the Coombs test was negative—and in the positive one the mother was O and the baby A.

It would therefore seem that no harm has been done by the procedure, but whether the giving of ante-partum treatment would eliminate the small failure rate remains to be seen. Big series are being investigated in Canada, Australia and Germany (Paper 47), but extremely large numbers are necessary before a valid comparison with the standard post-partum treatment can be made. It must be remembered that all Rh-negative women with Rh-positive husbands would have to be treated, as amnio-centesis is a procedure not to be undertaken as a routine, and without it one could not be sure whether a fetus was Rh-positive or Rh-negative.

From A. Zipursky and L. G. Israels (1967). Canad. Med. Assoc. J., 97, 1245-57. Copyright (1967), by kind permission of the authors and Canadian Medical Association

THE CANADIAN MEDICAL ASSOCIATION JOURNAL

LE JOURNAL DE L'ASSOCIATION MEDICALE CANADIENNE

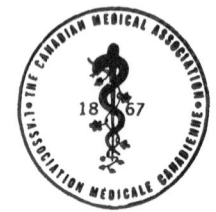

Volume 97 • Number 21 • November 18, 1967

The Pathogenesis and Prevention of Rh Immunization

ALVIN ZIPURSKY, M.D., F.R.C.P.[C]* and
LYONEL G. ISRAELS, M.D., F.R.C.P.[C],† *Winnipeg, Man.*

RH immunization of Rh-negative women during or subsequent to pregnancy is a response to the presence of fetal red cells in the mother. It has been the goal of several groups, including our own, to define this process of isoimmunization in Rh-negative women and to develop a rational program for its prevention.

Our earlier studies[1] and those of others[2,3] showed that fetal erythrocytes frequently are found in the blood of pregnant women during pregnancy; immediately following labour, larger numbers of fetal erythrocytes are found in the mother's blood than during the pregnancy.[4] Therefore it has been suggested that the delivery period is the time of maximum risk of immunization.[4] This proposal is supported by the recent studies of Woodrow *et al.*,[5] who showed that large transplacental hemorrhages at the time of birth are frequently followed by the development of Rh immunization. Furthermore, analysis of their data indicates that there is a direct relationship between the volume of circulating fetal cells in the mother immediately after delivery and the probability of subsequent Rh immunization. However, more than 50% of the women who subsequently became immunized had few or no fetal cells demonstrable in their blood at delivery. Cohen and Zuelzer[6] in their study of 127 Rh-negative women found that only one of the eight who subsequently developed antibodies had had a large transplacental hemor-

rhage at delivery. They suggested that Rh-negative women are at risk throughout pregnancy and that the delivery process is relatively unimportant in the pathogenesis of Rh isoimmunization. Similarly we have shown that primary isoimmunization may follow a pregnancy in which fetal erythrocytes had not been demonstrated post partum.[7]

The possibility that Rh immunization can result from the relatively small quantities of fetal erythrocytes entering the maternal circulation before labour is supported by the observation that Rh-negative subjects produced Rh antibodies following repeated injections of 0.1 ml. of Rh-positive fetal erythrocytes.[7] This provides support for the concept that isoimmunization can result either from the small volumes (less than 0.1 ml.) of fetal cells which frequently enter the maternal circulation throughout pregnancy[1,2] or from a large transplacental hemorrhage at delivery. In the present study the relative importance of these two possible mechanisms in the pathogenesis of Rh isoimmunization is examined. A program of prophylaxis in both antepartum and postpartum women has been undertaken. On the basis of these observations, we report here our initial studies in both antepartum and postpartum women on the development of a program for the prevention of Rh immunization.

METHODS

In our early studies fetal cells were demonstrated by a modification of the acid elution technique of Kleihauer, Braun and Betke.[8] More recently we have employed the original technique because, as pointed out by Cohen *et al.*,[2] the distinction between fetal and adult hemo-

From the Departments of Pediatrics and Medicine, University of Manitoba, Winnipeg, Manitoba.
This study was supported by a Public Health Grant (Canada) and a United States Public Health Grant (H-3238).
*Professor and Head, Department of Pediatrics, McMaster University, Hamilton, Ontario.
†Professor of Medicine, University of Manitoba, Winnipeg.
Reprint requests to: Dr. A. Zipursky, Department of Pediatrics, Faculty of Medicine, McMaster University, Hamilton, Ontario.

TABLE I.—INCIDENCE OF FETAL CELLS IN THE BLOOD OF Rh-NEGATIVE WOMEN IMMEDIATELY AFTER DELIVERY

Scan count*	Estimated volume of fetal red blood cells in maternal circulation (ml.)†	Total group		Baby Rh+		Baby Rh—	
		Number	%	Number	%	Number	%
0	0 - 0.02	980	82.4	613	82.3	267	82.5
1 - 4	0.02 - 0.1	149	12.5	97	13.0	52	11.7
5 - 20	0.1 - 0.2	34	2.8	20	2.7	14	3.1
>20	>0.2	27	2.3	15	2.0	12	2.7
Total		1190	100.0	745	100.0	445	100.0

*Number of cells found during a 10-minute scan of two blood smears.
†An approximation based on the number of cells seen per 10-minute scan (see Methods).

globin-containing cells is much clearer. In our hands, the *in vitro* sensitivity of the two techniques is similar. Recently we have further modified the technique to distinguish more clearly between fetal erythrocytes and leukocytes (see Appendix).

Using *in vitro* mixtures of fetal and adult cells, the lower limit of detection is one fetal cell in 100,000 adult red cells.[1] This is equivalent to about 0.04 ml. of fetal blood or 0.02 ml. of fetal erythrocytes in the maternal circulation. This order of *in vitro* sensitivity is valid *in vivo* as we have been able to detect fetal cells in four adults injected with 0.01 ml. of fetal cells. This is a 10-fold increase in sensitivity over that reported by us previously.[1]

We have used the counts of *in vitro* mixtures to calibrate the assay for estimating the volume of fetal cells in the maternal circulation.[1] We estimate that 5 to 20 cells per 10-minute scan represents 0.1-0.2 ml. of fetal cells and that more than 20 cells represents greater than 0.2 ml. in the maternal circulation. Woodrow *et al.*[5] consider that a "fetal-cell score" of five by their method represents 0.25 ml. of fetal blood or approximately 0.1 ml. of cells. It would appear that the techniques have the same sensitivity.

The presence of antibodies and their titres were determined by techniques referred to previously.[1] Erythrocyte-survival studies were done by either the ^{51}Cr technique or by the persistence of fetal cells by the acid elution method. With the latter technique the survival of fetal erythrocytes in the circulation of adult volunteers has been found to range from 56 to 105 days.[9]

RESULTS AND DISCUSSION

A. *The Pathogenesis of Rh Isoimmunization. The Incidence of Fetal Erythrocytes in the Circulation of Postpartum Women and the Subsequent Development of Rh Antibodies*

Blood for fetal cells was drawn within the first 24 hours post partum from 1190 Rh-negative women. The number of such cells seen during a 10-minute scan is designated in the tables as the "Scan Count". The subjects were then arbitrarily divided into four groups in accordance with the scan counts. Although it is only semi-quantitative, the method readily permits the identification of a group of women who have received unusually large numbers of fetal cells. In the present study we have arbitrarily selected a scan count of five or more cells (representing approximately 0.1 ml. or more of fetal erythrocytes in the maternal circulation) as indicative of a "large" transplacental hemorrhage. Table I shows that of the total group of 1190 Rh-negative women, 5.1% had a scan count of five or more. The incidence of scan counts in excess of five or more was 4.7% in those women with Rh-positive babies and 5.8% in those with Rh-negative babies. These differences are not statistically significant. The influence of ABO incompatibility on the incidence of fetal cells in the maternal circulation is shown in Table II. High scan counts (5 cells or more) clearly occurred more often in the ABO compatible group (59 out of 948) than in the incompatible group (2 out of 242). The incidence of lower scan counts (1 to 4 cells) was also greater in the ABO compatible group ($x^2 = 17.2$; $p < .001$).

TABLE II.—THE EFFECT OF ABO INCOMPATIBILITY ON THE PRESENCE OF FETAL CELLS POST PARTUM

Scan count	Volume of fetal red blood cells in maternal circulation (ml.)	ABO compatible		ABO incompatible	
		No. of women	%	No. of women	%
0	0 - 0.02	756	79.7	224	92.6
1 - 4	0.02 - 0.1	133	14.0	16	6.6
5 - 20	0.1 - 0.2	33	3.5	1	0.4
>20	>0.2	26	2.8	1	0.4
Total		948	100.0	242	100

These studies indicate that fetal erythrocytes in quantities of 0.1 ml. or more are found in 5.1% of postpartum women, and in highest frequency in ABO compatible pregnancies. This incidence is compared to those reported by others in Table III. The incidence of fetal cells in an unselected group in quantities greater than 0.10 ml. in the present series was compared to the postpartum cases reported by Woodrow

TABLE III.—Incidence of "Large" Numbers of Fetal Cells in the Blood of Women Immediately after Delivery

Author	Number of women	Approximate volume in ml.*	Number of instances	%	
A. ABO blood group of baby and mother not considered					
Woodrow et al[5] (Table II)	200	>0.12	17	8.5	$\chi^2 = 3.68$ (not significant)
Present study	1190	>0.10	61	5.1	
Woodrow and Finn[4]	692	>0.12	92	13.3	$\chi^2 = 37.4$ p = <.001
B. Baby and mother ABO compatible					
Woodrow et al.[5] (Table III)	216	>0.12	26	12.0	$\chi^2 = 8.78$ p = <0.01
Present study	948	>0.10	59	6.3	
Cohen et al.[2] (Table VI)	622	>0.20	52	8.4	$\chi^2 = 25.1$ p = <0.001
Present study	948	>0.20	26	2.8	

*In each instance the approximate volume was deduced from the fetal cell count. Woodrow et al.[5] and Cohen et al.[2] record their so-deduced volumes as volumes of whole blood. These have been converted to volumes of cells by dividing their figures by two.

et al.[5] (Table III); the two groups were not statistically different ($\chi^2 = 3.68$; p > .05). A more recent publication by Woodrow and Finn[4] reports that 19.8% of 692 postpartum samples had fetal-cell scans greater than three and 13.3% had fetal-cell scans of five or more (which they interpret to represent 0.25 ml. of blood[5]). This incidence of 13.3% is significantly greater ($\chi^2 = 37.4$; p < .001) than that of the present series. When ABO compatible pregnancies are compared (with reference to quantities greater than 0.1 ml.), the present series differs significantly from the early series of Woodrow et al.[5] ($\chi^2 = 8.78$; p < .01). In comparing hemorrhages of 0.2 ml. or more, Cohen et al.[2] reported a much higher incidence than the present series ($\chi^2 = 25.1$; p < .001). Because of the unstandardized and variable crude methods of estimating volumes of fetal cells in the maternal circulation, such comparisons are difficult. Nevertheless it is possible that the incidence of "large" transplacental hemorrhages may vary in different centres and these observations may, in part, explain the relatively high proportion of isoimmunization due to "large" transplacental hemorrhages in the Liverpool study as compared with our series (vide infra).

The time at which transplacental hemorrhage occurs has been studied recently by Woodrow and Finn.[4] They concluded that large transplacental hemorrhages (fetal-cell score of five or more) are more likely to occur at delivery than at any other time during pregnancy. Our own findings in a group of 87 women followed up during the last month of pregnancy (Table XIII) do not support their contention. In this series, labour played an insignificant role in the production of fetal hemorrhage. A similar conclusion was reached by Cohen et al.,[2] who

found that of 11 women whose blood contained an estimated 0.2 to 5.0 ml. of fetal cells after delivery, seven had had similar amounts present from 1 to 43 days earlier. However, they did find that fetal erythrocytes enter the maternal circulation in greater frequency as pregnancy progresses. They found that the incidence of fetal cells in the first, second and third trimesters increased progressively from 6.7 to 15.9 to 28.9%. Similar observations have been made by Clayton et al.[10] and by Woodrow and Finn.[4] It would appear therefore that transplacental hemorrhage is more likely to occur in the last weeks of pregnancy. The relative importance of labour in the frequency and quantity of transplacental hemorrhage is not yet clear.

Woodrow et al.[5] consider that those women who have received "large" (greater than 0.25 ml.) quantities of fetal blood at or near the time of labour are at the greatest risk of developing antibodies and that the incidence of immunization increases in direct relationship to the volume of fetal blood in circulation post partum. It is not known, however, what proportion of Rh immunization results from such "high risk" pregnancies. Thus Cohen and Zuelzer[6] reported that of eight women who had developed antibodies after a pregnancy, only one had had a "large" quantity of fetal erythrocytes in her circulation post partum. We previously reported two women in whom antibodies had developed in the absence of a "large" transplacental hemorrhage.[7]

To determine the relative importance of "large" and "small" bleeds in the pathogenesis of Rh immunization, 573 women (whose babies were Rh positive) have been observed post partum for the development of anti-D antibodies. Blood was drawn from these women 4

TABLE IV.—RELATIONSHIP OF THE VOLUME OF FETAL ERYTHROCYTES IN THE MATERNAL CIRCULATION POST PARTUM AND THE SUBSEQUENT DEVELOPMENT OF Rh ANTIBODIES

Cell scan	Approximate volume of fetal cells	Women immunized/total group	% immunized
0 - 4......	0 - 0.1	16/538	3.0
>4.......	>0.1	5/35	14.3

to 12 months post partum, and the serum was tested for antibodies. The results shown in Table IV demonstrate two significant points. The first is that those women whose fetal-cell scan immediately post partum was greater than four, had an incidence of Rh immunization of 14.3% compared to an incidence of 3% in the group with lower cell scans. This supports the contention of Woodrow et al.[5] regarding the relationship between the size of the fetal bleed and chance of subsequent Rh immunization and therefore the existence of a "high risk" group.

TABLE V.—WOMEN WHO DEVELOPED ANTIBODIES POST PARTUM

			Parity	
	Scan count		P	M
Infant ABO-compatible..	0 - 4	13	4	9
	>4	5	3	2
Infant ABO-incompatible....	0 - 4	3	1	2
	>4	0		

However, the data in Table IV also show that most Rh immunizations followed a pregnancy in which the postpartum cell scan was four or less, since 16 of the 21 immunized women were in this category. Of the women who were immunized, eight were primiparae, and five of these did not have a "large" volume of fetal erythrocytes in their blood post partum (Table V). In these women, the primary immunizing event must have been a transplacental hemorrhage which was either very small or occurred well before delivery.

These data, along with those of Cohen and Zuelzer[6] and of Woodrow et al.[5] as reported by McConnell,[11] are summarized in Table VI. Thus

of 51 women who developed antibodies following delivery, fetal cells were not demonstrable post partum in 22. An additional 13 had "small" quantities of cells and would therefore not have been recognized as a "high risk" group. Sixteen of the 39 women did have "large" bleeds demonstrable post partum. Thus, in 69% of the women in the three series, the development of antibodies must have resulted from an antigenic stimulus prior to labour or perhaps as a result of a "small", frequently undetectable hemorrhage during labour. Woodrow et al.[5] have criticized the data of Cohen and Zuelzer because the latter authors did not state whether their subjects were primiparae or multiparae, since if they had been multiparae the appearance of antibodies could have reflected a secondary stimulus. Eight patients in our study were primiparae (Table V) and in five there was no evidence of a "large" transplacental hemorrhage post partum. Furthermore, all of the subjects of Woodrow et al.[5] (Table V) were primiparae and 7 of 13 had not had a "large" bleed post partum. Therefore, it would appear that Rh isoimmunization occurs in women either as a result of a "large" transplacental hemorrhage at delivery or probably more often as a result of smaller, sometimes undetectable bleeds which occur at any time in pregnancy. Woodrow et al.[5] based their original studies of immunological protection on the identification of the "high risk" postpartum group. In the light of our experience this would protect only a minority of the Rh-negative women at risk. Any program of prophylaxis of Rh immunization must be based on these considerations and should include not only the "high risk" group but all Rh-negative women at risk.

B. *Studies on the Prevention of Rh Immunization. The Use of Rh-Immune Globulin*

RESULTS

Rh isoimmunization in volunteers receiving Rh-positive cells can be prevented by the administration of anti-Rh containing gamma globulin or serum.[12, 13] This suggested that a similar approach could be used for the prevention of

TABLE VI.—RELATIONSHIP BETWEEN THE PRESENCE OF FETAL ERYTHROCYTES IN THE CIRCULATION POST PARTUM AND THE SUBSEQUENT DEVELOPMENT OF ANTI-Rh ANTIBODIES
Quantity of fetal erythrocytes found in the maternal circulation post partum

	"Large" No. of women	Approx. vol.	"Small" (1-4) No. of women	Approx. vol.	None No. of women
Cohen and Zuelzer*[6]	1	(0.2 ml.)	3	(0.02-0.2 ml.)	4
McConnell[11]	10	(>0.12 ml.)	7	(<0.12 ml.)	5
Present series	5	(>0.1 ml.)	3	(<0.1 ml.)	13

*The original data in the authors' articles were expressed as numbers of fetal cells from which the amount of fetal *blood* was estimated. These estimates have been converted in this table to ml. of fetal *erythrocytes* by dividing by two.

Rh isoimmunization in pregnant women. Preliminary results of such studies have been reported by others and suggest that passive immunization, post partum, with anti-Rh antibody can prevent Rh isoimmunization.[11, 14] We have undertaken similar studies. Specifically we have: (1) examined the biological activity of a preparation of anti-Rh globulin ("Rh-Immune Globulin"); (2) studied the effect of this agent on newly delivered Rh-negative women whose blood contained Rh-positive fetal cells; and (3) studied the use of this preparation in Rh-negative women during pregnancy.

The results of these investigations follow.

1. THE BIOLOGICAL ACTIVITY OF A PREPARATION OF ANTI-RH (D) GAMMA GLOBULIN ("RH-IMMUNE GLOBULIN")

"Rh-Immune Globulin" was prepared by the Connaught Medical Research Laboratories, University of Toronto, from plasma obtained by repeated plasmaphereses of three Rh-negative women. We selected as our plasma donors women who had had at least one fetal death due to Rh hemolytic disease. We thought the response of the fetus a better index of the quality of antibody than the test-tube titre. Their antibody titres before and after plasmaphereses are shown in Table VII. Three lots were used successively in the present study. The first (Lot 1-1) contained 5% and the second and third (Lots 2-1 and 3-1) 16% gamma globulin. Antibody titres of Lot 3-1 are shown in Table VIII. The titres obtained by several laboratories are also listed in Table VIII. They demonstrate the difficulty in comparing antibody titres from one laboratory to those of another. The antibody titre of Lot 2-1 was similar to that of 3-1 but Lot 1-1 was lower, with a titre in albumin of 1 out of 320 and indirect Coombs of 1 out of 640. The anti-D content of Lot 3-1 was measured for us by Dr. N. C. Hughes-Jones (St. Mary's Hospital, London, England) and found to be 190 µg. per ml. The gamma globulin was administered as a deep intramuscular injection. No side effects were associated with its use.

TABLE VII.—ANTIBODY TITRES IN THE PLASMA USED AS A SOURCE OF ANTI-RH (D) GAMMA GLOBULIN

		Before plasmaphereses			After plasmaphereses		
		Antibody titre*				Antibody titre*	
Donor	Date	S	A	Number of plasmaphereses	Date	S	A
A	June, 63	1	128	17	Aug./64	1	64
B	June, 63	1	256	5	Aug./64	1	64
Br	Dec. 63	1	64	9	Aug./64	1	256

*S and A represent the reciprocal of the saline and albumin titres respectively.

TABLE VIII.—ANTI-D TITRATIONS OF LOT 3-1, RH IMMUNE GLOBULIN

	Technique	
	Albumin	Indirect Coombs
Rh Laboratory (Winnipeg)...	1/1024	1/6400
Medical Research Council Laboratories (London)....	1/5000	1/20,000
Dade Laboratories (Florida)..	1/4000	
Commonwealth Serum Laboratories (Australia)...	1/16,000	1/4000
St. Mary's Hospital (London).		1/4000

a. Anti-D Levels in Recipients Following an Injection of Rh-Immune Globulin

The appearance of anti-Rh (D) antibody in the circulation following intramuscular injection of 20 ml. of Lot 1-1 is shown in Fig. 1. Anti-D was found first after four hours, reached maximum levels in two days and persisted for over six weeks. The maximum levels of anti-D activity achieved after various doses are shown in Table IX.

TABLE IX.—MAXIMUM ANTI-D LEVELS IN CIRCULATION FOLLOWING INTRAMUSCULAR INJECTION OF RH-IMMUNE GLOBULIN

Rh immune globulin (ml.)		Maximum anti-D level attained*			
Lot 1-1 (5%)	Lot 2-1 (16%)	Saline	Papain	Albumin	Indirect Coombs
20.0		0	8	2	4
5.0		0	4	2	2
1.0		0	Tr	0	Tr.
	1.5	0	+	0	±
	0.4	0	0	0	0

*Antibody level is expressed as the reciprocal of antibody titre.
Tr = trace.
+ = antibody present, demonstrable in whole serum only.
± = antibody possibly present.

b. Effect of Rh-Immune Globulin on the Life Span of Rh-Positive Fetal Red Cells

(i) In Women After Delivery

The survival of fetal cells, as determined by the acid-elution technique, was followed in 11

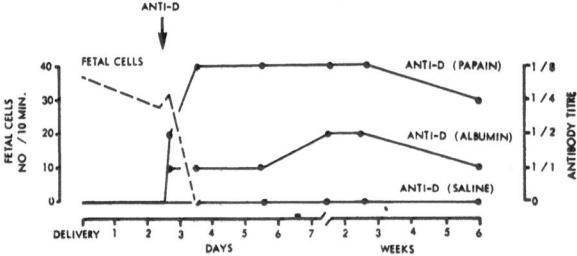

Fig. 1.—Patient S. Fetal erythrocytes were found in the circulation post partum and on repeat examination. Twenty ml. of 5% anti-D gamma globulin were given at 86 hours post partum. The disappearance of fetal cells as well as the appearance of antibodies is shown.

TABLE X.—Survival of Rh-Positive, ABO-Compatible, Fetal Erythrocytes in Postpartum Women after Injection of Rh-Immune Globulin

Subject	Time of injection (hours post partum)	Volume of injection (ml.)		Scan count					
				Prior to injection	After injection (hours)				
		Lot 1-1	Lot 2-1		24	48	72	96	120
S.	86	20		30*	0	0			
P.	64	20		2.6%†	82	1	0		
F.	120	5		530	63	0			
V.	24		1.5	31	2	6	0		
Ra.	51		1.5	46	0				
R.	27		1.5	52		5	0		
B.	40		1.5	215	140	0			
Mc.				190	253	65	1		
A.	140		1.5	784	420	28	0		
Pl.	72		1.5	3.2%†	2.0%	2.3%	2.0%	2.0%†	
D.	40		0.4	22			15	0	
St.	48		0.4	140			110		0

*All results are recorded as scan counts except for the pre-injection sample in patient "P" and all samples in patient "Pl", where results are recorded as percentage of cells in the patient's blood that were fetal.

†A second dose of 1.5 ml. (Lot 2-1) was given and when next tested six days later, no cells were found.

women who had received Rh-Immune Globulin post partum. The survival of fetal cells in one of these (Mrs. S.) is shown in Fig. 1 and all results are shown in Table X. When quantities of 5.0 ml. or more of Lot 1-1 or 1.5 ml. of Lot 2-1 were given, fetal cells were, with two exceptions, gone by 48 hours. In Mrs. R. fetal cells were still present at 48 hours but had disappeared by 72 hours. In Mrs. Pl. 3.2% of the cells in her circulation were fetal when she received her first injection of Rh-Immune Globulin after delivery. As this did not remove the Rh-positive cells over the next four days, she was given a second injection. Fetal cells had disappeared from her circulation when she was next studied six days later. The smallest dose administered, 0.4 ml. of Lot 2-1, appeared to remove fetal cells at a slower rate in two subjects since cells were still demonstrable at 72 hours, although they had disappeared when the blood was examined at 96 and 120 hours.

(ii) In Males Receiving Untagged Cells

Eighteen Rh-negative men were each given 2 ml. of Rh-positive cord erythrocytes intravenously. Forty-eight hours later, six received 5.0 ml. and six 1.0 ml. of Lot 1-1 Rh-Immune Globulin and six control subjects received 1.0 ml. of commercial gamma globulin. Fetal cell counts were done at 24-hour intervals beginning 48 hours before injection of the gamma globulin. In the group receiving 5 ml. there was a rapid disappearance of fetal cells, most of them being gone by 48 hours. The disappearance was slower in the group receiving 1.0 ml., although it was more rapid than in the control.

At one week no fetal cells were demonstrable in those receiving either 1.0 or 5.0 ml. anti-D gamma globulin, whereas in five of the six controls such cells were seen in numbers from 9 to 73% of the original (mean survival was 43%). Two weeks after injection there were no fetal cells demonstrable in the control group.

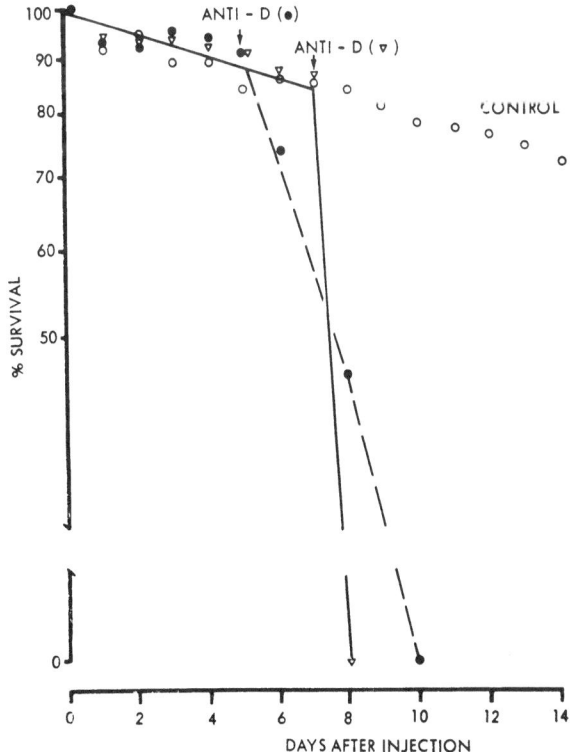

Fig. 2.—The survival of 51Cr-labelled Rh-positive cord erythrocytes in the circulation of three Rh-negative subjects. Each subject received 1.6 ml. cord erythrocytes on day 0. 0—control; ●—received 0.5 ml. 5% Immune Globulin on day 5; ▲—received 2.0 ml. 5% Rh Immune Globulin on day 8. A fourth subject (not shown), who received 1 ml. on day 5, had an erythrocyte survival that did not differ significantly from that of the control.

The reason for the disappearance of the fetal cells in this group is not clear, although it may be related to immunization of some of these subjects.

(iii) Males Receiving ^{51}Cr Labelled Cells

Four Rh-negative men each received, from one donor, 1.6 ml. of the same Group O Rh-positive compatible cord erythrocytes tagged with 100 microcuries of ^{51}Cr. All subjects were studied for five days to determine the cell survival over that period. On day 5, one subject received 1.0 ml. and one received 0.5 ml. of Lot 1-1 Rh-Immune Globulin. A third subject was given 2.0 ml. on day 8 while the fourth was retained as a control. The results (Fig. 2) show that the injected cells were rapidly removed from the circulation by an injection of 2.0 ml. of gamma globulin and at a slower rate by 0.5 ml. In one case not shown in this figure, a dose of 1.0 ml. was ineffective (the ^{51}Cr survival was identical with the control), suggesting that removal may not be solely a function of dose. Further studies using smaller volumes of fetal cells were done and the results are shown in Table XI.

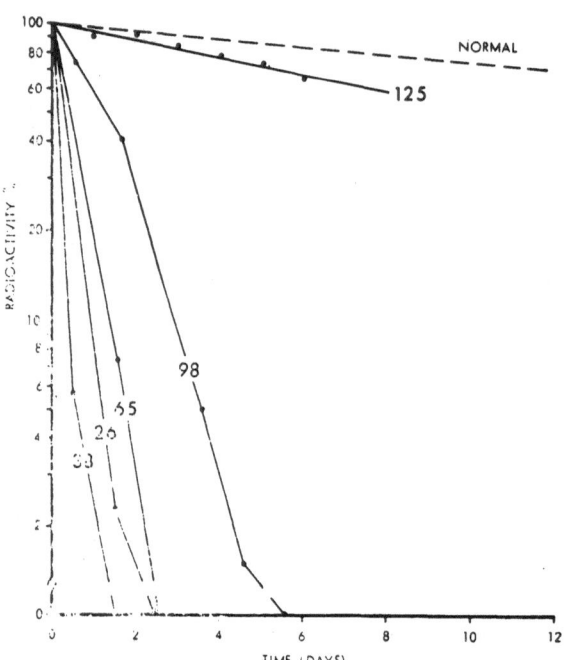

Fig. 3.—^{51}Cr survival studies at intervals following the administration of 0.5 ml. Rh-Immune Globulin. The dashed line represents a hypothetical survival curve for normal blood. The solid lines represent survival curves of ^{51}Cr-labelled erythrocytes (0.5 ml.) given at 26, 38, 65, 98 and 125 days following the administration of Rh-Immune Globulin.

TABLE XI.—Rh-Immune Globulin (Connaught) and Clearance of Rh-Positive Cord Erythrocytes from the Circulation of Rh-Negative Subjects

Experiment	Volume of cells (ml.)	Volume of 16% gamma globulin (ml.)	^{51}Cr survival (half-life) days
He.	0.5	0.5	<1
T.	0.5	0.5	<1
He.	0.34	0.1	2
SH.	0.34	0.02	3.5

In one subject, He., repeated ^{51}Cr erythrocyte survival studies were performed following the injection of 0.5 ml. of Rh-Immune Globulin (Fig. 3). As indicated in Table XI, erythrocyte survival immediately after the injection of 0.5 ml. gamma globulin was less than 24 hours. The survival of 0.5-ml. volumes of cord erythrocytes was still less than three days two months later, less than six days at three months, and it was only after four months that the ^{51}Cr survival of Rh-positive cord erythrocytes approached normal (Fig. 3). Assuming a half-life of Rh-immune globulin in circulation of 30 days, it can be estimated that 98 days after the injection of 0.5 ml. of Rh-Immune Globulin the amount remaining in circulation would be equivalent to an injection of approximately 0.06 ml. of Rh-Immune Globulin.

Thus these studies (Table XI and Fig. 3) indicate that 0.02 ml. to 0.06 ml. (3.8 to 11.4 micrograms of anti-D antibody) of Rh-Immune Globulin can effectively shorten the life span of 0.3 to 0.5 ml. volumes of Rh-positive cord erythrocytes. This is comparable to the data of Mollison and Hughes-Jones,[15] who found that one microgram of anti-D antibody decreased the half-life ^{51}Cr survival of 0.3 ml. of cells to 100 hours. In two experiments where five micrograms were given, the half-life was 39.5 and 43.5 hours respectively.

c. The Effect of Rh-Immune Globulin in Preventing Primary Rh Isoimmunization in Rh-Negative Subjects

This study is the continuation of that described in section b (ii). Eighteen Rh-negative men who did not have Rh antibodies were each given 2.0 ml. of Rh-positive cord blood intravenously. Subjects 1 to 8 received blood from one placenta, subjects 9 to 13 from a second and subjects 14 to 18 from a third. Forty-eight hours later, six (1 to 5 and subject 17) were injected intramuscularly with 5 ml. and six (6 to 10 and subject 16) with 1.0 ml. of Lot 1-1 Rh-Immune Globulin (5%), while six controls received 1.0 ml. of commercial gamma globulin (16%).

Three of the controls developed anti-D (Table XII), whereas none of the protected did. Six months after the initial injection 13 of the subjects received a second injection of 2.0 ml. of Rh-positive cells. Repeat injections were not given to four of the six in the 5.0 ml. group or to one of the six in the 1.0-ml. group. None of those who did not already have anti-D developed it during the three months following this second stimulus, but a significant rise in antibody titre took place in the three immunized subjects who already had anti-D (Table XII).

ary response. Had only the albumin technique been used in subjects M. and Mc., primary immunization would not have been detected on day 196.

These observations emphasize an important consideration in any study dealing with Rh immunization and its prevention. Reliance cannot be placed on a single method of detection when antibodies are being sought; further, serial examinations for antibodies should be carried out.

TABLE XII.—ANTIBODY RESPONSE OF THREE MALE SUBJECTS

Date	Day	Fetal red blood cells (vol.)	Anti-D antibody											
			Subject H.				Subject M.				Subject Mc.			
			S.	A.	P.	I.C.	S.	A.	P.	I.C.	S.	A.	P.	I.C.
Nov. 3, 1964	0	2.0 ml.	—	—	—	—	—	—	—	—	—	—	—	—
Dec. 10	38		—	—	—	—	+	—	—	—	—	—	—	—
Dec. 24	52		1	—	1	—	+	+	2	+	—	—	—	—
Jan. 25, 1965	84		1	1	2	1	1	1	4	2	—	—	—	—
Feb. 25	111		2	2	2	2	—	2	4	2	—	—	—	—
March 25	139		1	2	2	2	—	1	1	1	—	—	—	—
April 22	168	Day	1	4	8	4	—	—	2	1	—	—	Tr.	—
May 20	196	0 2.0 ml.	1	4	8	8	—	—	1	—	—	—	Tr.	Tr.
May 27	7		16	16	32	32	8	64	256	128	4	1	8	2
June 3	14		16	32	128	64	1	64	256	128	1	16	64	64
June 17	28		16	64	256	128	1	64	256	128	2	16	32	32
July 17	58		2	128	256	128	1	32	256	128	1	8	32	32
Aug. 22	92		1	128	512	128	1	64	256	128	1	4	8	8

*Antibody levels are expressed as the reciprocal of the antibody titre.
S = Saline, A = Albumin, P = Papain, I.C. = Indirect Coombs.
—No antibody demonstrable.
Tr. Trace of antibody.

The antibody responses (Table XII) of the three immunized men deserve individual comment. The response of subject H. is a "standard" response; thus, no antibody was demonstrable on day 38, but one, demonstrable by the saline and papain techniques, was present by day 52, and one demonstrable by all four techniques was present by the day 84. Thereafter the titre rose slowly to a peak at days 168 to 196. The secondary response was brisk, the saline titre falling away after day 28. In subject M, the primary response began a little earlier, but followed the same pattern of development, although at a lower level; by day 139 the response was beginning to fade and by day 196 the antibody could be demonstrated only by the papain method. If on this day this man had been tested only by the indirect Coombs technique, he would have been considered as unimmunized. Interestingly, in spite of the generally weak primary response, the secondary response was even brisker than that of subject H. In subject Mc. the only evidence of primary immunization was a very weak papain and Coombs reaction on day 196, and yet his response to the second stimulus is a classical, though low-level, second-

The final proof that primary immunization has not occurred is failure of the recipient to give a secondary response reaction to a second dose of antigen.

2. THE USE OF RH-IMMUNE GLOBULIN TO PREVENT PRIMARY RH IMMUNIZATION IN WOMEN WHOSE BLOOD CONTAINS RH-POSITIVE FETAL ERYTHROCYTES AFTER DELIVERY

Fifteen newly delivered Rh-negative women whose blood had scan counts of five or more, and whose babies were ABO-compatible and Rh-positive, received Rh-Immune Globulin and were followed up for three or more months post partum (nine have been followed for six or more months post partum). They received 1.5 ml. of 16% Rh-Immune Globulin with the exception of two who received 0.4 ml. of 16% and two received 5 and 20 ml., respectively, of 5% Rh-Immune Globulin. Antibodies are not demonstrable in any of these 15 women. To date 35 women who had scan counts of five or more after delivery and did not receive Rh-Immune

Globulin have been tested at four or more months post partum. Five had antibodies (Table IV).

3. THE USE OF RH-IMMUNE GLOBULIN DURING THE THIRD TRIMESTER OF PREGNANCY

The data outlined in the previous sections suggest that many if not most cases of primary Rh immunization result from transplacental passage of fetal cells at some time before the onset of labour. Accordingly, it seemed necessary to develop a technique whereby Rh-Immune Globulin could be given during pregnancy. That this seemed feasible was suggested by the findings noted earlier, which indicated that small doses of Rh-Immune Globulin were adequate to destroy fetal erythrocytes and prevent Rh immunization (see Section B.1). Nevertheless, it seemed possible that even these small quantities of a lethal antibody might cause harm to the fetus. Accordingly, before proceeding with the injection of pregnant women we attempted to simulate the condition in the fetus, by examining the effect of Rh-Immune Globulin on the life span of Rh-positive erythrocytes in Rh-positive subjects.

Two Rh-positive infants, R. (aged 2 months and weighing 8 pounds) and M (aged 18 months and weighing 18 pounds), were each given 5.0 ml. of ^{51}Cr-tagged autologous blood. Forty-eight hours later each received 0.5 ml. of Rh-Immune Globulin (Lot 1-1) while M. received a second dose of 0.5 ml. one week later. The erythrocyte ^{51}Cr life span in M. is shown in Fig. 4. The calculated half-life for red-cell survival in R. and M. was found to be 21 and 31 days, respectively. (A half-life of 21 days is normal for the erythrocytes of an infant of 2 months.[17])

Thus, quantities of antibody far in excess of those which a fetus would likely receive if the mother were given a "protective" dose of Rh-Immune Globulin did not appear to shorten erythrocyte life span. We concluded that it would be safe to give such doses of antibody to mothers during pregnancy. Still proceeding with caution, we at first gave the globulin at various times during the last trimester (Series A).

We started by giving a single dose of 0.4 ml. one week before delivery. Later we increased this to a single dose of 1 ml. one week before delivery. Our final program consisted of 1 ml. given at what was judged to be the 28th week followed by two 0.4 ml. doses four weeks apart.

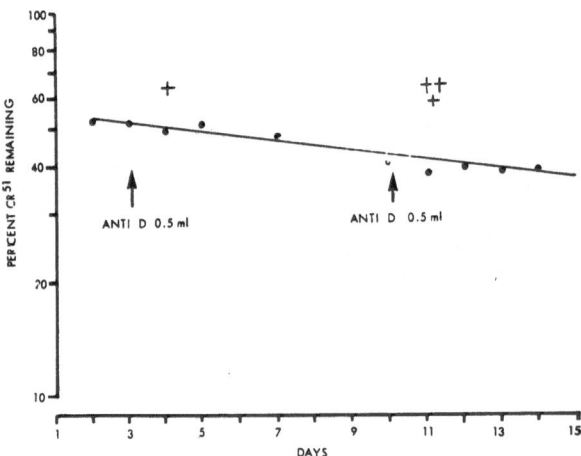

Fig. 4.—^{51}Cr survival of autologous cells in an 18-month, Rh-positive experimental subject. On day 3, the subject received 0.5 ml. of 5% anti-D (Rh-Immune Globulin). This was repeated on day 10.

+ =Direct Coombs test weakly positive.
+++=Direct Coombs test strongly positive.

a. SERIES A

(i) Anti-D Levels Following the Injection of Anti-D Gamma Globulin During Pregnancy

Forty-seven pregnant women received Rh-Immune Globulin and were studied serially thereafter for antibodies in their serum. Only two of the women given a dose of 0.4 ml. had demonstrable antibodies in their serum, but antibodies were demonstrable in three of seven, of those receiving a single injection of 1.0 ml. In those women receiving multiple injections, antibodies were demonstrable in all but two of the 23 cases studied. In all cases in which they were found, antibodies were demonstrable only by the papain technique and were never more than "weakly positive".

(ii) The Effect on the Fetus of Anti-Rh Administration to the Mother

Immediately after birth the following hematological studies were performed on all babies: hemoglobin concentration, hematocrit, reticulocyte count, white blood count and differential. All babies were followed for evidence of hyperbilirubinemia in the first five days of life. Thirty-five of the babies were Rh-positive. The direct Coombs test was "weakly positive" in five of these infants. Two of these five were ABO-incompatible, which may explain the positive test. In one of these (born one day after receiving 0.4 ml. anti-Rh gamma globulin) the bilirubin rose to 14.0 mg. % by day 3 (this was considered to represent a case of ABO-incompatibility—hemolytic disease). All infants were well and there was no evidence of hematological abnormalities related to the administration of Rh-Immune Globulin to the mother.

(iii) The Incidence of Fetal Erythrocytes in the Circulation of Mothers Receiving Rh-Immune Globulin

The blood of 34 women who subsequently delivered Rh-positive infants was examined for fetal cells immediately before the administration of Rh-Immune Globulin. In six or 17.5%, fetal cells were demonstrable. In five of these, studied within a week after injection, fetal cells were no longer found.

Fetal cells were found for the first time following injection in four of 10 women receiving 0.4 ml., in one of seven receiving 1.0 ml. and in five of the 18 who received multiple injections.

(iv) The Development of Antibodies in Women Receiving Rh-Immune Globulin

Twenty-five women have been followed up for longer than four months (20 for more than six months). None have developed antibodies. Six of the group received 0.4 ml., one 0.8 ml. and the remainder 1 ml. or more. Four of the group were ABO-incompatible.

b. SERIES B

In the second antepartum study (Series B), Rh-negative pregnant women were divided into three groups. One received 1.5 ml. Rh-Immune Globulin at the 36th week of gestation; one received 1.5 ml. immediately postpartum and one acted as the control group.

(i) The Incidence of Fetal Erythrocytes

These observations during the last month of pregnancy are shown in Table XIII. It is evident that large volumes of fetal erythrocytes are less frequently found in the circulation of women who received 1.5 ml. Rh-Immune Globulin at the 36th week of gestation. The frequency of small transplacental bleeds did not differ significantly in the groups studied.

(ii) The Newborn Infant

All infants were hematologically normal and with one exception the Coombs test was negative; in that patient, the mother was group O and the infant was group A.

(iii) The Development of Antibodies

Blood samples obtained six months postpartum, or longer, were examined for anti-D antibodies. In the unprotected group 1 of 21

TABLE XIII.—SCAN COUNTS OF FETAL CELLS IN CIRCULATION DURING THE LAST MONTH OF PREGNANCY IN SERIES B

a. The entire group at 36 weeks and the untreated thereafter

		Scan counts			
	Total	0	5	5 - 20	20
36 weeks.......	87	75	8	4	0
37 weeks.......	54	45	7	1	1
38 weeks.......	43	33	5	4	1
Labour: 1st stage	47	38	7	1	1
After 3rd stage..	57	44	8	3	1

b. Women who received 1.5 ml. Rh-Immune Globulin at 36 weeks

		Scan counts			
	Total	0	5	5 - 20	20
37 weeks.......	24	20	4	0	0
38 weeks.......	16	12	4	0	0
Labour: 1st stage	15	15	0	0	0
After 3rd stage..	24	19	5	0	0

developed an anti-D antibody. In the group who received Rh-Immune Globulin at delivery (20) and at 36 weeks' gestation (20) none developed antibodies. ABO-incompatibility between mother and fetus was found in two of 21 unprotected, four of 20 injected post partum and five of 20 injected at 36 weeks.

GENERAL DISCUSSION

The present studies were undertaken on the thesis that Rh isoimmunization during pregnancy results from the transplacental passage of fetal erythrocytes and that active immunization can be prevented by passive immunization with anti-Rh antibodies. This hypothesis has been presented by others[12, 13] and preliminary observations by these groups offer support for the rationale of this approach.[11, 14]

The Rh-Immune Globulin used in the present study has been prepared in three lots; initially a 5% preparation (Lot 1-1) and later 16% gamma globulin preparations (Lots 2-1 and 3-1). All three have incomplete antibody activity demonstrable in vitro (Table VIII) and in vivo (Table IX, Fig. 1). The absence of complete (saline) antibodies is in part due to the selection of donors (Table VII) who had very low levels of saline antibodies and in part to the method of preparation of concentrate which removes most of the macroglobulin (IgM) antibodies. The antibody titre of our anti-Rh gamma globulin, as we have measured it, is considerably lower than that used by others.[5, 13] The donors had been selected not primarily because of their antibody titre but because in all cases the antibody appeared to be capable of producing severe hemolytic disease. This was evidenced by a history of fetal death (due to Rh disease) in all women.

We have demonstrated in volunteers that as little as 0.02 ml. of Rh-Immune Globulin can significantly shorten the life span of 0.34 ml. of Rh-positive cord erythrocytes. These findings are supported by the observations in pregnant women whose blood contained fetal erythrocytes (Table X). In these cases it appeared that 1.5 ml. was effective in removing small quantities of fetal cells; it is likely also that in two women, D. and St., a dose of 0.4 ml. caused a less distinct, but significant shortening of erythrocyte life span. However, when the quantity of Rh-positive erythrocytes in circulation is large, greater volumes of antibody must be used to effect removal. This is clearly evident in subject Pl. (Table X). This woman was found to have 3.2% fetal cells in her blood, which would represent about 125 ml. of fetal blood in her circulation. This quantity of blood was not removed by the administration of 1.5 ml. anti-Rh gamma globulin (Lot 2-1), but did disappear after a second dose. In subject P. a large dose of 20.0 ml. (Lot 1-1) quickly removed a similar volume of fetal erythrocytes. These observations suggest that the removal of small quantities (2.0 ml. or less) of fetal Rh-positive erythrocytes from the maternal circulation, in most instances, was effected by the administration of 0.4-1.5 ml. (Lot 2-1) anti-Rh gamma globulin.

Although it is evident that this preparation destroys fetal Rh-positive erythrocytes, its biological effectiveness must be judged by its ability to prevent primary isoimmunization of Rh-negative subjects by Rh-positive erythrocytes. That these two effects (on life span and on antigenicity) are interrelated has been suggested by the original studies of Clarke et al.[12] Nevertheless, it remained to be determined whether our anti-Rh gamma globulin preparation could prevent primary Rh isoimmunization in experimental subjects and pregnant women. The 12 "protected" subjects in Section B (1,c,) did not develop primary immunization. Seven were restimulated six months later and did not show a secondary or booster response. Three of the six "unprotected" subjects developed antibodies and showed a classical secondary response when restimulated. Thus doses of 1.0 ml. and 5.0 ml. of 5% gamma globulin were effective in preventing primary immunization. This quantity of antibody is considerably less than that used by Woodrow et al.[5] and Freda, Gorman and Pollack[13] to prevent primary isoimmunization. However, neither of these groups attempted to establish the minimum effective dose. Recently, however, Clarke et al.[16] presented evidence which suggested that as little as 0.5 ml. anti-D gamma globulin is capable of

preventing Rh immunization. Gorman's data suggest that 100 μg. of anti-D could prevent Rh immunization following the injection of 6.0 ml. of Rh-positive erythrocytes.[17] His findings are comparable to those of the present study, in which it was found that as little as 1.0 ml. of 5% Immune Globulin prevented Rh immunization. This volume is assumed to contain approximately 60 μg. anti-D on the assumption that its content would be 5/16 of that in the 16% preparation. Gorman,[17] however, found that 10 μg. was not protective. This suggests that the minimum dose for the prevention of Rh immunization is between 10 and 100 μg. of anti-D antibody.

Our studies to date in postpartum women suggest that our preparation is effective in preventing primary immunization in Rh-negative mothers. Thus 15 mothers who had had "large" transplacental hemorrhages and received anti-Rh gamma globulin have been followed up for more than three months and none have developed antibodies. In contrast, 35 women in the present series who had "large" transplacental hemorrhages have been followed up for more than four months and five have already developed antibodies.

The Liverpool group have held that most cases of Rh immunization result from a "large" transplacental hemorrhage occurring during labour. They have identified these women and studied the effectiveness of their preparation of anti-D containing gamma globulin in preventing immunization. Their most recent results in this high-risk group are encouraging and indicate that these women can be protected.[18] However, the evidence presented in this paper (Section A) and by others[6] suggests that identification and protection of the "high risk" group will not prevent the majority of cases of Rh immunization. We believe that Rh immunization can result from the smaller bleeds which occur so frequently during pregnancy. For this reason we considered the possibility of treating women during pregnancy. It is evident from our studies that such a procedure is feasible and does not harm the fetus and that "protective" doses of Rh Immune Globulin can be given safely during pregnancy.

Freda, Gorman and Pollack[14] have approached the problem in another way. They reasoned that since antibodies rarely appear during the immunizing pregnancy, passive immunization should be effective if given immediately post partum. In their study, anti-Rh antibodies are administered to Rh-negative women post partum if the infant is Rh-positive, ABO-compatible, irrespective of the presence or absence of fetal cells in the maternal circulation. Their most recent findings strongly support this approach. Thus 37 of 318 controls became immunized, whereas none of 369 women who had received protection developed antibodies.[17]

These results all represent postpartum follow-up studies in which women have been observed for the appearance of Rh antibodies. The lack of antibody formation strongly suggests that Rh immunization has been prevented; however, for the reasons given, these studies must be continued into subsequent pregnancies to determine that the protected women have not indeed been sensitized and whether or not antibodies will appear during their next Rh-positive pregnancy. However, preliminary observations from both the Liverpool and Columbia groups[14, 17] indicate that the protected women do *not* develop antibodies during a subsequent pregnancy. It would appear therefore that the protection is real and that postpartum passive immunization with Rh antibodies is an effective means of preventing Rh immunization. Accordingly many centres are now actively studying the value of their own anti-Rh antibody preparation in the prevention of Rh immunization.

In Canada, the Connaught Medical Research Laboratories of the University of Toronto have prepared Rh-Immune Globulin, as used in the present study. This material is now being used in a number of centres throughout Canada as part of a co-ordinated program which will lead to the availability of a simple and practical means of preventing Rh immunization.

Summary The relation between transplacental hemorrhage and the development of Rh immunization has been studied.

Rh immunization developed more frequently in women whose blood contained relatively large volumes of fetal erythrocytes post partum. Nevertheless this high-risk group accounted for only a small proportion of women developing Rh antibodies post partum. It is suggested, therefore, that all Rh-negative women, whose infants are Rh-positive, ABO-compatible, are at risk of developing antibodies.

Rh-Immune Globulin (Connaught), with anti-D activity demonstrable *in vitro* and *in vivo*, can destroy Rh-positive erythrocytes and appears to prevent Rh immunization in experimental subjects and postpartum women.

Rh-Immune Globulin has been given to Rh-negative women, ante partum and post partum, with no ill effect. It is likely, therefore, that this preparation will prove to be an effective means of preventing Rh immunization.

Résumé Cet article aborde la question de la relation entre l'hémorragie transplacentaire et l'apparition de l'iso-immunisation Rh.

L'iso-immunisation Rh apparaît plus fréquemment chez les femmes dont le sang contient des quantités relativement importantes d'hématies fétales durant le post-partum. Pourtant, ce groupe de sujets, bien qu'il constitue un "risque élevé", n'a représenté qu'une faible proportion des femmes qui ont présenté des anticorps Rh au cours du post-partum. On estime donc que toutes les femmes à Rh-négatif, dont les enfants ont un Rh-positif avec compatibilité ABO, courent le risque de former des anticorps.

La globuline immunisante Rh (Connaught), dotée d'une activité anti-D décelable *in vitro* et *in vivo*, peut détruire les érythrocytes Rh-positifs et permet de prévenir l'iso-immunisation Rh chez des sujets d'expérience et chez les femmes durant le post-partum.

On a administré la globuline immunisante Rh à des femmes Rh-négatives, tant *ante-partum* que *post-partum*, sans déclencher de réactions défavorables. Il est donc probable que ce produit se révélera comme un moyen efficace de prévenir l'iso-immunisation Rh.

The authors gratefully acknowledge the assistance of Dr. Bruce Chown, who took part in so many discussions leading toward the completion of this paper, and whose criticisms were of such great value. The assistance of Dr. Rebecca Yeow, Miss Helen Peters, Miss Catherine Anderson, Miss Janet Pollock and Mrs. Judy Decker is also gratefully acknowledged. Thanks are also due the Canadian Red Cross Blood Transfusion Service, Manitoba Depot, Warden F. S. Harris, his staff and the volunteers at Stoney Mountain Penitentiary and to Dr. G. H. Lowther and his staff at the Manitoba School in Portage la Prairie.

REFERENCES

1. ZIPURSKY, A. et al.: *Lancet*, 2: 489, 1963.
2. COHEN, F. et al.: *Blood*, 23: 621, 1964.
3. FREESE, U. E. AND TITEL, J. H.: *Obstet. Gynec.*, 22: 527, 1963.
4. WOODROW, J. C. AND FINN, R.: *Brit. J. Haemat.*, 12: 297, 1966.
5. WOODROW, J. C. et al.: *Brit. Med. J.*, 1: 279, 1965.
6. COHEN, F. AND ZUELZER, W. W.: *Vox Sang.*, 9: 75, 1964.
7. ZIPURSKY, A. et al.: *Birth Defects Original Article Series*, 1: 84, 1965.
8. KLEIHAUER, E., BRAUN, H. AND BETKE, K.: *Klin. Wschr.* 35: 637, 1957.
9. ZIPURSKY, A.: *Seminars Hemat.*, 2: 167, 1965.
10. CLAYTON, E. M., JR. et al.: *Obstet. Gynec.*, 28: 194, 1966.
11. McCONNELL, R. B.: *Ann. Rev. Med.*, 17: 291, 1966.
12. CLARKE, C. A. et al.: *Brit. Med. J.*, 1: 979, 1963.
13. FREDA, V. J., GORMAN, J. G. AND POLLACK, W.: *Transfusion*, 4: 26, 1964.
14. Idem: *Science*, 151: 828, 1966.
15. MOLLISON, P. L. AND HUGHES-JONES, N. C.: *Immunology*, 12: 63, 1967.
16. CLARKE, C. A. et al.: *Brit. Med. J.*, 1: 213, 1966.
17. GORMAN, J.: Personal communication.
18. CLARKE, C. A. et al.: *Brit. Med. J.*, 2: 907, 1966.

APPENDIX

THE ACID ELUTION TECHNIQUE FOR THE DEMONSTRATION OF FETAL ERYTHROCYTES

Reagents:

1. *Hematoxylin solution*

Hematoxylin crystals	5 g.
Alcohol—absolute	50 ml.
Ammonium or potassium alum	100 g.
Mercuric oxide	2.5 g.
Distilled water	1000 ml.

Dissolve the hematoxylin in the alcohol and the alum in the water with the aid of heat. Remove from heat and mix the two solutions. Bring to a boil as rapidly as possible. Remove from heat and add the mercuric oxide slowly. Reheat until it becomes dark purple, remove from flame immediately and plunge the vessel into a basin of cold water until cool.

The stain is ready for use as soon as it cools. Addition of 2 to 4 ml. of glacial acetic acid per 100 ml. of solution increases the intensity of the nuclear stain. Filter before use.

2. *Eosin solution* (0.5%)
Eosin (water soluble, yellow shade)   5 g.
Distilled water................. 1000 ml.
Filter before storing.

3. *Buffer*
Prepare immediately before use:
75.4 ml. of 0.1M citric acid

24.6 ml. of 0.2M sodium phosphate
pH should be 3.2 - 3.3

Technique:

Fresh clotted blood is preferred; however, heparinized blood may be used. Alcohol-cleaned slides must be used. Mix, on the slide, two drops of serum with one drop of blood and prepare a thin blood smear. Air-dry for 30 - 60 minutes.

Slides are fixed in 80% alcohol for five minutes. Wash thoroughly under running cold tap water. Place in buffer (at 30°C.) for five minutes. Wash slides again under running tap water for five minutes. Stain for five minutes with eosin. Wash eosin off with running water. Stain slides with freshly filtered hematoxylin for two to three minutes. Wash and dry in air.

Papers 41 & 42

41. Leading article. (1967). Prevention of Rh-haemolytic disease *Med. J. Aust.*, *2*, 1035-6.
42. Leading article. (1969). Prevention of Rh-haemolytic disease—1969. *Med. J. Aust.*, *1*, 1034-6.

Commentary

The Australians were quick to recognise the potentialities of preventing Rh HDN (Paper 41) and their Red Cross Organisation set up a special committee to consider the matter. As early as 1967 it recommended to the National Executive of the Red Cross Society that the treatment should be carried out routinely in Australia, and within three months the gammaglobulin was available on a national basis free of charge.

The second article (Paper 42) shows how quickly all mothers at risk were able to receive the therapy, and it pointed out that 'the potential benefits to the individual mother and to the community are enormous'. What has happened since that time in Australia is indicated in Paper 47, but accurate information as to how far the immunisation rate has been lowered is still awaited.

Paper 41

THE MEDICAL JOURNAL OF AUSTRALIA

SATURDAY, AUGUST 5, 1967

PREVENTION OF Rh–HAEMOLYTIC DISEASE

RH-HÆMOLYTIC DISEASE of the newborn occurs when antibodies present in the mother's circulation cross the placenta and damage the baby's red cells.

The rhesus blood group system contains a number of antigens which can be differentiated by their reactions with specific antisera. Clinically, the D-antigen is the most important member of the rhesus antigen complex, and testing for the presence of this D-antigen determines whether a blood sample is typed as Rh(D)-positive or Rh(D)-negative.

The clinical problem in Rh-sensitization arises from the relative ease with which an Rh-negative person can be stimulated to produce rhesus antibodies. This may occur as the result of transfusion with Rh-positive blood or from the introduction of Rh-positive cells by transplacental hæmorrhage during pregnancy with an Rh-positive fœtus.

Two main types of rhesus antibody—"complete" and "incomplete"—have been identified. The "complete" or "saline" antibody is capable of causing direct agglutination of Rh-positive erythrocytes in saline. It is an immunoglobulin of high molecular weight, the so-called 19S or IgM type of antibody, which appears usually as an early response to immunization, does not cross the placenta, and is not a factor in the pathogenesis of hæmolytic disease of the newborn. The other type of rhesus antibody is described as an "incomplete" antibody. It does not agglutinate erythrocytes in saline directly. Although adsorbed to Rh-positive cells, the antibody will cause agglutination only under special laboratory conditions. This antibody is of the 7S or IgG type, with a relatively low molecular weight, and crosses the placenta readily. It usually appears later in the immunization process and is the important factor in Rh-hæmolytic disease of the fœtus and newborn infant.

Until a few years ago, Rh-hæmolytic disease could be managed only by treating the affected infant, but recent advances in immunology are opening the way to means of effective prevention. It has been known for many years that passive antibody is capable of specific immunosuppression, and consequently it was reasoned that it might be possible to protect Rh-negative mothers from sensitization if preformed antibody could be administered at the same time as the antigen, i.e., when fœtal Rh-positive cells were present in the maternal circulation. It had also been noted that if the Rh-positive fœtus had an ABO group incompatible with that of the mother the likelihood of Rh immunization occurring was much diminished, possibly because the fœtal cells are rapidly removed from the maternal circulation. Experimental studies on Rh-negative male volunteers injected with Rh-positive cells followed by anti-D antibody have shown that the "foreign" cells were rapidly cleared from the circulation, and no endogenous antibody was subsequently formed; furthermore, it was shown that the initial complete protection by anti-D could be repeated at the next Rh-positive stimulus.

However, before Rh-negative mothers could be protected by anti-D administration it was necessary to know answers to two questions relating to the natural history of sensitization: whether fœto-maternal hæmorrhages do occur, and if so, when; and whether it is possible to time the antibody injection to nullify the effects of such occurrences. There is now a substantial body of evidence that leakage of fœtal red cells into the maternal circulation is of quite frequent occurrence. Fœtal cells can be distinguished in the maternal circulation by differential staining methods, and by means of such techniques it has been shown that the majority of transplacental hæmorrhages occur during parturition. Furthermore, there is a direct relationship between the size of the transplacental hæmorrhage and the likelihood of sensitization of the mother.

Since the early 1960's a number of clinical trials have been conducted in England, the U.S.A. and Germany. Rh-negative mothers who had borne an Rh-positive fœtus were randomly allocated to "treatment" and "control" groups, the former being given an injection of anti-D gamma globulin within 72 hours of delivery, and the latter receiving no treatment. Both groups were subsequently studied to determine whether or not antibodies developed. A major landmark in this work was the publication in October last year of the results of a combined study[1] carried out at centres in England (Liverpool, Sheffield, Leeds and Bradford) and Baltimore. This involved 156 Rh-negative primiparas, half of whom received 5 ml. of gamma globulin containing a very high titre of incomplete anti-D soon after parturition. The results were extremely encouraging, and suggested that nearly all cases of Rh immunization can be prevented by the injection after delivery of high-titre incomplete anti-D gamma globulin. More recently, a report[2] by workers at the Columbia-Presbyterian Medical Center in New York, and at the Memorial Hospital of Long Beach, California, summarizes the progress of 666 mothers involved in their own and other trials. These include the English-Baltimore combined study, the Freiburg (Germany) study, and another New York series. Not one of the 329 mothers in these studies who received anti-D gamma globulin developed antibodies, whereas in 46 of the 337 controls antibody was detected. Fifty-eight women have completed their second pregnancy

[1] *Brit. med. J.*, 1966, 2 : 907 (October 15).
[2] *J. Amer. med. Ass.*, 1967, 199 : 390 (February 6).

268

THE MEDICAL JOURNAL OF AUSTRALIA   August 5, 1967

carrying an Rh-positive, ABO-compatible fœtus, and again, none of 31 previously protected mothers developed antibodies, whereas 11 of the 27 controls had antibodies and babies with Rh disease.

The results to date clearly show that the administration of "incomplete" anti-D antibody to mothers at risk effectively prevents their sensitization by Rh-positive fœtal cells. The exact mechanism by which the preformed antibody prevents the development of endogenous antibodies is not understood, but is presumably related to the very rapid disappearance of fœtal red cells from the maternal circulation which it produces. The prophylactic anti-D antibody must be administered to the mother within 72 hours of delivery to be effective, and a similar injection must be repeated after each subsequent delivery of an Rh-positive baby. Anti-D antibodies do not occur naturally and the first Rh-positive baby of an Rh-negative mother is therefore usually unaffected.

What are the sources of anti-D gamma globulin and how much is needed? The anti-D antibody is present in the circulation of Rh-negative mothers who have borne one or more Rh-affected children, and in the occasional Rh-negative person who has received Rh-positive blood. It has been estimated that to protect all the mothers at risk in Australia it will be necessary to provide some 20,000 protective doses of anti-D gamma globulin annually. Since the treatment is obviously effective, the number of sensitized mothers will decrease and so this source of the antibody will eventually disappear. In the meantime, such mothers are being asked to become voluntary blood donors to the Australian Red Cross Society so that their plasma may be fractionated and high-titre anti-D gamma globulin prepared at the Commonwealth Serum Laboratories in Melbourne. Small supplies of this material will shortly be made available for use in the most urgent cases.

The Australian Red Cross has set up a special subcommittee, comprising representatives of all interested bodies, to advise on ways in which the supply of anti-D plasma can be increased to meet all current and future demands. If this campaign proves successful, it is hoped that at an early date, sufficient supplies will be available to protect all Rh-negative mothers against sensitization by Rh-positive cells. When this stage is reached, Rh-hæmolytic disease will become a medical curiosity.

This Committee[3] met on May 17, 1967, in the Council Room, of the Australian Medical Association, and considered the medical, moral and legal implications of the use of anti-D gamma globulin in the prevention of Rh-hæmolytic disease. It was agreed that the following recommendations be forwarded to the National Executive of the Australian Red Cross Society.

General

1. That this form of medical treatment should be carried out in Australia.

2. That Phase 1 of any programme to produce an anti-D globulin here should be to utilize women volunteers with existing antibodies (i.e., those who have had Rh-affected babies).

Moral and Legal Considerations

3. The Committee regards hyperimmunization for this purpose as morally right, provided that the donor is made aware of all the implications and that ample and continuing provision is made for the donor's safety for the remainder of his life. (The need to explain the position individually and carefully to each potential donor is emphasized.)

4. (a) that the programme must be adequately covered legally.

(b) that the Red Cross should seek legal advice to see that the interests of the donor are covered and that if the Red Cross should become involved it is adequately covered so as to ensure that the donor will not suffer hardship.

These recommendations will be considered by the National Executive of the Australian Red Cross Society at its meeting in August, 1967.

The descriptive leaflet included as a loose supplement in this issue has been prepared by the National Red Cross Blood Transfusion Committee and is issued jointly by the Australian Red Cross Society and the Australian Medical Association.

---

[3] The members of the Committee were as follows: Dr. Edgar Thomson, Chairman; Dr. R. H. Macdonald (Australian Medical Association); Dr. B. Mathieson (Commonwealth Department of Health); Dr. S. E. L. Stening (Australian Pædiatric Association); Dr. Ella Macknight (Australian Council of the Royal College of Obstetricians and Gynæcologists); Dr. Peter Schiff (Commonwealth Serum Laboratories); Dr. Judith Hay and Dr. J. P. Morris (National Blood Transfusion Committee); Miss N. Minogue (Australian Red Cross Society); Dr. G. Archer (Director N.S.W. Blood Transfusion Service—observer).

THE MEDICAL JOURNAL OF AUSTRALIA

SATURDAY, MAY 17, 1969

PREVENTION OF Rh-HAEMOLYTIC DISEASE—1969

CONSIDERABLE advances have taken place in the prevention of Rh-hæmolytic disease since the subject was last reviewed in these columns.[1] Recent overseas reports[2-4] have confirmed the efficacy of this form of prophylactic therapy and relatively few failures have been noted.[3]

Because of considerable changes which have occurred in the procurement of anti-D plasma and in the supply of anti-Rh(D) gamma globulin since 1967, it is desirable to review the present position, particularly as far as Australia is concerned.

The mechanism of Rh(D)-sensitization is now well known. Fœtal cells from an Rh-positive baby may cross the placenta and enter the maternal circulation. Such an occurrence is referred to as a fœto-maternal hæmorrhage and most frequently takes place at or about the time of delivery; occasionally, however, it may precede the time of confinement by a considerable period. The Rh-positive cells are an antigenic stimulus to the mother's immune mechanism and as such may initiate the production of the mother's own (endogenous) anti-Rh(D) antibody. This iso-immune, incomplete antibody can subsequently cross the placenta in the reverse direction during a following Rh-positive pregnancy, damaging the fœtal erythropoietic system, which, in turn, leads to the development of hæmolytic disease of the newborn.

The initial experiments and trials designed to prevent Rh-hæmolytic disease were based on two observations. One, made by Levine in 1943[5] showed that Rh-sensitization of the mother was much less likely to occur if the fœtal cells were ABO-incompatible as well as Rh-incompatible. The second fact, which had been well-known to immunologists for many years, is that passively administered antibody will prevent primary immunization (or sensitization) of an experimental animal if it is administered together with or shortly after the antigen.

The interesting initial experiments which were carried out by Professor Clarke's group in Liverpool and by Freda, Gorman and Pollack in the United States, and the subsequent numerous clinical trials carried out in many centres, are too well known to be described here in detail. The reader is referred to previous reviews[1,6] for the historical summary. The results have been remarkable and have convincingly shown the efficacy of passive immunization with anti-D antibody in the prevention of

Rh-sensitization. Dr Schneider from Freiburg reviewed world-wide results available in September, 1968, and was able to show a protection rate of 93·2% in Rh-negative mothers who were tested for the development of Rh antibodies four to six months after the birth of an Rh-positive child. In other words, about 93 out of every 100 women who would have been sensitized before the availability of anti-D immunoglobulin can now be adequately protected against this eventuality. Furthermore, the protection rate after a second Rh-positive pregnancy can be maintained at approximately this level provided a further dose of anti-Rh(D) gamma globulin is again administered within 72 hours of delivery. This indicates that passive antibody is not merely masking the development of the mother's own endogenous antibody.

Why has the protection rate not been maintained at 100%, as it appeared to be in the early reports of clinical trials? The answer is not immediately obvious, and much effort is now being directed toward its elucidation. In the case of the multiparous mother, she may have been sensitized by a previous Rh-positive pregnancy even though no anti-D antibodies can be found by the most sensitive techniques presently in use. Presumably, either the antibodies are present in the maternal circulation at sub-threshold levels, or the immune mechanism has been "triggered" but will "fire" only after the stimulus of a further Rh-positive pregnancy. A different explanation is required for the occasional woman who becomes immunized during her first pregnancy, assuming, of course, that previous contact with the D antigen can be completely excluded. In these cases a large fœto-maternal hæmorrhage or a series of repeated small bleeds well before the onset of labour seems the most likely stimulus to primary immunization.

The programme to supply anti-Rh(D) gamma globulin for Australian requirements was initiated at a meeting held in May, 1967, between representatives of the Commonwealth Department of Health, the National Blood Transfusion Committee of the Australian Red Cross Society, the Commonwealth Serum Laboratories, the Australian Medical Association, the Australian Council of the Royal College of Obstetricians and Gynæcologists and the Australian Pædiatric Association. The meeting made certain recommendations to the National Executive of the Australian Red Cross Society, the most important being "that this form of medical treatment should be carried out in Australia". The National Executive accepted the challenge, and within three months (August, 1967) the first material for therapeutic use on an

[1] MED. J. AUST., 1967, 2: 261 (August 5).
[2] J. Amer. med. Ass., 1967, 199: 390 (February 6).
[3] Brit. med. J., 1967, 4: 7 (October 7).
[4] Lancet, 1968, 2: 1 (July 6).
[5] J. Hered., 1943, 34: 71.
[6] Scientific American, 1968, 219: 46 (November).

THE MEDICAL JOURNAL OF AUSTRALIA   MAY 17, 1969

Australia-wide basis was distributed to State blood banks from the Commonwealth Serum Laboratories. The National Blood Transfusion Committee was given the task of procuring adequate supplies of suitable plasma for the production of this new therapeutic agent.

Initially, supplies of plasma with suitable titres of incomplete anti-D antibody were available only from donors who had been previously sensitized by an Rh-positive pregnancy or as the result of transfusion of Rh-positive blood to an Rh-negative recipient. It soon became evident that these sources of supply would be insufficient if protection was to be given to all mothers at risk (presently estimated to require 25,000-30,000 doses per annum), and late in 1967 the Blood Transfusion Services commenced an immunization programme to augment existing supplies. Rh-negative volunteers (mostly males) are now immunized to the Rh(D) antigen by the injection of carefully screened Rh-positive cells, and when the incomplete anti-D titre reaches a suitable level in the serum of these individuals, blood donations are obtained and the plasma sent to C.S.L. for processing. Frequently, plasmapheresis is employed. This technique has the advantage that the red cells are returned to the donor. Thus, plasma may be obtained from the one donor at more frequent intervals whilst the number of immunized volunteers required for the programme is kept to a minimum.

Australia can be proud of the fact that it was one of the first countries to make anti-Rh(D) gamma globulin available on a national basis, free of charge, and that within the relatively short period of 20 months sufficient plasma supplies have been built up to enable all mothers at risk to receive this therapy. Initially, anti-Rh(D) gamma globulin was available only for Rh-negative primiparæ who gave birth to an Rh-positive, ABO-incompatible infant. Later it became possible to ease restrictions to include all Rh-negative mothers who had such babies. Since January of this year it has been possible to further relax the requirements which qualify a mother for this form of immunoprophylactic therapy. The following conditions now apply: (i) The mother shall be Rh negative. (ii) In the case of live births the baby shall be Rh positive. (iii) There shall be an absence of antibodies (D) detectable by an appropriately sensitive technique in a sample of maternal blood taken at the time of delivery or miscarriage. (iv) The material shall be made available to all Rh-negative women who abort or miscarry after eight weeks, unless it is known with certainty that the father is Rh negative also.

In all instances, the recipient must be shown to be free of anti-D antibodies by an appropriately sensitive technique (e.g. papain) as closely as possible to the time when the immunoglobulin injection is planned. There is no value in administering passive antibody once Rh(D) endogenous antibody formation has commenced. Although passive antibody can reduce the level of the primary or secondary response in the experimental animal, the doses required are relatively enormous, and its practical value in the human has yet to be established.

Although the mechanism whereby anti-D immunoglobulin prevents sensitization has not yet been fully elucidated, the efficacy of this form of preventive medicine has been clearly established. The therapy is virtually without risk, and the potential benefits both to the individual mother and to the community are enormous. Every medical practitioner should be thoroughly familiar with this form of therapy and the indications for it; it is his duty to ensure that every mother at risk receives adequate protection. Further details are readily available from the quoted literature, from the National Blood Transfusion Committee of the Australian Red Cross Society and from Directors of the Blood Transfusion Services, who are also responsible for the issue of anti-Rh(D) gamma globulin on request from practitioners or hospitals.

Paper 43

43. Pollack, W., Ascari, W. Q., Kochesky, R. J., O'Connor, R. R., Ho, T. Y. and Tripodi, D. (1971). Studies on Rh prophylaxis; 1. Relationship between doses of anti-Rh and size of antigenic stimulus. *Transfusion, 11,* 333-9.

Commentary

It will be clear from a quick scan of this paper that its primary object is to establish (in Rh-negative male volunteers) the maximum amount of Rh-incompatible blood which can be 'neutralised' by the standard USA dose of anti-D (267 μg)—and the short answer is about 35 ml of blood (13.4 ml of packed red cells) (see Table 2). Furthermore, the overall findings are that, in immunologically susceptible people, the bigger the dose of red cells the more likely is immunisation to occur. Nevertheless, as might be expected, some antibody preparations are more efficient than others, and this can be tested by measuring the concentration, equilibrium constant and index of heterogeneity, terms which are explained in Paper 37. Another way by which potency could be assessed would be to find the volume of Rh-positive cells which can be "neutralised" by 1 ml of the preparation being investigated, but as this would have to be done in volunteers it would take a very long time. Therefore it seems preferable, using 'case law', to find out which equilibrium constants and heterogeneity indices are most effective in protection.

There are other important points in this paper. The data show that even when 100 ml of blood (37·5 ml of packed red cells) are given, only 65% of the controls become immunised, even after challenge with 0·2 ml of blood from the original donor. This supports the view that a considerable proportion of the population are 'non-responders'. Pollack *et al.* however, make the point that it cannot be inferred from their findings that such people are genetically incapable of being immunised. (It seems to us that the best way to test this genetic hypothesis would be by family studies, looking at the immunisation rates in suitable Rh-negative sisters of propositi who were 'responders' and 'non-responders' respectively).

Another point concerns the immunisation rate in the Rh-negative volunteers after the breakdown in protection begins (i.e. after 35 ml of blood). The authors feel that if passively administered antibody acted merely to reduce the concentration of antigen reaching immunocompetent cells, the slopes of the lines in Figures 2 and 3 ought to be the same. In fact, the immunisation rate in the treated never gets anywhere near the 65% in the controls, and this may be because the antibody acts on some target organ (e.g. the macrophage) to interfere with processing. Perhaps it is that even though the antigen sites are very incompletely coated (when large volumes of blood are involved) yet there is enough blocking of the sites to render the processing by macrophages less efficient than normal.

Note: In the paper the term 'asymptotic' is frequently used. Definition: An asymptote is 'a line which approaches nearer and nearer to a given curve but does not meet it within a finite distance'.

From W. Pollack et al. (1972). Transfusion, 11, 333-9. Copyright (1972), by kind permission of the authors and J. B. Lippincott, Co

Studies on Rh Prophylaxis

1. Relationship between Doses of Anti-Rh and Size of Antigenic Stimulus

W. POLLACK, W. Q. ASCARI, R. J. KOCHESKY, R. R. O'CONNOR, T. Y. HO, AND D. TRIPODI

From the Divisions of Diagnostics and Immunology, Ortho Research Foundation, Raritan, New Jersey

One hundred and seventy-eight (178) Rh-negative volunteers, distributed into a treated and control series of six groups each, were studied to establish: (i) approximately 70 per cent of Rh-negative individuals are susceptible to being immunized by a single injection of Rh-positive blood; (ii) that, for immunologically susceptible individuals, the frequency of immunization increases with the volume of Rh-positive erythrocytes administered; and (iii) that a possible relationship exists between potency of Rh immune globulin and effectivity. This relationship can be used to calculate an effective dose of Rh immune globulin in the treatment of large feto-maternal hemorrhages or accidental tranfusions of Rh-positive blood to Rh-negative women.

THE USE of passively administered antibody to prevent primary immune induction has gained wide acceptance for the prophylaxis of Rh immunization. Nevertheless, there still remain several unanswered questions, not the least of which is the dose of antibody to give for a known volume of circulating Rh-positive red blood cells. This question arises most commonly when it becomes apparent that a large feto–maternal hemorrhage has occurred or when Rh-positive blood is administered inadvertently to young Rh-negative women and it is suspected that a single dose of about 300 μg of anti-Rh immune globulin will not prevent immunization.

There is today an increasing tendency to use "rules of thumb" in estimating the appropriate dose of antibody to give in such cases. One rule that appears to be gaining acceptance is the ratio of the amount of antibody in μg to the volume of red blood cells or whole blood in ml. However, these estimates appear to range from 5 μg/ml to 30 μg/ml, depending on the particular male volunteer study used to establish the ratio. Such a rule is based on several implied assumptions some of which are (i) that antibody binds to the red blood cells *in vivo* to bring about its immunosuppressive effect; (ii) that the variation in the Rh antigen content from different individuals is unimportant; and (iii) that all antibody preparations are equally effective providing the same number of micrograms of antibody are given to the patient.

The correctness of these assumptions have yet to be demonstrated. Nevertheless, previous data[2, 4, 5, 7, 8] can be used to argue that a relationship does exist between the dose of antibody and suppression and, therefore, that antibody must first combine with the foreign red blood cells *in vivo* before exerting its immunosuppressive (or augmentation) effects. Further, if antibody binds to the red blood cells, it presumably binds to the Rh antigen, inasmuch as immunosuppression is highly specific for the Rh factor. Thus, the concentration of Rh antigen *in vivo* might be a more critical factor than the volume of red blood cells, since the amount of antibody bound must comply with the law of mass action.

Compliance with the mass law means that the binding of antibody to antigen must conform to some physical adsorption isotherm equation. Both Hughes-Jones[3] and Pollack and Kochesky[9] have described assays of anti-Rh preparations in which the binding data can be interpreted as fitting a modification of the Freundlich adsorption isotherm described by Sips[10] over relatively narrow ranges of reactant concentrations.

Received for publication March 29, 1971; accepted July 28, 1971.

TABLE 1. *Donors Used to Provide Blood for Volunteer Study (1969–1970)*
(Total No. of Donors: 30)

No.	Genotype	Mean Rh_o (D) Antigen Concentration of Erythrocytes (Picomoles/ml)	Rh Antigen Range
6	$R_o r$	259	179–312
3	$R_1 r$	204	154–251
3	$R_2 r$	360	265–453
10	$R_1 R_1$	286	137–456
4	$R_1 R_2$	337	313–368
2	$R_2 R_2$	473	460–487

NOTE: Assays were not conducted on two $R_1 R_1$ donors. Average antigen content used for all volunteers = 300 p-moles/ml. 95 per cent confidence interval = 183–417 p-moles/ml.

This equation takes the form:

$$\frac{[Ag\,Ab]}{[Ab]\,[ag]^a} = K_o^a$$

where [Ag Ab] is the equilibrium concentration of bound antigen (or antibody); [Ab] and [Ag] are the equilibrium free concentration of antibody and antigen, respectively; K_o is the average equilibrium association constant, and α is the index of heterogeneity of antibody.

Other adsorption equations may also be used and may better fit the data. Nevertheless, the use of the Sips equation to define an antibody preparation in terms of concentration, average equilibrium constant, and index of heterogeneity, while intellectually satisfying, does not simplify the problem of selecting an appropriate dose of antibody to treat a large feto–maternal hemorrhage. Because of this, Pollack and Kochesky[9] suggested that potency be expressed as the average circulating Rh-positive red blood cell volume that can be "neutralized" by one ml of the preparation; the volume is computed from the appropriate adsorption equation *in vitro* and is based on an appropriate male volunteer study.

The original aim of this study was to attempt to provide a definite answer to the question of the appropriate dose to give for a large circulating Rh-positive red blood cell volume as well as to explore the possibility of expressing potency in terms of red blood cell volumes based on the Sips equation. However, to do this, it is necessary to determine the assay equilibrium

ratio of bound to free antigen that results in complete suppression. In this calculation, the volume element in which the antigen–antibody reaction takes place must be known, since the influence of the equilibrium association (binding) constant is greater for larger volumes than for smaller. This volume element is not known; it could correspond to the intra-and extravascular space (about six liters) or it may be much smaller (*e.g.* the total volume of the intracellular space where the erythrocytes are finally sequestered). Further, it is unlikely that equilibrium is ever achieved *in vivo* nor can it be assumed that the equilibrium constant obtained for an assay milieu *in vitro* will be identical to that *in vivo*.

Because of these considerations the data obtained from the present volunteer study has been used only to determine the most appropriate dose in terms of μg.

Methods and Materials
Volunteers

Volunteer candidates were recruited from three prisons as well as from normal life. Two hundred men and two post-menopausal women were selected who were in normal health, Rho(D)- and Du-negative, and with no detectable atypical antibodies in their sera. The mean age of the volunteers was 37 years; the range was 20 to 65 years.

The volunteers were distributed into six groups according to the volume of packed Rh-positive red blood cells they received. Each group consisted of a control and a treated series. The volunteers in each group received a single intravenous injection of blood equivalent to a starting volume of 11.6 ml. Later injections were increased to 37.5 ml of packed erythrocytes.

Donor Blood

Blood for stimulation was obtained from 30 group O, Rho (D)-positive donors who fulfilled the criteria for whole blood donation as recommended by the AABB. In addition, each donor was required to have donated blood at least twice during the previous six months with no evidence of hepatitis in the recipients. Using conventional methods, blood was drawn from the donors into plastic bags containing 67.5 ml of ACD solution (NIH Formula A). The donor cells were typed, and prior to use the hematocrit was corrected for trapped plasma and red blood cell swelling by multiplying the observed packed cell volume by 0.91. Triplicate antigen analyses were performed on 28 of the 30 blood donors by the method described previously.[9]

Stimulation and Follow-Up

Compatibility testing of sera from volunteers was performed on the blood to be injected to insure maximum safety and to prevent the inclusion of a previously immunized volunteer. All volunteer sera were found to be compatible by saline, albumin and antiglobulin technics.

After adequate mixing of the donor packs, blood was withdrawn by syringe for hematocrit and for injection into the volunteers in the prescribed volumes. On the same day, the volunteers were also injected intramuscularly with the contents (approximately one ml) of the coded vial of immune globulin.

The volunteers were carefully followed serologically at monthly intervals. At the end of six months, those volunteers whose sera showed no detectable antibody were then challenged with 0.2 ml of whole blood from the same donor. One week later a serum sample was obtained from all volunteers and serologic analysis was used to determine the outcome of the whole experiment.

Immune Globulin

The immune globulin preparations used in this study were prepared by the same modification of the Cohn alcohol procedure used for the production of RhoGAM*, Rho (D) Immune Globulin (Human). The control γ globulin solution was prepared from the plasma of Rh-positive blood donors, while the anti-Rh γ globulin was prepared from recently immunized Rh-negative volunteers and contained anti-Rho (D) as the only blood group antibody. Both preparations were otherwise identical with respect to total protein content (150 mg ± 15 mg/ml) and volume in the vial (1.1 ml). In all other respects, the immune globulin preparations complied with the minimum standards of the Division of Biologics Standards, N.I.H. The vials

* Trademark of Ortho Diagnostics, Raritan, New Jersey 08869.

TABLE 2. *Incidence of Immunization in Groups of Volunteers Given Varying Volumes of Rh-positive Blood Showing 95 Per Cent Confidence Ranges of Fraction Immunized* (1969-1970 Study)

	Mean Volume of Packed Erythrocytes Given (ml)					
	11.6 (range 10.9-12.4)	13.4 (range 12.6-14.6)	18.1 (range 16.6-19.6)	21.2 (range 20.8-21.3)	30.1 (range 28.4-32.3)	37.5 (range 35.9-41.7)
Untreated group Amount immunized						
Fraction	7/16	6/12	11/19	5/8	7/11	13/20
Per cent	(43.8%)	(50.0%)	(57.9%)	(62.5%)	(63.6%)	(65.0%)
95 per cent confidence range	0.190-0.702	0.211-0.789	0.335-0.798	0.215-0.915	0.308-0.891	0.107-0.816
Treated group Amount immunized						
Fraction	0/19	0/18	3/18	2/8	4/12	6/17
Per cent	(0%)	(0%)	(16.7%)	(25.0%)	(33.3%)	(35.3%)
95 per cent confidence range	0-0.177	0-0.186	0.034-0.414	0.082-0.651	0.099-0.651	0.142-0.614

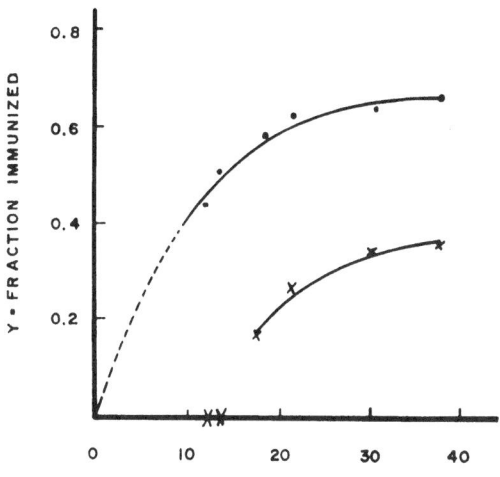

FIG. 1. Fraction of male volunteers immunized (Y) for various volumes of packed Rh + red blood cells (V). • = control groups. $Y_1 = 0.679$ $(1 - e^{0.094V})$. X = treated groups. $Y_2 = 0.357 - 6.61e^{0.193V}$.

of both control and anti-Rh-containing preparations were coded according to a random number sequence so that the total study could be completed under a "double blind" format.

The anti-Rh preparation was assayed several times, both before and at the completion of the experiment as previously described,[9] and was found to contain a total anti-D content of 267 ± 3 μg/ml. During the course of the study, neither preparation showed any evidence of physicochemical deterioration and both preparations contained less than one per cent aggregates as judged by analytic ultracentrifugation methods.

Serologic Methods

Serologic analyses of the volunteers' sera were carried out in two laboratories. The tests at the Ortho Research Foundation included trypsinized screening and panel cells as well as untrypsinized cells. All analyses were otherwise conventional and in accordance with recommendations of the AABB technical procedures manual. There were no sera that showed discrepancies between the two participating laboratories, nor were there differences in results between the various serological methods used.

Results

Analysis of Donor Blood Used for Stimulation

Of the 30 blood donors used in this study, only 28 were analyzed for antigen content by radioimmune assay. The probable Rh genotype and ranges of antigen concentration/ml of red blood cells is shown in Table 1. The average antigen content for the 28 donors was found to be 300 picomoles/ml with a 95 per cent confidence interval of 183–417 picomoles/ml. While

there is some overlap in antigen concentrations, in general, R_2 cells tend to have a higher antigen content than R_1 cells and R_0 cells show a slightly higher antigen content than R_1 cells.

Results of Male Volunteer Study

Of the 202 volunteers who entered the study, 178 (176 males and two postmenopausal females) remained until the experiment was completed. No adverse reactions were experienced by any of the volunteers in either the control or treated series.

Results of serologic analysis for both the treated and control series are shown in Table 2. Frequency of Rh immunization in the treated series of groups is consistently lower than for the corresponding groups in the control series. However, the differences are statistically significant at or greater than the 95 per cent confidence level only for the groups given 11.6 ml through 18.1 ml. In the treated volunteers given 11.6 ml and 13.4 ml of packed erythrocytes, the observed frequency of immunization was zero, although the total number of volunteers in each group was relatively small. If passive immunization acts by reducing the actual dose of antigen, the probability of immunization would decrease in volunteers given Rh immune globulin, but not necessarily to a zero frequency at the 11.6 and 13.4 ml level. In other words, the frequency of immunization might be too low to expect to observe any immunized subjects among the total number in these two experimental groups.

To determine the maximum quantity of Rh-positive red blood cells that could be rendered nonimmunogenic by the single dose of anti-Rh immune globulin used in this study, the data was examined to see whether it conformed to a mathematical model that seemed applicable to immunization by this antigen. The data was therefore resolved into the graph shown in Figure 1. In this graph the abscissa (v) is the volume of packed erythrocytes administered, and the ordinate (y) is the fraction of volunteers immunized. The dose–response relationship is obvious for both the control and treated series: as the volume of red blood cells given increases, the fraction of the total number of subjects immunized also increases.

In determining the correct regression equations for these two sets of data it is apparent that for the control series, as v (the volume of cells) becomes infinitely small, y (the fraction of men immunized) must tend to zero. However, for the treated series we expect y to reach zero as the volume of cells reaches a limiting low value where the dose of antibody provides absolute immune suppression. At the other extreme, as the volume of red blood cells becomes infinitely large we should expect both curves to plateau at a value of y at or less than unity.

One regression equation that satisfactorily

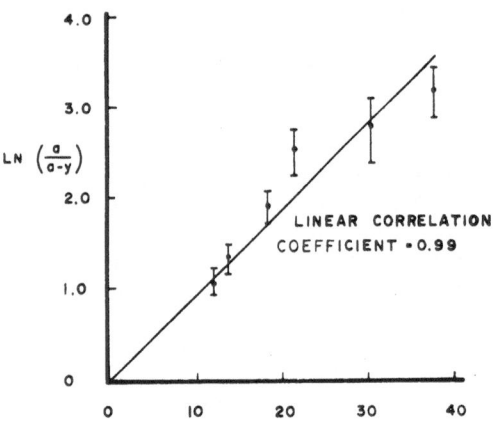

FIG. 2. Control series. Linear transformation of Y_1 in which $\mathrm{LN}\left(\frac{a}{a-y}\right) = bV$ where $a = 0.679$ and $b = 0.094$. Graph shows 95 per cent confidence intervals.

describes these boundary conditions takes the form:

$$y(v) = A - Be^{-cv}$$

where A is the asymptotic value and B and c are constants. For the control series, $B = A$ since the regression line must pass through the origin. The values for these constants are shown in Figure 1 for both sets of data. Since there is no algebraic solution for this equation, an iterative procedure based on Taylor's theorem was used and the results were obtained by computer.

The asymptotic value for the control series was found to be 0.679. This implies that no more than 68 per cent of volunteers can be immunized by a single injection of Rh-positive blood regardless of how large a volume is given. The asymptotic value for the treated series was found to be 0.357, a value that is significantly different from the control value of 0.679. It would be tempting to speculate on the immunologic significance of the difference between the asymptotic values for the control and treated series were it not for the fact that the iterative procedure used to obtain these values is very sensitive to small changes in the fraction of the men immunized by the larger volumes of blood. Therefore, it is wiser to leave such speculation until data are obtained on a larger group of volunteers injected with volumes of blood in excess of those used in this study.

Nevertheless, from any set of data, when the asymptotic values are known and if the equation chosen is the true one, it should be possible to linearize the exponential equation by logarithmic transformation. The data for the control series are shown in Figure 2 along with the confidence limits. As expected, extrapolation passes through the origin and the data are

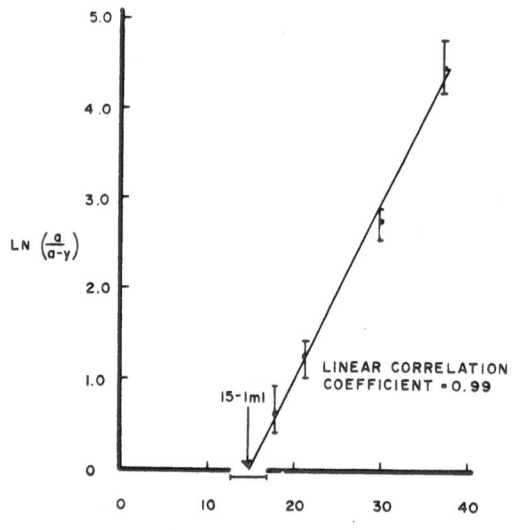

FIG. 3. Treated series. Linear transformation of Y_2 in which $\mathrm{LN}\left(\frac{a}{a-y}\right) = \mathrm{LN}\left(\frac{a}{b}\right) + CV$ where $a = 0.357$, $b = 6.610$ and $c = 0.193$. Graph shows 95 per cent confidence intervals.

shown to be approximated very closely by the linear regression line, as shown by the linear correlation coefficient.

Figure 3 shows the logarithmic transformation of the data from the treated series. The extrapolated intercept to the abscissa is shown to be 15.1 ml, with confidence limits from 13 to 17 ml. This mean value of 15.1 ml represents the maximum volume of Rh-positive red blood cells that could be "neutralized" in vivo by one vial of this experimental lot of anti-Rh immune globulin.

Conclusions

Two conclusions may be drawn from these data. The first is that not all Rh-negative individuals are susceptible to being immunized by a single injection of Rh-positive red blood cells, no matter how large. These observations are in substantial agreement with the data of Archer et al.[1] and Mollison et al.[6] However the data presented here differ in one important respect by establishing that the probability of a susceptible Rh-negative individual forming detectable antibody rises with the dose of Rh antigen given. However, it is impossible to conclude from these data that 20 to 30 per cent of all Rh-negative individuals are genetically incapable of being immunized. The asymptotic value of 68 per cent for the control series may have resulted from the limit of two exponential equations, one representing immunization and the other, tolerogenic doses of red blood cells.

The second conclusion stems from the linearity of the transformed data and the difference between the slopes of the transformed control and treated series. One would have expected that if passively administered antibody acted merely to reduce the concentration of antigen reaching immunocompetent cells, the slopes ought to have been the same. That is, the graph of Figure 3 for the treated series would have been identical to the graph of Figure 2 for the control series, except that the point of origin in the former would be at 15.1 ml red blood cells. One possible explanation is that antibody acts on some target organ (*e.g.*, the macrophage) to interfere with processing, for the significance of change in slope is that the immunogenicity of the red blood cells has been reduced. Such a mechanism will also explain the differences between the asymptotic values for the control and treated series, if this is confirmed by a larger study.

The extrapolation value of 15.1 ml of erythrocytes shown in Figure 3 is the maximum average volume that could be rendered nonimmunogenic by one ml of the anti-Rh preparation used. If the assumption is valid that the effectiveness of a preparation can be related to the potency by the use of the "rule of thumb" ratio of μg of antibody to volume of red blood cells, then the lower value of the 95 per cent confidence interval should be used, *i.e.*, 13 ml. Thus, the ratio we were seeking is 267/13 or 20 μg/ml of red blood cells.

Employment of this constant for any IgG anti-Rh preparation that has been assayed according to the methods previously described leads to a simple method of reporting potency of anti-Rh preparations in terms of the number of ml of Rh-positive red blood cells that can be effectively neutralized by one vial of the preparation. It still remains to be demonstrated that

this ratio will hold true for other anti-Rh preparations and larger volumes of erythrocytes. Nevertheless, there is some comfort in the knowledge that most commercial preparations of anti-Rh globulins are manufactured from much larger pools of plasma obtained from hyperimmunized donors than was used for the preparation in this study.

By choosing this value instead of the mean, we are safe in using the average value for the antigen content for all the red blood cell donors used in this study.

If this suggested method of reporting potency is used, it will allow physicians to prescribe the correct dose of antibody to give for excessively large feto–maternal hemorrhages. It is not suggested that it be used to reduce the amount of immune globulin for microhemorrhages, since such small volumes for circulating fetal blood cannot be quantitated with the same precision as the larger volumes.

References

1. Archer, G. T., B. R. Cooke, K. Mitchel, and P. Parry: Hyperimmunisation des donneurs de sang pour la production des gamma-globulines anti Rh (D). Rev. Franc. Transfusion 12: 341, 1969.

2. Dudok de Wit, C., and E. Borst-Eilers: Failure of anti-D immunoglobulin injection to protect against rhesus immunization after massive foetal maternal haemorrhage. Report of four cases. Brit. Med. J. 1: 152, 1968.

3. Hughes-Jones, N. C.: The estimation of the concentration and equilibrium constant of anti-D. Immunology 12: 567, 1967.

4. ———, and P. L. Mollison: Failure of a relatively small dose of passively administered anti-Rh to suppress primary immunization by a relatively large dose of Rh-positive red cells. Brit. Med. J. 1: 150, 1968.

5. Mollison, P. L., and Hughes-Jones, N. C.: Clearance of Rh-positive red cells by low concentrations of Rh antibody. Immunology 12: 63, 1967.

6. ———, M. Frame, and M. E. Ross: Differences between Rh (D) negative subjects in response to Rh (D) antigen. Brit. J. Haemat. 19: 257, 1970.

7. Pollack, W., J. G. Gorman, H. J. Hager, V. J. Freda, and D. Tripodi: Antibody-mediated immune suppression to the Rh factor: Animal models suggesting mechanism of action. Transfusion 8: 134, 1968.

8. ———, J. G. Gorman, and V. J. Freda: Preven-

tion of Rh hemolytic disease. E. B. Brown and C. V. Moore, Eds., Progr. Hemat. 6: 121, 1969.

9. ———, and R. J. Kochesky: The importance of antibody concentration, binding constant, and heterogeneity in the suppression of immunity to the Rh factor. Int. Arch. Allerg. 38: 320, 1970.

10. Sips, R.: On the structure of a catalyst surface. J. Chem. Physics 16: 490, 1949.

11. Unpublished observations from this laboratory.

W. Pollack, Ph.D., Director of Research, Diagnostics, Ortho Research Foundation, Raritan, New Jersey 08869. (Correspondence)

W. Q. Ascari, M.D., Division of Diagnostics, Ortho Research Foundation. Present address: Associate Pathologist, Department of Pathology, Somerset Hospital, Somerville, New Jersey 08876.

R. J. Kochesky, B.S., Assistant Scientist, Division of Immunology, Diagnostics, Ortho Research Foundation.

R. R. O'Connor, B.S., Assistant Manager of Field Studies, Research Services, Diagnostics, Ortho Research Foundation.

T. Y. Ho, M.S., Associate Mathematician, Research Services, Diagnostics, Ortho Research Foundation.

D. Tripodi, Ph.D., Director, Division of Immunology, Diagnostics, Ortho Research Foundation.

Paper 44

44.   Prevention of Rh-haemolytic disease: final results of the "high-risk" clinical trial. A combined study from centres in England and Baltimore. (1971). *Brit. Med. J.*, *ii*, 607-609.

Commentary

This paper is a follow-up of the Rh-negative primiparae who had been treated by 1,000 µg of anti-D shortly after the delivery of their first baby (Paper 34). As already stated, it was very important to follow these women through their next Rh-positive pregnancy, since it was possible that this second baby might make the antibodies overt and this would mean that immunisation had only been temporarily suppressed after the first pregnancy. It will be seen from this paper that the fear was unfounded, antibodies rarely appearing in the next Rh-positive pregnancy, and in general treated Rh-negative mothers started their second pregnancy 'immunologically virgin'. The failure rate in the treated was only 2·3%, whereas 30·7% of the controls were immunised after the second Rh-positive baby. The reason for the high immunisation rate in both classes was because these women were a high risk group, as judged by the number of fetal cells found in the mother's circulation after delivery of the first baby.

With regard to the last paragraph of the paper (the question of dosage) other papers (Papers 43 and 46), amply confirm the view that 1,000 µg is an unnecessarily high dose for the majority of mothers.

From C. A. Clarke et al. (1971), Brit. Med. J. ii, 607-9. Copyright (1971), by kind permission of the authors and the British Medical Association

Prevention of Rh-Haemolytic Disease: Final Results of the "High-Risk" Clinical Trial

A Combined Study from Centres in England and Baltimore*

Summary

The final results are reported of a trial of about 1,000 μg of anti-D gammaglobulin given intramuscularly to a selected high-risk group of Rh-negative primiparae just delivered of an ABO-compatible Rh-positive baby, the aim being to prevent them becoming immunized to Rh. Six months after delivery only 1 out of 173 treated mothers had been immunized as against 38 out of 176 controls. The crucial test of the prophylactic therapy depends on the presence or otherwise of anti-D at the end of a second Rh-positive pregnancy. Of 86 treated mothers two had antibodies at this time compared with 20 out of 65 controls.

The results show a high degree of protection in this group of mothers.

Introduction

In a previous report on the prevention of Rh immunization (Combined Study, 1966) we described the results of a clinical trial from four different centres aimed at testing the effectiveness of administering 5 ml of anti-D gammaglobulin to selected Rh-negative women immediately after the delivery of their first Rh-positive ABO-compatible child. The results, and the conclusions derived from them, were largely based on a test for Rh antibodies carried out on the mothers six months or later after delivery. Only a few of the mothers had at that time had second pregnancies and we noted that definite proof that Rh immunization can be prevented by this method must rest on the immunological state of the treated mothers at the delivery of a subsequent Rh-positive baby.

Since the earlier report the study has been continued and a considerable number of mothers included in the trial have been followed through second pregnancies. The results of this enlarged trial are presented here.

Selection of Patients and Methods

The relevant details were given in the earlier paper. In summary, the mothers were all Rh-negative (rr) primiparae, free of antibodies, who had just been delivered of ABO-compatible Rh-positive babies, and in each case a sample of maternal blood had shown the presence of 0·2 ml or more of circulating fetal blood as judged by the acid-elution test of Kleihauer et al. (1957). Mothers with this degree of feto-maternal haemorrhage had been shown to have, in the absence of any treatment, about a 20% risk of developing immune anti-D within six months (Woodrow et al., 1965).

The following took part in the study:
Liverpool Group: C. A. Clarke, M.D., F.R.C.P., F.R.S.; W. T. A. Donohoe, A.I.M.L.T.; R. Finn, M.D., M.R.C.P.; D. Lehane, M.B., F.R.C.PATH.; R. B. McConnell, M.D., F.R.C.P.; P. M. Sheppard, D.PHIL., F.R.S.; Shona H. Towers, M.D., M.R.C.O.G.; J. C. Woodrow, M.D., F.R.C.P.
Sheffield Group: C. C. Bowley, F.R.C.O.G., F.R.C.PATH.
Leeds and Bradford Group: L. A. D. Tovey, M.D.
Baltimore Group: Wilma B. Bias, PH.D.; J. R. Krevans, M.D.

*From the Nuffield Unit of Medical Genetics, Department of Medicine, University of Liverpool; the Sheffield Regional Blood Transfusion Service; the Leeds Regional Transfusion Laboratory; the Baltimore City Hospitals.

In the treated group the mothers were given, as a rule within 36 hours of delivery, 5 ml of anti-D gammaglobulin containing, in the British centres, about 1,000 μg of IgG anti-D. (In Baltimore the dose was higher and possibly as high as 5,000 μg.) Control mothers were not treated and so far as possible treated and control mothers were alternated.

The Kleihauer-Betke technique as applied in this trial and the methods for testing for antibodies were described in the previous report. Samples of serum were obtained from treated and control mothers six months after delivery and sometimes at later dates as well. The details of the methods used in Liverpool for ascertaining second pregnancies have been described (Woodrow and Donohoe, 1968). Follow-up in the other centres has varied from this in detail, but in each case the aim was to ascertain as many second pregnancies as possible, while giving each pregnancy, whether treated or control, an equal chance of coming to notice. Maternal blood samples were obtained for antibody testing both during the second pregnancy and at delivery. Cord blood samples were tested for ABO and Rh blood groups and by Coombs tests in the hospital clinical laboratories.

Problem of Passive Versus Active Immunity

The length of time for which anti-D can be detected in maternal serum after administration of gammaglobulin showed pronounced differences, due partly to inherent variability between recipient mothers and partly because methods of testing for antibodies varied in sensitivity. Thus at the time of the previous report (Combined Study, 1966) two of the mothers treated in Sheffield still showed positive reactions when their sera were tested by a very sensitive papain technique eight months after delivery, but subsequent tests were negative. We now consider that these mothers were not actively immunized. When such a sequence of events was observed the mothers are categorized as "not immunized" at six months after delivery.

Results

TEST FOR ANTIBODY AT SIX MONTHS

A total of 349 mothers (176 controls and 173 treated) were tested six months after delivery. The results of tests for Rh antibodies at this time are given in Table I. There is no evidence of heterogeneity between the different centres. The results confirm the marked protective effect of 1,000 μg of anti-D in this group of mothers.

TABLE I—*Results of Testing for Rh Antibodies Six Months after Delivery*

Centre	No.	Not Immunized	Immunized
	Controls		
Liverpool	92	72	20
Baltimore	31	23	8
Sheffield	41	31	10
Leeds and Bradford ..	12	12	0
Total ..	176	138	38 (21·6%)
	Treated		
Liverpool	94	93	1
Baltimore	26	26	0
Sheffield	39	39	0
Leeds and Bradford ..	14	14	0
Total ..	173	172	1 (0·6%)

There was one failure of prophylaxis. The patient had had, so far as could be ascertained, neither previous pregnancies nor blood transfusion. She was blood group O and was delivered of a group O Rh-positive infant. There was evidence of about 1·2 ml of circulating fetal blood after delivery, and within 24 hours of the delivery she received 1,000 µg of anti-D. This produced quite a severe local reaction at the site of injection (none is usually observed), and a tender swelling with erythema persisted for three days. Six months later her serum showed anti-D by saline, albumin, and indirect Coombs techniques. She subsequently delivered a severely affected infant which died.

The pretreatment delivery serum was carefully checked for antibodies and none were found. On reviewing the history it was discovered that when two months pregnant she had been given a prophylactic dose of gammaglobulin against rubella and we thought she might have made antibodies to this which would perhaps have inactivated the anti-D given later. This view was reinforced when we heard of the failure in a treated multipara in an Irish trial using Ortho-gammaglobulin. This patient had received an antirubella injection at the 11th week of her second pregnancy and made anti-D at the end of her third pregnancy (Walsh et al., 1968). However, in our patient no anti-Gm antibodies were detected (Sylvia D. Lawler, personal communication, 1967) and skin tests to gammaglobulin were negative.

We did in fact carry out in Liverpool a wider investigation of the incidence of anti-Gm antibodies. We found that 1 out of 75 controls had developed a new anti-Gm antibody six months after delivery. This finding compares with four instances of anti-Gm antibodies in 62 treated cases, the difference not being significant ($\chi_1^2 = 2·33$; $P > 0·10$).

The largest volumes of transplacental haemorrhage encountered in the group treated with 1,000 µg were estimated to be 170, 46, and 31 ml respectively. The first case has been reported in detail (Woodrow et al., 1968), and it is of interest that this patient had delivered a second Rh-positive baby and that a sample of blood taken after this delivery was free of antibodies.

SECOND PREGNANCY TESTS

The results of antibody tests carried out after the second Rh-positive pregnancies (both ABO compatible and incompatible) are given in Table II; 20 out of 65 control mothers (30·7%) had anti-D by this time. Of these, 12 had developed antibodies within six months after the first pregnancy and the remaining eight did so during their second pregnancy.

TABLE II—Results of Testing for Rh Antibodies at the end of the Second Rh-Positive Pregnancies

Centre	No.	Not Immunized	Immunized
	Controls		
Liverpool	38	30	8 (7)
Baltimore	4	3	1
Sheffield	19	10	9 (5)
Leeds and Bradford	4	2	2
Total	65	45	20 (12) (30·7%)
	Treated		
Liverpool	59	57	2 (1)
Baltimore	12	12	0
Sheffield	10	10	0
Leeds and Bradford	7	7	0
Total	88	86	2 (1) (2·3%)

The number of mothers who had developed antibodies after the first pregnancy are given in parentheses. They are *included* in the larger number.

Of the 88 treated mothers two had antibody, one being the failure described above. The other patient was recorded as showing a fetal cell score of 6, implying about 0·2 ml of circulating fetal blood, but intermediate cells were present and accurate counting was impossible. She was free of antibodies six months after delivery and at the beginning of the second pregnancy but developed anti-D during the last few weeks of this pregnancy, the baby being only mildly affected.

Discussion

The most important conclusion to be drawn from this trial is that the protection against Rh immunization provided by the anti-D gammaglobulin is evident not only at the period after the first pregnancy but also during the crucial subsequent Rh-positive pregnancy. This rules out any idea that antibody production in the period after the first delivery has merely been temporarily suppressed, because if this had been so one would have expected a considerable number of the treated mothers to have developed antibodies in the second pregnancy. Complete protection by the administered anti-D will have been obtained if, indeed, the treated mothers showing no antibodies at the end of the second Rh-positive pregnancy are virtually in the same state as that obtaining at the end of the first pregnancy. If further protection is required a second dose of anti-D must now be given.

It will be recalled that the original aim of this trial was to see whether Rh immunization by pregnancy can be prevented to an appreciable degree by giving anti-D gammaglobulin after delivery, in the same way that experimental immunization had been prevented (Clarke et al., 1963). This has been unequivocally shown to be true.

Degree of Protection.—The failure rate of this prophylactic therapy can be expressed as the incidence of antibodies in treated mothers as a percentage of that in controls. Tests at the end of the second pregnancy show a failure rate of about 7%, though, because of the low incidence of failure, the confidence limits for this value must be wide. There was thus obtained in this group of mothers a 93% suppression of immunization.

Two Failures.—The reason for the two instances of failure is not apparent. Mention has already been made of antigammaglobulin antibodies, and Ascari et al. (1969), thinking along different lines, speculated that gammaglobulin used for rubella prophylaxis might contain a small amount of IgG anti-D, and that this might have an enhancing effect in the sense, presumably, that any Rh-positive fetal cells entering the maternal circulation at the time of the injection might be more likely to immunize the mother. However, various batches of pooled gammaglobulin used for general prophylactic purposes have since been examined (K. L. G. Goldsmith, personal communication, 1970) and no definite evidence of anti-D has been found in any of them. Moreover, a general inquiry into the administration of previous gammaglobulin to the treated mothers in Liverpool does not lend any support to the idea.

It is of some importance to note that the selection for this trial of mothers with 0·2 ml or more of circulating fetal blood probably implies that the mothers had most likely had a very recent transplacental haemorrhage and had not been primed at the time anti-D was given (otherwise the fetal cells would have been cleared), and this is ideal for complete protection. Where no or very few fetal cells are present at delivery the situation is different and a trial of preventive treatment in these mothers has been carried out in Liverpool and is reported separately (Woodrow et al., 1971).

Other Clinical Trials.—The results of clinical trials have been reported from Australia, Canada, Federal Republic of Germany, Finland, Netherlands, Sweden, U.K., and U.S.A. (Woodrow, 1970). These are not exactly comparable with the trial reported here as they often include multiparae, selection according to fetal cell score was not part of the design, and mothers have been treated after ABO-incompatible as well as ABO-compatible pregnancies. There is, however, general agreement that the success rate is high. Ignoring the heterogeneity of this material and combining the results of antibody tests in the post-delivery period, 354 (5·3%) out of 6,701 controls have developed anti-D, while 47 (0·31%) out of 15,114 treated mothers had antibody at this time. The overall success rate is about 94%. Tests during subsequent pregnancies show that 81 (11·4%) out of 712 untreated mothers had anti-D at this time compared with 15 (1·2%) out of 1,265 treated mothers (these figures are cumulative and include mothers who developed antibodies after the first pregnancy observed). The overall success rate at this time is thus of the order of 90%.

Question of Dosage.—Though our 5-ml trial throws no light on the question of dosage, data from elsewhere make it certain that 1,000 µg is an unnecessarily large amount for the majority of mothers. Information from most trials suggests that 200 to 300 µg of anti-D is adequate for about 99·8% of all transplacental haemorrhages, a breakdown of protection occurring only if the volume of fetal red cells in the maternal circulation is 10 ml or above. Where this is so, apparent protection has been obtained with doses ranging from 4 to 50 µg of anti-D per ml of fetal red cells, with a mean ratio of 25 µg: 1 ml, while failures have been reported with doses ranging from 2 to 20 µg of anti-D per ml of fetal red cells, the mean ratio being 8 µg:1 ml (W.H.O., 1971).

We wish to record our gratitude to the women who took part in this trial and to the blood donors whose plasma was used as the source of anti-D. For the supply and preparation of the anti-D gammaglobulin we are indebted to Dr. W. d'A. Maycock and Mr. L. Vallet, of the Lister Institute of Preventitive Medicine. The continuation of the trial has been made possible by the co-operation of Professor Sir Norman Jeffcoate and his consultant colleagues, and the medical, nursing, and laboratory staffs of the Liverpool Maternity Hospital and Mill Road, Broadgreen, Sefton General, and Fazakerley Hospitals. The technical staff in the various laboratories involved in this work have continued to give valuable assistance.

This research has been made possible by generous grants from the Nuffield Foundation and from the Research Committee of the United Liverpool Hospitals.

References

Ascari, W. Q., Levine, P., and Pollack, W. (1969). *British Medical Journal*, 1, 399.
Combined Study from Centres in England and Baltimore (1966). *British Medical Journal*, 2, 907.
Clarke, C. A., *et al.* (1963). *British Medical Journal*, 1, 979.
Kleihauer, E., Braum, H., and Betke, K. (1957). *Klinische Wochenschrift*, 35, 637.
Walsh, N. P., Peter, S., Sr., and Hewitt, S. R. (1968). *Journal of the Irish Medical Association*, 61, 315.
Woodrow, J. C. (1970). *Series Haematologica*, 3, No. 3.
Woodrow, J. C., *et al.* (1965). *British Medical Journal*, 1, 279.
Woodrow, J. C., Bowley, C. C., Gilliver, B. E., and Strong, S. J. (1968). *British Medical Journal*, 1, 148.
Woodrow, J. C., Clarke, C. A., McConnell, R. B., Towers, Shona H., and Donohoe, W. T. A. (1971). *British Medical Journal*, 2, 610.
Woodrow, J. C., and Donohoe, W. T. A. (1968). *British Medical Journal*, 4, 139.
World Health Organization. (1971). *Bulletin*. In press.

Paper 45

45. Woodrow, J. C., Clarke, C. A., McConnell, R. B., Towers, S. H. and Donohoe, W. T. A. (1971). Prevention of Rh-haemolytic disease: results of the Liverpool "low-risk" clinical trial. *Brit. Med. J., ii,* 610-612.

Commentary

The results of the 'low risk' trial make interesting comparison with Paper 44. A 'low-risk' mother was defined as one in whose circulation either no or very few fetal cells were present after the birth of her first Rh-positive baby. In this trial, the dose of anti-D given was $200\mu g$.

It will be seen that though the results of treatment were very good, yet the incidence of immunisation in the second Rh-positive pregnancy was slightly but not significantly higher than in the high risk trial. The reason for this may be that 'primed' mothers are more likely to get into the low-risk trial since the number of fetal cells may be zero or low because of concealed anti-D antibody which eliminates them.

From J. C. Woodrow et al. (1971). Brit. Med. J., ii, 610-2. Copyright (1971), by kind permission of the authors and the British Medical Association

610   BRITISH MEDICAL JOURNAL   12 JUNE 1971

Prevention of Rh-haemolytic Disease: Results of the Liverpool "Low-risk" Clinical Trial

J. C. WOODROW,   C. A. CLARKE,   R. B. McCONNELL,   SHONA H. TOWERS,   W. T. A. DONOHOE

British Medical Journal, 1971, 2, 610–612

Summary

A clinical trial is reported in which Rh-negative primiparae, just delivered of an Rh-positive ABO-compatible infant and in whom fetal cell counts after delivery suggested less than 0·2 ml of circulating fetal blood, were treated with about 200 μg of anti-D gammaglobulin. Three (0·36%) out of 844 women thus treated developed anti-D in the subsequent six months; this is 10% of the incidence in untreated controls. Three (1·8%) out of 171 treated mothers had anti-D at the end of the second Rh-positive pregnancy, and this is 18% of the incidence in controls.

Possible reasons for the occasional failure of the treatment are discussed and the results of this trial are compared with those of a previous trial in which 1,000 μg or more of anti-D was given to a different group of mothers. The combined results of the two trials lead to the conclusion that the passive administration of anti-D gammaglobulin after delivery affords in this population of Rh-negative women a 95% protection rate in the post-delivery period and an 89% protection rate by the end of the subsequent pregnancy.

Introduction

In our report of a clinical trial to test the effectiveness of about 1,000 μg of anti-D gammaglobulin in preventing Rh immunization of Rh-negative primiparae (Combined Study, 1966) it was noted that a further trial had been initiated in Liverpool. The plan of this second one was to treat mothers showing less than an estimated 0·2 ml of Rh-positive fetal blood in their circulation after delivery with about 200 μg of anti-D gammaglobulin. The results of this trial are presented here and some implications discussed.

Design of trial

In general the design of the trial was similar to that described for the 1,000-μg trial. Rh-negative primiparae were ascertained in five maternity units immediately after the delivery of ABO-compatible Rh-positive infants. Maternal blood samples were tested by the Kleihauer-Betke technique (Kleihauer et al., 1957), the scoring system previously described being used (Combined Study, 1966). Mothers were selected for the trial in whom a fetal cell score of 0–4 was found, suggesting less than

Nuffield Unit of Medical Genetics, Department of Medicine, University of Liverpool, Liverpool L69 3BX
J. C. WOODROW, M.D., F.R.C.P., Senior Lecturer in Medicine
C. A. CLARKE, M.D., F.R.C.P., F.R.S., Professor of Medicine and Director of the Nuffield Unit of Medical Genetics
R. B. McCONNELL, M.D., F.R.C.P., Research Fellow
W. T. A. DONOHOE, A.I.M.L.T., Chief Technician

Chester Royal Infirmary, Chester
SHONA H. TOWERS, M.D., M.R.C.O.G., Consultant Obstetrician and Gynaecologist

0·2 ml of circulating fetal blood. In the absence of treatment the incidence of anti-D six months after delivery in this group was about 6%. Alternate cases were treated by administering intramuscularly 1 ml of a gammaglobulin solution containing 200 μg of anti-D (N. C. Hughes-Jones, personal communication, 1967). (At this time mothers showing 0·2 ml or more of fetal blood were being treated with 1,000 μg of anti-D (Combined Study, 1971).) The aim was to administer the anti-D by intramuscular injection within 36 hours of delivery, but in some instances this could not be done and delays of up to three to five days occasionally occurred. The untreated cases served as controls.

Tests for antibodies

Control and treated mothers were visited at home about six months after delivery and samples of venous blood obtained. Various methods were used in order to ascertain the occurrence of subsequent pregnancies, and further samples of blood were obtained immediately after this second delivery. In many instances blood was also taken at about 35 weeks of this second pregnancy.

The sera were tested for antibodies in saline and albumin and by antiglobulin and papain methods.

Results

The results of testing six months after delivery are shown in Table I. Thirteen (3·6%) out of 362 control mothers had developed anti-D at this time. None of 353 treated mothers showed antibodies.

The results of testing 255 of these women for antibodies at the end of the second Rh-positive pregnancy are given in Table II. Included are cases in which the second baby was either ABO compatible or incompatible. Thirteen out of 127 control mothers had anti-D, four having developed it previously within six months of the first delivery. Thus nine

TABLE I—Results of Tests for Antibodies Six Months after Delivery

			No.	Not Immunized	Immunized
Controls	..	..	362	349	13 (3·6%)
Treated	..	..	353	353	0
Total	..	..	715	702	13

TABLE II—Results of Tests for Antibodies at End of Second Rh-positive Pregnancies

			No.	Not Immunized	Immunized
Controls	..	..	127	114	13 (4*) (10·2%)
Treated	..	..	128	125	3 (2·3%)
Total	..	..	255	239	16

*Number of mothers who had developed antibodies after the first pregnancy. They are included in the larger number.

BRITISH MEDICAL JOURNAL   12 JUNE 1971   **611**

controls developed antibodies during this second pregnancy as against 3 out of 128 in the treated group. The following are the details of these failures of prophylaxis.

Case 1.—A group O Rh-negative mother was treated about 24 hours after the delivery of a group O Rh-positive infant, a fetal cell score of 1 being found (a score of 5 implies approximately 0·2 ml of circulating fetal blood). No antibodies were found on testing six months later, and she became pregnant again. A routine test at 34 weeks of this second pregnancy showed no antibodies, but at delivery her serum showed anti-D + C by saline and antiglobulin techniques. The infant was group O Rh-positive, direct Coombs positive, but was only very mildly affected.

Case 2.—A group B Rh-negative mother was treated about 24 hours after delivery of a group O Rh-positive infant, the fetal cell score being 1. Tests for antibodies were negative six months later, and at this time she was already three months pregnant again. Routine antenatal testing at 20 weeks of pregnancy was negative, but at 34 weeks anti-D was detected by saline, albumin, and antiglobulin techniques. She was induced at 38 weeks, and a group B Rh-positive infant was delivered showing a positive direct Coombs test. The haemoglobin at birth was 115% but fell to 60% subsequently. The child did well without transfusion.

Case 3.—A group O Rh-negative mother showed no circulating fetal cells after delivery of a group O Rh-positive infant and was treated with anti-D about 24 hours after delivery. Tests were made for antibodies and were negative six months later. She became pregnant again a year after this. A routine test at 30 weeks of pregnancy showed no antibodies, but anti-D in saline and albumin was present at delivery. A group O Rh-positive infant was delivered at home and appeared healthy. No clinical observations suggesting the presence of neonatal anaemia or jaundice were made but a direct Coombs test was not carried out.

FURTHER TREATED MOTHERS

When the controlled trial ended it was decided that all mothers at risk should be treated and we have data on 491 further women selected in the same way and who were given 200 μg of anti-D after delivery. Three were found to have anti-D six months later, demonstrable by saline, albumin, and antiglobulin methods. The fetal cell scores in these women after delivery were 0, 1, and 3 respectively. It may be relevant that in two mothers the anti-D was not given until the third and fifth day after delivery. The total incidence of anti-D six months after delivery in all treated mothers is, therefore, 3 out of 844 (0·36%). This is exactly 10% of the incidence in the controls and indicates a 90% protection rate.

Some time after the controlled trial ended we decided to treat, with 200 μg, women with a fetal cell score of 5 to 25—that is, 0·2 to 1·0 ml of circulating fetal blood. So far we have followed for six months 48 women in this series, none of whom has developed antibodies.

Forty-three mothers treated after the end of the controlled trial have had second Rh-positive pregnancies and none showed anti-D at the end of this pregnancy. Thus out of a total of 171 treated mothers 3 (1·8%) had anti-D at the end of the subsequent pregnancy. This is about 18% of the incidence of antibodies after a second pregnancy in the control women. In other words the degree of protection achieved was 82%.

MOTHERS WITH ANTIBODIES AT DELIVERY

In order to avoid delay in the administration of anti-D it was not routine practice to test for antibodies the pretreatment maternal blood samples before the administration of the anti-D gammaglobulin. It therefore happened that seven mothers who received anti-D gammaglobulin were found on later testing to have anti-D in their pretreatment sera. All showed anti-D in the samples taken six months after delivery. In five instances both baseline and six-month samples showed strong activity by albumin and Coombs techniques. In two mothers the baseline samples showed activity only by an enzyme method and their

six-month samples showed no significant change in the behaviour of these antibodies.

Discussion

The results of this trial show the efficiency of the preventive treatment, and there are some interesting comparisons to be made with a first and larger dose trial carried out in Liverpool and other centres (Combined Study, 1971). The trial described here differs from the first one in two respects. Firstly, the dose of anti-D is of the order of 200 μg while that in the first trial was 1,000 μg or more. Present evidence suggests, however, that for most treated women in the two trials this difference in dosage was of no significance. Secondly, selection of mothers for this present trial was based on zero or very low count of fetal cells after delivery, while a substantial count of fetal cells was a requisite for the inclusion of a mother in the first trial. A superficial consideration of the matter might lead one to expect that the failure rate would be lower in the present trial since the amount of Rh-positive fetal blood in the maternal circulation at the time of treatment was smaller. In fact, there is a suggestion of a somewhat higher incidence of failure in the present trial as judged both by antibody tests six months after delivery (if mothers treated after the end of the controlled trial are included the rate of protection is 90%) and by tests at the end of the subsequent pregnancy (protection rate 82%). These figures can be compared with those for the first trial—that is, 97% and 93% respectively (Combined Study, 1971).

The question must be posed of why failures of therapy occurred in this present trial when the amount of anti-D given might have been expected easily to protect against the volumes of Rh-positive blood present in the maternal circulation at the time of treatment. Indeed, in two instances *no* fetal cells were counted in maternal blood samples after delivery. The most likely explanation is that transplacental haemorrhage, possibly of substantial size, had occurred some time before delivery and that a primary immune response with total or partial clearance of the fetal cells had occurred by the time of delivery. In other words, when the anti-D was given the primary immune response had already begun, and the anti-D was too late to prevent the further development of the immune response. That Rh-positive red cells can be cleared at a stage in the immune response when there is no demonstrable antibody has been shown by Mollison *et al* (1969). They injected 34 Rh-negative male volunteers with Rh-positive red cells, giving some anti-D as well, and challenged them later with ⁵¹Cr Rh-positive red cells. By serological testing only two of the 13 subjects who initially received red cells alone (no anti-D) developed antibody, but five other controls showed subnormal cell survival at 7 to 10 days after they had been challenged, indicating that priming had occurred. Woodrow *et al* (1969) carried out similar studies in volunteers from which again it was evident that rapid clearance of Rh-positive cells took place after challenge even though there was no detectable antibody present in volunteers who made conventional antibodies later.

In contrast to the above situation, the presence of a more substantial volume of fetal blood at delivery in the first trial would favour protection in that the immune response is less likely to have begun in these mothers, and in many cases the transplacental haemorrhage occurred either very late in pregnancy or during labour.

Because of the risk of priming during a first pregnancy Canadian workers have been, and are now, treating women during the third trimester (Zipursky and Israels, 1967; Buchanan *et al.*, 1969; Bowman, 1970). We await the results of the extensive Manitoba trial with interest. This approach might be expected to prevent most failures since priming during the latter part of pregnancy seems to be a commoner cause of the failure of postpartum treatment than is the occurrence of unusually large transplacental haemorrhages.

BRITISH MEDICAL JOURNAL   12 JUNE 1971

GENERAL ASSESSMENT OF Rh PROPHYLAXIS

If one assumes that the difference in dosage of anti-D used in the present trial and that used in the first one (Combined Study, 1971) is irrelevant, it is of interest to combine the data from the two trials in order to make an overall assessment of the degree of success achieved. Women coming within the category of this present trial are a little over four times as common in our population as those in the first trial category. If this is taken into account, the overall incidence of antibodies developing in the six months after treatment can be estimated to be 0·4%. This is 4·9% of the expected 8·2% incidence of antibodies six months after first ABO-compatible pregnancies (Woodrow, 1970). This represents, therefore, a 95% protection rate at this time.

The cumulative incidence of antibodies at the end of the second pregnancies subsequent to treatment is estimated to be 1·9% overall. This is 11% of the expected 17·3% incidence of anti-D at this time. The protection rate at this stage is thus 89%.

Two points are worth making in relation to this latter figure. Firstly, in four instances of failure which have occurred in the two trials the anti-D has not appeared until relatively late in the second pregnancy. Experience in Liverpool suggests that 0·8% of Rh-negative women develop antibodies during the first Rh-positive pregnancy, and it seems quite likely that in many instances this represents a primary response. It may well be that a similar event occasionally occurs in the Rh-positive pregnancy following treatment, and in these circumstances it cannot be expected that the anti-D administered after the previous pregnancy will prevent the appearance of antibodies at this time.

Secondly, the crude incidences of antibodies may not quite tell the whole story. It is possible that some women who without treatment would develop anti-D in the months after the first pregnancy are prevented from doing so by the administration of anti-D gammaglobulin, but because the immune response is not totally suppressed they start the second pregnancy in a primed state and are thus at risk of developing antibodies later during this second pregnancy. Though such a case would be counted as a failure, the treatment may in fact have been of considerable benefit to the second Rh-positive infant which, instead of being exposed throughout the period of pregnancy to maternal anti-D, is exposed to antibody only during the latter part of the pregnancy, the antibodies, in addition, probably being of lower affinity.

PROBLEM OF IMMUNIZED MOTHERS

No definite effect of the administration of 200 µg of anti-D was seen in the seven mothers who had antibody in the pre-treatment samples. Though the fact that the two mothers showing papain-active anti-D (negative in saline, albumin, and by Coombs test) before treatment still showed the same type of antibody six months later, we can draw no firm conclusions because another mother showing similar antibody at delivery was given 1,000 µg of anti-D, and in spite of this a strong albumin and Coombs-positive anti-D was found six months later.

In general it is not to be expected that mothers who have demonstrable antibody in their blood can be helped by the administration of anti-D gammaglobulin. An attempt to prevent the further development of the immune response in mothers with very weak anti-D at delivery has been made by Godel et al. (1968). These weak antibodies could sometimes be detected only by using ficin or protease treated -D-/-D- cells, and in five out of nine untreated mothers the antibody could not be found six months later. Thus the fact that only 1 of their 13 treated mothers showing this type of antibody at delivery still had a positive test six months later is difficult to assess. However, as the authors argue, the immune response in the mothers may have been only in the form of IgM antibody at the time anti-D was given and the further development of the response with the appearance of IgG anti-D may have been prevented. Further results are awaited with interest, and it remains to be seen whether these observations have an important practical bearing.

This trial would not have been possible without the help of numerous individuals and these are detailed in the report of a previous clinical trial (see Combined Study, 1971).

References

Bowman, J. M. (1970). *British Journal of Haematology,* **19,** 653.
Buchanan, D. I., Bell, R. E., Beck, R. P., and Taylor, W. C. (1969). *Lancet,* **2,** 288.
Combined Study from Centres in England and Baltimore (1966). *British Medical Journal,* **2,** 907.
Combined Study from Centres in England and Baltimore (1971). *British Medical Journal,* **2,** 607.
Godel, J. C., Buchanan, D. I., Jarosch, Jean M., and McHugh, Maureen (1968). *British Medical Journal,* **4,** 479.
Kleihauer, E., Braun, H., and Betke, K. (1957). *Klinische Wochenschrift,* **35,** 637.
Mollison, P. L., Hughes-Jones, N. C., Lindsay, M., and Wessely, J. (1969). *Vox Sanguinis,* 16 421.
Woodrow, J. C. (1970). *Series Haematologica,* **3,** No. 3.
Woodrow, J. C., Finn, R., and Krevans, J. R. (1969). *Vox Sanguinis,* **17,** 349.
Zipursky, A., and Israels, L. G. (1967). *Canadian Medical Association Journal,* **97,** 1245.

Paper 46

---

46. Report of MRC Anti-D Working Party. (1974). Controlled trial of various anti-D dosages in suppression of sensitisation following pregnancy. *Brit. Med. J., ii,*75-80.

Commentary

There will never be another trial quite like this. At the time that it was designed there was a shortage of gammaglobulin and one of the reasons why it was carried out was to see if a smaller than standard dose (this was $200\,\mu g$ when it was started) would be equally effective. There were some grounds for thinking that this might be so from cell survival studies carried out by Mollison *et al.* (Paper 38). In these experiments as little as $15\,\mu g$ of anti-D largely suppressed immunisation by a challenge given six months after the original stimulus.

As will be seen from Paper 46, there were about 1,600 Rh-negative primiparae in the trial and they were randomly given one of four doses of anti-D gammaglobulin after the birth of their first Rh-positive, ABO compatible baby. Those administering the injection had no idea whether they were giving, $200\mu g$, $100\mu g$, $50\mu g$, or $20\mu g$. When the design of the trial was first being considered the question of a proper control (i.e. no treatment at all) was discussed, but this was thought unethical as even at this time there was good evidence that anti-D did protect against Rh immunisation.

The overall results of the trial were not unexpected (i.e. a high degree of protection was obtained) but two points call for comment.

The first is that $20\mu g$, although not so efficient as the higher doses, nevertheless achieved a considerable degree of protection. (The usual figures in Rh-negative primiparae in the UK are about 8% of women at risk immunised at six months and a further 9% at the end of the next Rh-positive pregnancy, i.e. about 17% in all if no prophylaxis is given).

The second point concerns the detection of passive antibody. Detractors of anti-D therapy had surmised that enzyme antibodies heralded the formation of conventional antibodies, whereas those who favoured the treatment had thought that most enzyme antibodies in treated women were the remains of the injected antibody, and that they would disappear in time. Reference to Tables II and III strongly supports this latter view, for if enzyme antibodies mean immunisation then one would expect more of them with dose 4 ($20\mu g$) than with dose 1 ($200\mu g$). The reverse was found to be the case and all the 'passives' had disappeared in group 1 by the end of the second Rh-positive pregnancy. All in all, the trial confirms the effectiveness of anti-D, the immunisation rate being cut by about 90%.

An interesting sideline is that in the failures, as judged by a positive Coombs test in the cord blood of the second D-positive infant, there was evidence that those mothers who had received the lowest dose of anti-D after the last pregnancy had babies more severely affected than the rest. If this is not just due to chance, it would suggest that prophylaxis is of some use even if immunisation occurs in spite of it. This could be due to overt antibody only appearing late in the second pregnancy, the injected anti-D having held the immune antibody in check at the priming level.

From M. R. C. Working Party (1974). Brit. Med. J., ii, 75-80. Copyright (1974), by kind permission of the authors and the British Medical Association

BRITISH MEDICAL JOURNAL   13 APRIL 1974

Controlled Trial of Various Anti-D Dosages in Suppression of Rh Sensitization following Pregnancy

Report to the Medical Research Council by the Working Party on the Use of Anti-D Immunoglobulin for the Prevention of Isoimmunization of Rh-negative Women During Pregnancy

Summary

In a controlled trial phials containing 200 μg, 100 μg, 50 μg, or 20 μg of IgG anti-D were given to nearly 2,000 D-negative primiparae whose infants were D-positive and ABO-compatible. Only mothers whose serum lacked anti-D were included and the dose of anti-D was always given within 36 hours of delivery. Each phial contained the same total volume of immunoglobulin and the particular dose given to any patient was not known to the clinician. The anti-D content of the phials was estimated three times during the course of the trials and remained fairly constant. Six months after delivery the incidence of a positive indirect antiglobulin test result, indicating the presence of anti-D, in the four dose groups (with about 450 women in each group) was as follows: 0·22%, 0·23%, 0·44%, and 1·35%. The trend towards an increase in the frequency of failures as the dose decreases was significant at the level of P=0·02.

In each dose group about 200 women were followed to the end of a second pregnancy with a D-positive infant. The failure rates (in order of decreasing dosage) as judged by a positive indirect antiglobulin test result at the second delivery were as follows: 1·5%, 1·1%, 1·5% and 2·9%. The differences between the dose groups were not statistically significant. The overall failure rate (1·7%) was about one-tenth of that expected in an untreated series. Though the results failed to prove any differences in success rates between doses of 200, 100, 50, and 20 μg of anti-D, they do suggest, in conformity with other evidence, that a dose of 20 μg is suboptimal for routine use. The results support the belief that a dose of 100 μg is adequate.

Introduction

By the beginning of 1966 evidence was growing that Rh sensitization, which would otherwise follow pregnancy in a proportion of D-negative women, could probably be prevented by giving the mother an injection of anti-D immediately after delivery, though it was realized that the effectiveness of the treatment could not be properly assessed until the outcome of second pregnancies with D-positive infants was known (Clarke, 1967). Meanwhile it seemed important to standardize the dose of anti-D and to define the minimum dose which was likely to be effective. Accordingly a working party was set up by the Medical Research Council to consider what further trials could usefully be carried out and to initiate such trials.

In late 1966 the working party began a controlled trial in which only half the subjects were to be treated with anti-D, but within a year evidence of the effectiveness of treatment had become so much stronger that the trial was converted to one of dosage, and the control group, instead of getting no treatment, received a relatively small but potentially effective dose of anti-D. This small-scale trial was made up of 28 untreated patients, 76 on 260 μg anti-D, and 29 on 20 μg anti-D, was ended in late 1967. Since the results of this preliminary trial added nothing material to those obtained in the main trial they are not referred to further.

Members of the Working Party: Professor P. L. Mollison, Chairman; Mr. S. L. Barron; Dr. C. C. Bowley; Professor J. C. McClure Browne; Professor Sir Cyril Clarke; Professor Sir Richard Doll; Dr. K. L. G. Goldsmith; Dr. C. A. Holman; Dr. N. C. Hughes-Jones; Dr. J. H. Humphrey; Professor R. J. Kellar; Dr. W. d'A Maycock; Dr. J. G. Robertson; Dr. G. H. Tovey; Dr. W. Walker; Dr. J. Wallace; Dr. M. L. N. Willoughby; Professor P. J. Huntingford, Secretary from 1966-71; Dr. W. J. Jenkins, Secretary since 1971.

The planning of a larger trial began in mid-1967. At this time there was only enough anti-D available in the United Kingdom to treat about 12% of the primiparae at risk or about 5% of the total number of D-negative women in the population who might benefit from it. We therefore thought it essential, and justifiable, to determine the lowest dose of anti-D which was capable of suppressing Rh sensitization in recently delivered women. Accordingly a trial was planned in which four doses would be used—200 μg, 100 μg, 50 μg, and 20 μg of anti-D referred to as doses 1, 2, 3, and 4 respectively. Each dose was made up to 2 ml with immunoglobulin free from anti-D so that the user could not tell by simple inspection of the phials which dose they contained. Each phial carried a serial number coded to the actual dose present.

This second trial was begun at the end of 1967 and all the 2,000 available phials (500 each of the four doses) had been given before the end of 1970. As well as testing the serum of all treated women for anti-D about six months after delivery of their first infant, as many as possible of the treated women were followed up to discover the outcome of their next pregnancy with a D-positive infant. The follow-up ended on 31 January 1973.

Patients and Methods

SELECTION OF PATIENTS

Women were selected according to the following criteria: (a) they had to be D-negative primiparae whose serum had no detectable anti-D at the time of delivery of their first infant, (b) the infant had to be D-positive and ABO-compatible, (c) there had to be no history of abortion or blood transfusion, (d) the patient had to be married (in view of the difficulty of following up single women), (e) the patient had to be white (in view of the low incidence of Rh sensitization among non-whites), (f) it had to be possible to give the dose of anti-D immunoglobulin within 36 hours of delivery.

Once these criteria had been met a coded serial number was used to select the phial to be given. Each woman was told that the injection was being given as part of an investigation to find the best way of preventing Rh immunization and that if she agreed to receive the injection she would be asked to give further blood samples and to collaborate by providing information about later pregnancies.

From the total number of patients considered for the trial 1,006 were excluded because they failed to satisfy one or more of the criteria. In addition there were seven women who satisfied all the criteria but were excluded because of the results of the test for fetal red cells in their blood (see below). During the later phase of the trial, when anti-D immunoglobulin had become freely available, women with D-positive infants who had been excluded from the trial received a dose of anti-D from other sources.

TABLE I—*Assays of Anti-D Concentration in Four 2-ml doses*

Dose	Expected Anti-D Concentration (μg/ml)	Original Assay Oct. 1967 (μg/ml)	Later Assays		
			Jan. 1969 (μg/ml)	Jan. 1970 (μg/ml)	June 1972 (μg/ml)
1	100	134	140	87*	75†
2	50	55	60	60	43†
3	25	21	28	30	
4	10	11	13	10	

*Average of two estimates.
†Average of four estimates in four laboratories (see text).

The mother's blood was in all cases examined for the presence of fetal red cells though it was intended that the information should be used only retrospectively. The seven women excluded as a result of a test for fetal red cells included two who were considered by the centre at which they were treated to have such a large transplacental haemorrhage (estimated to be 10 ml and 18 ml red cells respectively) that they would not be treated adequately should they happen to receive one of the smaller doses of anti-D. The other five women were treated at a second centre which was at one period looking for cases with detectable fetal cells to test the effect of some new batches of anti-D immunoglobulin; only one of these five cases were estimated to have a transplacental haemorrhage exceeding 4 ml red cells. The possible effect of excluding these cases is considered below.

PREPARATION OF ANTI-D IMMUNOGLOBULIN

Anti-D immunoglobulin was prepared by the cold ethanol fractionation process from pooled plasma, obtained mainly from women immunized by pregnancy and partly from deliberately immunized D-negative men volunteers. Most of the individual plasma samples from which the pool was derived had anti-D titres (estimated by agglutination in albumin) between 64 and 512. Most of the batches did not agglutinate D-positive red cells suspended in saline. The final dried product was dissolved in 0·1 mol NaCl/l. containing 1:10,000 thiomersal to prepare a stock solution of immunoglobulin containing 135 g protein/l. Examination by gel diffusion using specific antisera* gave the following results (mg/100 ml): IgG 12,800; IgM 15; IgA 400; IgD 10. The anti-D concentration of this stock solution, estimated by the direct and indirect methods (Hughes-Jones and Stevenson, 1968), was 288 µg/ml. Solutions planned to contain 100 µg/ml, 50 µg/ml, 25 µg/ml, and 10 µg/ml were prepared by diluting the stock solution with 0·15 mol NaCl/l. containing 1:10,000 thiomersal and adding a solution of normal human immunoglobulin free from anti-D to produce a final total protein concentration of 50 g/l.

Phials containing exactly 2 ml of each of the four doses were prepared and a list was made in which each of the doses at each of the four dose levels was assigned randomly to a number in the range 1 to 2.000. The numbers were then sorted into four groups according to dosage and the appropriate labels attached to the ampoules and to their cardboard containers. Frequent checks were made to ensure that the phials were correctly labelled.

The anti-D concentrations in the four doses were assayed at the W.H.O. International Reference Centre on three occasions between 1967 and 1970 and that of doses 1 and 2 was assayed again in July 1972 by four laboratories in a W.H.O. collaborative trial (table I). With the method used the confidence limits (P=0·05) of a single assay are 66-150% and this explains the variability of individual results. All the assays can be analysed together, however, to give a more accurate estimate of the original concentration of anti-D in the different doses and the rate of fall of anti-D concentration with time. The confidence limits (P=0·05) for the concentration in each dose in October 1967 were as follows: dose 1, 108-131 µg/ml; dose 2, 54-65 µg/ml; dose 3, 27-32 µg/ml; and dose 4, 11-13 µg/ml. These calculations assume that the dilutions of the original stock solution were correctly made. The analysis also indicates that the anti-D concentration fell at about 4% a year so that in late 1970 when the trials were concluded the concentrations of anti-D in the various doses were about 12% less than the values given above.

Thus the doses actually given may have been about 20% greater initially than the nominal values of 200, 100, 50, and 20 µg and are unlikely to have been lower than the nominal values by the time the trials were concluded. Since not quite the whole contents of a phial can be injected the nominal values seem to be satisfactory descriptions of the doses actually used in the trial.

*Estimates made by Dr. R. A. Thompson.

STANDARDIZATION OF TESTS FOR ANTI-D

Sera from all women were tested immediately after delivery and six months later, using the indirect antiglobulin test (I.A.G.T.) and an agglutination test with enzyme-treated red cells. Twice during the trial coded samples of serum were distributed to all participating laboratories to estimate the sensitivity and reliability of testing. Some of the samples contained various concentrations of anti-D, prepared by diluting anti-D immunoglobulin in AB serum, but most consisted only of "inert" AB serum. The highest dilutions of anti-D that could be detected by the different laboratories were 0·008-0·2 µg/ml when using the I.A.G.T. and 0·001-0·02 µg/ml when using enzyme-treated cells. Different laboratories differed considerably in their ability to detect trace amounts of anti-D, and while an enzyme technique was the most sensitive for the detection of anti-D it was prone to produce false positive reactions. When the antiglobulin technique was used, however, not one false positive result was recorded at any of the 12 laboratories in two surveys.

STANDARDIZATION OF ACID-ELUTION COUNTS

All the laboratories prepared blood films by the method of Betke and Kleihauer (1958) or some modification of it. To assess the accuracy and precision of estimates of fetal red cells samples containing known proportions of fetal to adult red cells were distributed to all centres five times between 1966 and 1971. At the first distribution some laboratories simply counted the number of darkly staining cells in a given number of low-power fields, but analysis of the results showed that to compensate for the varying numbers of adult red cells scanned due to the varying thickness of blood films it was necessary to relate the number of fetal cells to the number of maternal cells scanned. Most centres reported their results as a ratio of darkly stained to unstained cells though a few centres did not adopt this method until about December 1969.

When the accuracy and precision of the method was finally evaluated in June 1971 it was found that when the number of fetal red cells corresponded to a transplacental haemorrhage of about 1 ml red cells most centres estimated the amount to within a factor of 2, though when the amount of fetal red cells present corresponded to a transplacental haemorrhage of 0·1 ml or less estimates varied by a factor of almost 10.

Results

RESULTS OBTAINED

Of the 2,000 phials issued 600 were used at Sheffield; about 350 each at Bristol and at Law Hospital (County of Lanark); 150-200 each at Brentwood, Newcastle, and Glasgow; and 30-50 each at three London hospitals—Hammersmith, Lewisham, and St. Mary's. Results in only 1,800 cases were suitable for analysis. The remaining cases had to be excluded because follow-up examinations were not carried out after six months (75 cases), the mother or child were found not to satisfy the criteria for inclusion after the dose had been given (27 cases), records of the use of the phial were missing (88 cases), or more than one dose was given to the mother (10 cases).

Of the 1,800 women 807 had a second pregnancy with a D-positive infant before 1 February 1973 and the results of tests for the presence of anti-D in the serum are known. Of the remaining 993 women 357 were known to have had a second pregnancy before 1 February 1973 but in 233 cases the infant was D-negative and in the remaining 124 cases samples of blood were not obtained from either the mother or the baby at delivery; 294 women were known not to have become pregnant for the second time before 1 February 1973 or, if they had become pregnant, were not expecting their infant before that date. There remained 342 women who were

III—*Results Six Months after First Pregnancy related to Results at End of Second D-positive Pregnancy*

Dose	No. of Cases	Six Months after First Pregnancy	End of Second Pregnancy		
			No Anti-D	I.A.G.T.* Positive	Enzyme-only† Positive
1	206	No Anti-D 194	193	1 ⎫	0
		I.A.G.T.* Positive 1	0	1 ⎬ 1·5%	0
		Enzyme-only† Positive 11	10	1 ⎭	0
2	189	No Anti-D 186	184	2 ⎫	0
		I.A.G.T. Positive 0	0	0 ⎬ 1·1%	0
		Enzyme-only Positive 3	3	0 ⎭	0
3	207	No Anti-D 202	200	2 ⎫	0
		I.A.G.T. Positive 0	0	0 ⎬ 1·5%	0
		Enzyme-only Positive 5	3	1 ⎭	1
4	205	No Anti-D 196	193	0 ⎫	3
		I.A.G.T. Positive 5	0	5 ⎬ 2·9%	0
		Enzyme-only Positive 4	2	1 ⎭	1
Total	807	No Anti-D 778	770	5 ⎫	3
		I.A.G.T. Positive 6	0	6 ⎬ 1·7%	0
		Enzyme-only Positive 23	18	3 ⎭	2

*Indirect antiglobulin test.
†Result positive only with enzyme-treated red cells.

lost to follow-up after being examined six months after their first pregnancy. Examination of the distribution of these women by dose and follow-up results at six months provided no evidence to suggest that failure to complete the follow-up had biased the results.

In most cases the injection of anti-D was given within 24 hours of delivery and in all cases was given within 36 hours.

FAILURES DETECTED SIX MONTHS AFTER FIRST PREGNANCY

The incidence of anti-D six months after delivery of the first infant is shown in table II. In 56 of the 66 women in whom anti-D was detected the result was positive only with enzyme-treated red cells, usually only with undiluted serum. In many of these 56 cases the positive results were probably due to the persistence of passively administered anti-D since the incidence was greatest in those women who had received the highest dose. Indeed, the number of positive cases (25) in the group which received the highest dose was almost as great as in the other three groups put together (31).

TABLE II—*Number of Cases in which Anti-D was detected Six Months after First Delivery*

Dose	Amount (µg/2 ml)	No. of Cases Tested	I.A.G.T.* Positive	"Enzyme-only"† Positive
1	200	459	1 (0·22%)	25
2	100	443	1 (0·23%)	13
3	50	452	2 (0·44%)	13
4	20	446	6 (1·35%)	5
Total		1,800	10	56

*Indirect antiglobulin test.
†Result was positive only with enzyme-treated red cells.
Test of difference between frequency of I.A.G.T.-positive results in groups receiving doses 1 and 4: P = 0.06 (exact test).
Test of significance of trend in frequency of I.A.G.T.-positive results from doses 1 to 4 through doses 2 and 3: χ^2 = 5·25; n = 1; P = 0·02.

FOLLOW-UP STUDIES IN SECOND PREGNANCIES

Of the 56 women whose serum contained anti-D detectable only with enzyme-treated red cells six months after their first D-positive infant, 23 were followed through a second pregnancy with a D-positive infant (see table III). Three of these 23 at the time of the second delivery had anti-D detectable by the I.A.G.T. and in two more the antibody could be detected only with enzyme-treated cells. Thus in 18 out of 23 cases it seemed that the positive result with enzyme-treated cells six months after the end of the first pregnancy must have been due either to the presence of passively administered antibody or to some artefact. A positive finding six months after the first pregnancy was almost certainly due in some cases to persistence of passively administered antibody but in

the women who received the smallest doses of anti-D it seems likely that the positive results at six months were either due to active immunization, but with too little antibody to be detected by the I.A.G.T., or were false positives.

There were only 10 out of 1,800 cases in which anti-D could be detected by the I.A.G.T. six months after the first delivery (see table II), but by the end of the second D-positive pregnancy (see table III) anti-D could be detected by the I.A.G.T. in 14 out of 807 cases. In nine of these 14 anti-D had also been detectable six months after the first pregnancy (by the I.A.G.T. in six and only by a test with enzyme-treated cells in three). There were an additional five cases in which anti-D was detectable at the end of the second pregnancy but only by using enzyme-treated red cells; in two of these cases anti-D had been detectable only with enzyme-treated cells after the first pregnancy while in three it had not been detected at all.

All six women in whom the results of the I.A.G.T. were positive six months after the first pregnancy and who had a second pregnancy with a D-positive infant had positive I.A.G.T. results at the time of the second delivery (see table III). Of the 23 women in whom anti-D was detected only with enzyme-treated cells six months after a first pregnancy, however, only three gave a positive response to the I.A.G.T. at the time of delivery of a second D-positive infant.

The risk of having anti-D (as proved by an I.A.G.T.) after a second D-positive pregnancy was 0·64% (5 out of 778) in women who showed no evidence of antibody six months after their first pregnancy, 13% (3 out of 23) in women who were positive only with the enzyme test six months after their first pregnancy, and 100% (6 out of 6) in women who had positive I.A.G.T. results six months after their first pregnancy. To correct for the slight bias (evident in tables II and III) against those groups in which more women who had anti-D six months after their first pregnancy were known to have become pregnant again with a D-positive fetus revised figures were calculated, on the assumption that all the women admitted to the trial had a second pregnancy and that in all cases the predictive significance of the results at six months was the same (see table IV).

TRANSPLACENTAL HAEMORRHAGE AND INCIDENCE OF IMMUNIZATION

The estimated extent of transplacental haemorrhage in 1,844 women initially accepted for the trial and in whom acid-elution tests were carried out is shown in table V. Transplacental haemorrhage was over 0·5 ml in 4·15% of all women examined. The relation between the size of transplacental haemorrhage and the time of appearance of anti-D (as proved by an I.A.G.T.) is considered for the four dose categories in table VI. There was a suggestion that, as judged by a positive I.A.G.T. result six months after the first pregnancy, the increased failure rate with dose 4 was associated with relatively large transplacental bleeds; four of the six failures associated with transplacental haemorrhages of 1 ml or more occurred with dose 4.

The association between relatively large transplacental haemorrhages and increased failures with dose 4 was not due simply to an increased incidence of relatively large transplacental haemorrhages in this group; the numbers of women who had a transplacental haemorrhage of more than 4 ml after their first pregnancy and who subsequently had a second pregnancy were 3, 1, 0, and 2 in dose groups 1, 2, 3, and 4 respectively. Nevertheless, only those women who received dose 4 formed anti-D.

There were three women who were estimated to have had a transplacental haemorrhage exceeding 4 ml who should have been included in the trial but who were in fact excluded. The number of women initially included in the trial in whom the extent of transplacental haemorrhage was estimated to be 4 ml or more was 12 out of the 1,844 cases in which a satisfactory test was done. The possible effect on the results of excluding the three women is considered below.

TABLE IV—*Failure Rates (expressed as a Percentage of Patients) as judged by a Positive Indirect Antiglobulin Test Result*

| Dose | Six Months after First Pregnancy | End of Second Pregnancy | |
		Observed*	Predicted†
1	0.2 "	1.5 "	1.5 "
2	0.2 "	1.1 "	1.2 "
3	0.4 "	1.5 "	1.4 "
4	1.4 "	2.9 "	2.1 "

*Test of difference between frequency of I.A.G.T.-positive results at end of second pregnancy in groups receiving doses 1 and 4; P = 0.4 (exact test). Test of significance of trend in frequency of I.A.G.T.-positive results at end of second pregnancy from doses 1 to 4 through doses 2 and 3: $\chi^2 = 0.62$; n = 1; $0.3 < P < 0.5$.
†Predicted on the assumption that all women admitted to the trial had had a second pregnancy and antibody results six months after a first pregnancy had the same predictive significance in all cases (see text).

TABLE V—*Estimates of Transplacental Haemorrhage (ml Fetal Red Cells) in 1,844 Women examined after Birth of First Infant*

Haemorrhage	Nil*	≤0.5	>0.5-1.0	>1.0-4.0	>4.0
Proportion of Women	42.25 "	53.6 "	2.15 "	1.35 "	0.65 "

*Includes cases in which not more than two darkly stained cells were seen.

CLINICAL CONDITION OF SECOND D-POSITIVE INFANTS

In the five cases where anti-D was detected in the mother's serum only with enzyme-treated red cells at the time of delivery of the second D-positive infant none of the infants appeared to suffer from haemolytic disease; all had negative results of direct antiglobulin tests and were clinically normal. In 14 cases in which anti-D was detected by the I.A.G.T. at the time of delivery of the second D-positive infant there was evidence that those infants born to mothers who had received

the lowest dose of anti-D were more severely affected than the rest. Of the six infants born to mothers who had received dose 4 only two needed no treatment; of the remaining four, one needed a single exchange transfusion, two needed two exchange transfusions, and one received an intrauterine transfusion followed by one postnatal exchange transfusion. Of the eight infants born to mothers who had been treated with doses 1, 2, or 3, however, six needed no treatment and two needed only a single exchange transfusion. All 14 affected infants made a satisfactory recovery.

Discussion

The aim of treatment with passively administered antibody is to prevent the D-negative subject from forming anti-D. When the interval between treatment and examination of the patient's serum for anti-D is relatively short—for example; six months—the problem arises of distinguishing between passively administered antibody and actively produced antibody. It is therefore necessary to consider how long passively administered antibody may be detectable in the recipient's plasma after the administration of a given dose.

After the intramuscular injection of radioiodine-labelled IgG the maximum plasma level, corresponding to the presence in the plasma of about 40% of the injected dose, is reached two to four days after injection (Smith *et al.*, 1972). Between about seven and 28 days after injection the plasma level declines with a $t\frac{1}{2}$ of about 21 days, but between 28 and 63 days after injection the $t\frac{1}{2}$ is about 28 days (Tee and Watkins, 1967). There is no evidence that the uptake and catabolism of anti-D molecules differ from those of pooled normal IgG. For example, Smith *et al.* (1972) found no significant difference in the uptake rate of anti-D and of ^{125}I-labelled IgG. Wallace (1971) injected 1,000 µg anti-D intramuscularly into a number of D-negative volunteers and found that the maximum plasma level (as estimated in an AutoAnalyzer) was reached in about two days. He also measured the rate of disappearance of anti-D from the plasma and found that over a five-month period the rate could be described by a simple exponential with a $t\frac{1}{2}$ of the order of 26 days. After an injection of 1,000 µg anti-D the average plasma concentration six months later was 0.0025 µg/ml—that is, about 1/100 the level observed 48 hours after injection. Using the AutoAnalyzer, antibody could still be detected in three out of eight subjects at nine months.

The maximum level of anti-D in the plasma after dose 1 (200 µg) would be expected to be about 0.04 µg/ml; six months later the level would be expected to be about 0.0004 µg/ml. Such a level is just within the sensitivity of the AutoAnalyzer, but it is almost certainly below the level which can be detected reliably by manual methods using enzyme-treated cells and is certainly below the level which can be detected by the I.A.G.T. Nevertheless, when tests were made with enzyme-treated cells six months after the administration of passively administered antibody positive results were observed

TABLE VI—*Time of First Appearance of Anti-D in Relation to Dose of Immunoglobulin and Size of Transplacental Haemorrhage in 18 Immunized Women*

| Dose | No. of Cases | First Appearance of Anti-D | Estimate of Transplacental Haemorrhage | | | | | |
			Not Done	Nil*	≤0.5	>0.5-1.0	>1.0-4.0	>4.0
1	3	Six months ater 1st delivery			1			
		In 2nd D-positive pregnancy	1†				1	
2	3	Six months after 1st delivery		1				
		In 2nd D-positive pregnancy		1	1			
3	5	Six months after 1st delivery			1			1
		In 2nd D-positive pregnancy		2	1			
4	7	Six months after 1st delivery			2		2	2
		In 2nd D-positive pregnancy		1				

*Includes cases in which not more than two darkly stained cells were seen.
†Many "intermediately stained" cells. No estimate attempted.

far more often in women who had had the highest dose of anti-D (see table II) though at the time the laboratories carrying out the test did not know which dose had been given to which women. It is possible that there is considerable variation in the rate of catabolism of anti-D and that this is one factor which leads to the detection of traces of the antibody in some subjects at a time when the concentration is expected to be too low to be detectable. Whether the same explanation can be extended to account for those cases in which anti-D was detected six months after a dose of 100 μg (dose 2) or even less is a matter for speculation.

Of the women in whom the results of a second pregnancy with a D-positive infant were known 23 had anti-D detectable only with enzyme-treated cells six months after a first pregnancy, and of these 23 only three had a positive I.A.G.T. result at the time of their second delivery. In these three cases the positive result with enzyme-treated cells after the first pregnancy may have been due to the presence six months after the first pregnancy of a concentration of antibody too low to be detected by the I.A.G.T. In the remaining 20 cases the positive results with enzyme-treated cells were presumably due either to the detection of passively administered antibody or to false positives. When these 20 women were tested after their second pregnancy a positive result was reported in only two cases, suggesting that when the result was positive only with enzyme-treated cells it was usually due to a previous injection of anti-D.

In the five women who had anti-D detectable only with enzyme-treated cells at the time of delivery of their second infant the results evidently could not have been due to the detection of passively administered antibody. In two cases anti-D had already been detected only with enzyme-treated cells six months after the first delivery and perhaps these two women should be regarded as having been weakly immunized. In the other three cases the finding may have been due to the development of anti-D during the second pregnancy. In all five cases it is of course possible that some or all of the results are false-positives. In any case the infants of these five mothers showed no evidence of haemolytic disease of the newborn.

As assessed by the I.A.G.T. six months after the first pregnancy the results indicated a trend towards a lower failure rate as the dose of anti-D increased (table II). When the results of second D-positive pregnancies were examined (table III) no significant trend was apparent though, as with the results at six months, there was a suggestion of a higher failure rate with the lowest dose. Similarly, the predicted failure rates at the end of a second pregnancy, based on the results six months after the first pregnancy, pointed to a failure rate slightly greater with dose 4 than with the other doses (see table IV). Finally, the severity of haemolytic disease in infants born to women who had received dose 4 seemed to be slightly greater than in the other infants.

In the light of information which has accumulated since the trial began the failure rates that might be expected with the different doses employed may be considered. There is evidence that the dose needed for the suppression of Rh sensitization is of the order of 25 μg antibody per ml D-positive red cells (W.H.O., 1971). Furthermore, reasonable agreement has been achieved on measurements of the extent of transplacental haemorrhage found immediately after delivery (see review by Mollison (1972) whose figures for the incidence of transplacental haemorrhage are used below). When any particular dose of anti-D is given to recently delivered women it is therefore possible to predict the number of cases in which the dose is expected to be too small to suppress immunization. If it is assumed that only 70% of D-negative subjects are responders (Mollison, 1972) and that all responders form anti-D when they receive a dose of D-positive red cells which is not fully "covered" by 25 μg anti-D per ml of cells the overall failure rate due to undertreatment from any particular dose of anti-D can be predicted. For example, 200 μg (dose 1) should protect against 8 ml D-positive cells; transplacental

haemorrhages of this amount or more are found in about 0·4% of women. Allowing for the fact that only 70% of D-negative women are responders the expected failure rate is thus calculated to be about 0·3%. Similiarly, with 20 μg (dose 4) the expected failure rate due to undertreatment is about 2·5%. These calculations suggest that the failure rate might be about 2% higher with dose 4 than with dose 1. The observed difference (about 1·5%) was in reasonable agreement.

There was evidence of an association between transplacental haemorrhages of 4 ml or more and failures with dose 4. Twelve women had an estimated transplacental haemorrhage of 4 ml or more after a first pregnancy, and there were three additional women with a transplacental haemorrhage of this extent who were excluded from the trial. If it is assumed that these three women would, if they had been included, have distributed themselves at random among the dose groups then there would have been only about one additional woman with a transplacental haemorrhage of 4 ml or more treated with dose 4. It seems evident that this could not have had any substantial effect upon the results.

The fact that the observed failure rate with a dose of 200-300 μg anti-D seemed to be about 1-2% by the end of a second D-positive pregnancy, as shown by the present trial and by several other series (for example, Eklund and Nevanlinna, 1973), suggests that many apparent failures of treatment when anti-D is given at the time of delivery are due to the occurrence of Rh sensitization before delivery.

Unless "failures" are carefully defined estimates of the failure rate are bound to vary from one series to another. For example, in the present series women whose serum contained anti-D at the end of their first pregnancy were excluded. No accurate estimate is available of the number of such women excluded but published data suggest that the figure would be about 0·5% (Woodrow, 1970; Eklund and Nevanlinna, 1973). On the same reasoning it may be assumed that about 0·5% of women develop anti-D at the end of the second pregnancy as a result of primary immunization in that pregnancy. Such women will falsely be included as failures of treatment.

The criterion of "serologically detectable anti-D" must also affect the reported failure rate. In the present series only women who developed a positive I.A.G.T. result were counted as failures. The five women with anti-D detectable only with enzyme-treated cells at the end of their second pregnancy were not counted as failures. Nevertheless, even if they had been included the overall failure rate would have risen by less than 1%.

In the United Kingdom and in a few other countries a dose of 100 μg anti-D has for some time been used for routine administration to unimmunized D-negative women recently delivered of a D-positive infant. Our results support the contention that this dose has a success rate which is not appreciably different from that observed with a dose of 200-300 μg. Whatever standard dose is adopted it is desirable to perform a screening test to detect large transplacental haemorrhages because it is likely that in such cases the risk of Rh immunization can be reduced by giving an appropriately increased dose of anti-D.

Requests for reprints to: M.R.C. Experimental Haematology Unit, St. Mary's Hospital Medical School, London W2 1PG.

References

Betke, K., and Kleihauer, E. (1958). *Blut*, 4, 241.
Clarke, C. A. (1967). *British Medical Journal*, 4, 7.
Eklund, J., and Nevanlinna, H. R. (1973). *Journal of Medical Genetics*, 10, 1-7.
Hughes-Jones, N. C., and Stevenson, Mary. (1968). *Vox Sanguinis*, 14, 401.
Mollison, P. L. (1972). *Blood Transfusion in Clinical Medicine*, 5th edn., Oxford, Blackwell Scientific Publications.
Smith, G. N., Mollison, D. P., Griffiths, B., and Mollison, P. L. (1972). *Lancet*, 1, 1208.
Tee, D. E. H., and Watkins, J. (1967). *British Medical Journal*, 4, 210.
Wallace, J. (1971). Personal communication.
World Health Organization. (1971). *Prevention of Rh Sensitization*. Technical Report Series, No. 468, p. 29, Geneva, W.H.O.
Woodrow, J. C. (1970). *Series Haematologica*, 3, 3.

Paper 47

47. Woodrow J. C. Effectiveness of Rh Prophylaxis. Paper given at Bonn Working Party, 1973. Haematoliga, (1974), 8, 281-290.

Commentary

This is a review of the experiences of anti-D prophylaxis in different parts of the world. It is based on a paper given at Bonn in 1973 at an anti-D working party and round table conference.

One of the reasons for a variable failure rate is that the tests used to detect antibody are of different sensitivity. Notable in this connexion is the absence of failures in the Canadian trial and it is here that there is the highest incidence of antibodies detected at the end of the first pregnancy—in other words, it is likely that more women were excluded from this trial.

Details of trials with intravenous anti-D (as gammaglobulin in Germany and plasma in South Africa) are described, and there seems no doubt that Rh-positive fetal cells are cleared more quickly by this route, and if the mother is very sensitive the time factor may be important. In Canada and Australia ante-partum prophylaxis is being tried and some preliminary results are given in Table 6. It seems however that a very large series would be needed to show that it was more effective than when given after delivery in the standard way.

Finally, some interesting data from California are reported which show how the infant mortality due to Rh HDN has fallen, particularly since the introduction of Rho-GAM (Hawes and Mordaunt, 1973).

From J. C. Woodrow **(1974)**, *Haematologia*, **8, 281-290.** *Copyright* **(1974)** *by kind permission of the author and Kultura.*

Woodrow J. C. (1974). Effectiveness of Rh Prophylaxis. Paper given at Bonn Working Party, 1973. *Haematologia*, 8, 281-290.

J. C. WOODROW,
Department of Medicine,
University of Liverpool.

When experimental studies had shown that it was possible to prevent Rh immunization by administering IgG anti-D and clinical trials were started, it was not anticipated that complete success would be achieved. The degree of optimism about the likely results of giving anti-D postpartum depended on how important one thought primary immunization to be during the months of pregnancy, for it seemed likely that primary immunization occurring as the result of a stimulus during labour should be entirely preventable but priming during pregnancy might not be. The use in recent years of Rh prophylaxis on a wide clinical scale makes possible an assessment of the degree of success which can be achieved. When one looks at the results reported from several centres throughout the world two main questions can be asked. First, what is the general effectiveness of the prophylactic treatment? Secondly, are there any important differences from one centre to another and, if so, what is their significance?

Before looking at the actual data it is profitable to review briefly the picture of Rh immunization as it occurs in the absence of treatment and to relate tests for antibody before and after treatment to this. Fig. 1 shows a sequence of two Rh-positive pregnancies which might, for example, be the first and the second.

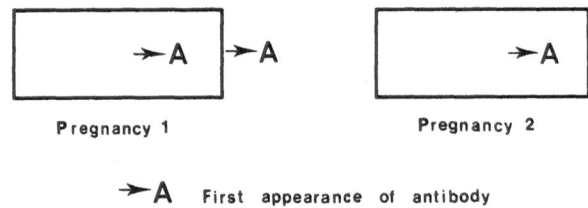

Pregnancy 1   Pregnancy 2

➤A   First appearance of antibody

Fig. 1   Sequence of two Rh-positive pregnancies, e.g. the first and second, with the times at which antibody commonly appears for the first time.

Antibodies may appear in the first pregnancy and in a proportion of cases there may have been a previous Rh-positive transfusion or an abortion. Hindemann (1) has put forward evidence to suggest that in some instances there has been priming of the Rh-negative mother when she herself was *in utero,* resulting from materno-foetal transfusion from her own own Rh-positive mother. However, in some instances primary immunization during the first pregnancy might be responsible. We might also expect that some mothers may have become primed before delivery but without antibodies being detectable. The actual figures for the incidence of antibodies during this first pregnancy vary from centre to centre and it is likely that the methods of antibody testing used could have an appreciable effect on the inclusion of cases in a clinical trial. A very weak antibody might be detected at one centre and the mother excluded from a trial but missed at another centre, the mother being treated, with the likelihood of failure resulting.

Antibodies may of course appear in the months subsequent to delivery, being about ten times more frequent where this first pregnancy is ABO-compatible than where it is incompatible. One common problem in treated women is that of distinguishing active from passive antibody at this time. Although the

T½ of IgG anti-D is of the order of 26 days, there is some evidence of considerable variation from individual to individual and what is later decided to have been passive antibody may be found by sensitive methods six months after treatment with 100-200 μg antibody. Clearly, differences in the way in which these antibodies are tested for, assessed and recorded, may make an appreciable difference when comparing one centre with another. When weak enzyme-active antibodies are found it is only a long follow follow-up that a firm decision as to their significance can be made.

Antibodies may appear for the first time during the second pregnancy. Comparison of the incidence in untreated mothers with that for the first pregnancy strongly indicates that in most instances we are dealing with a secondary response, priming having occurred as a result of the first pregnancy. For example, our own studies on untreated mothers in Liverpool showed that 0.95 per cent of mothers developed antibodies during their first Rh-positive ABO-compatible pregnancy and that approximately 10 per cent did so during the second Rh-positive ABO-compatible pregnancy. Assuming that the incidences of primary antibody formation in the two pregnancies were the same, the marked increase of antibody development during the second pregnancy must have been due to mothers being primed by the first pregnancy but showing no detectable antibody during the first part of the second pregnancy. A small foeto-maternal transfusion during this second pregnancy would then lead to a secondary response with antibody becoming detectable. However, some instances of antibody development during the second pregnancy are likely to be due to a primary response and it is not to be expected that these would be preventable by anti-D given after the first pregnancy. Differences in the interpretation put on the appearance of antibody during the pregnancy subsequent to treatment may occur between different centres.

A detailed account of the appearance of antibodies at this time in untreated mothers was given by Bishop and Krieger (2) who described two main patterns of response. In one there was the late development of an antibody active only by enzyme techniques with a negative direct Coombs test on the baby. At the other end of the scale there was the earlier development of an antibody, positive by antiglobulin methods, and often associated with a positive direct Coombs test on cord blood. It seems likely that the first pattern is typical of a primary response and the second of a secondary response. However there is some doubt that one can always be dogmatic in separating these two patterns because the responsiveness of Rh-negative individuals is very variable.

Two other points are worth noting. Apart from differences in the routine dose of anti-D used in the trials, it is often the case that where an unusually large foeto-maternal transfusion is detected, a dose of anti-D much larger than the standard one for the trial is given. The extent to which such cases are ascertained and the technical methods used to detect them vary from centre to centre. This may have an influence on the results of a clinical trial. Secondly, there is the possibility of differences in the natural history of Rh immunization from one area of the world to another. For example, the incidence of antibody after ABO-compatible pregnancies appears to be lower for West Germany (4.9%) (3) and Finland (4.3%) (4) than that found in other Western countries where the incidence is of the order of 8%.

The possible variables to be considered in assessing the results of clinical trials are listed in Table 1.

Table 1 Variables associated with Rh trials

A. SELECTION OF CASES
   (1) ABO compatibility
   (2) Parity
   (3) Antibody tests before treatment

B. TESTS FOR IMMUNIZATION AFTER TREATMENT
   (1) Passive—Active
   (2) In subsequent pregnancy

C. DOSAGE

D. VARIATIONS IN NATURAL HISTORY (?)

Table 2 Rh. Controlled clinical trials: Results of tests in the months after delivery

Centre	Controls			Treated		
	No.	present	Per cent Anti-D with Anti-D	No.	present	Per cent Anti-D with Anti-D
Liverpool Group						
1000 μg trial	176	38	21.6	173	1	0.58
200 μg trial	362	13	3.6	353	0	0.0
U.S.A.	1476	102	6.9	3389	6	0.18
West Canada	500	36	7.2	2247	0	0.0
Holland	329	17	5.2	1563	7	0.45
West Germany	2458	96	3.9	3091	15	0.49
Finland						
ABO Compatible	792	34	4.3	9569	12	0.13
ABO Incompatible	220	1	0.5	3151	5	0.16
Sweden	595	25	4.2	2214	8	0.36

Table 3 Rh. Uncontrolled clinical trials: Results of tests in the months after delivery

Centre	Total Tested	No. with Anti-D	Per cent with Anti-D
Liverpool*	980	4	0.4
Ministry of Health (England and Wales)	5693	26	0.46
Canada (low protein)	677	2	0.3
Australia	3706	16	0.42
Edmonton	574	3	0.52
Belgium	1548	5	0.32

* Total experience with treated mothers—includes results of controlled trial

THE RESULTS

Antibodies in the Post-Delivery Period

Table 2 gives the results for controlled clinical trials, based on tests for antibody in the months subsequent to treatment. The overall picture is of a 95 per cent reduction in the incidence of antibodies in treated mothers as compared to controls, i.e. a 5 per cent failure rate. Notable is the absence of failures in the Canadian trial. It is this group (5) which reports a relatively high incidence of antibodies at the end of the first pregnancy, often detectable only by sensitive enzyme methods and it is reasonable to speculate that instances of weak primary immunization are being detected and excluded from the trial. There is a suggestion in the Finnish data that treatment after ABO-incompatible pregnancies is relatively less successful but this has not been found by other groups.

Table 3 gives the corresponding results for uncontrolled trials. The overall incidence of antibodies six months after treatment is approximately 0.4 per cent.

Table 4 Rh. Controlled clinical trials: Results of tests in subsequent pregnancy

Centre	Controls			Treated		
	No.	Anti -D present	Per cent with Anti-D	No.	Anti -D present	Per cent with Anti-D
Liverpool						
1000 μg	65	20	30.7	88	2	2.4
200 μg	127	13	10.2	128	3	2.3
U.S.A.	179	24	13.4	438	5	1.1
West Germany	373	29	7.8	138	0	0.0

Antibodies in the Subsequent Pregnancy

In Table 4 are shown the results of testing for antibody in the Rh-positive pregnancy subsequent to treatment in those trials where controls have been used. The incidence of antibodies in treated mothers is, overall, approximately 9 per cent of that in controls.

The corresponding results of the uncontrolled trials are shown in Table 5. The average incidence of antibodies is 1.6 per cent. Taking into account the variation in the selection of mothers for the trials, this represents a little over 10 per cent of the expected incidence.

Table 5 Rh. Uncontrolled clinical trials: Results at end of subsequent pregnancies

Centre	Total Tested	No. with Anti-D	Per cent with Anti-D
Liverpool*	439	7	1.6
Holland	98	2	2.0
Australia	1218	13	1.1
Canada	483	8	1.7
Finland	1027	10	0.97
Sweden	75	1	1.3
S. Africa	587	15	2.5
Leeds	437	7	1.6
St. Louis	240	3	1.3

* Total experience with treated mothers: figures include those for controlled trial

Bowman (6) has suggested that it is likely that all the antibodies appearing in pregnancies subsequent to treatment in the Canadian trial are examples of primary responses but there is perhaps room for some doubt about this. In their analysis of the Finnish data, Eklund and Nevanlinna (4) estimated that of the 1 per cent of mothers developing antibody during the subsequent pregnancy, 0.35 per cent might be primary and 0.65 per cent secondary responses (this assumes that the incidence of primary responses was the same in this subsequent second as in the first pregnancy, i.e. 0.35 per cent). In Liverpool 1.2 per cent of mothers developed antibody during the pregnancy subsequent to treatment, and of these it is estimated that something like 0.5 per cent were primary and 0.7 per cent were secondary responses.

It is not easy to determine with certainty the causes of the apparent differences between centres. It is to be doubted whether differences in dosage have had a very marked effect on the results. In most centres 200-300 μg anti-D was being given. Sometimes an increased dose was given where unusually large foeto-maternal transfusions were detected and as mentioned above this might have had some relevance in this context. In some instances of apparent failure a comment was made that there was delay in administering the anti-D. It is possible that where a substantial stimulus has occurred and the mother is very sensitive, the time factor may be important.

In the series from West Germany there is included a proportion of mothers given anti-D immunoglobulin by the intravenous rather than by the usual intramuscular route. Schneider (3) reported that 4 of 1032 (0.39 per cent) mothers treated by intravenous anti-D developed antibody compared to 10 of 1444 (0.69 per cent) given intramuscular anti-D. Of a series of 3697 mothers given anti-D intravenously in doses varying according to the foetal cell count after delivery, 2 were reported as immunized during the subsequent months (7). There is thus a suggestion of a somewhat lower failure rate when anti-D is given intravenously but because of the difficulties mentioned above in relating results from different centres this question can only be resolved with a degree of certainty by a well controlled trial carried out at one centre with the aim of comparing the two methods of administration. If intravenous treatment is somewhat more effective in some instances it might be in mothers who have been weakly primed just before delivery and who then received a further stimulus during labour. The very rapid build up of antibody in the tissues might be crucial in such a situation.

In those centres where foetal cell counts after delivery are done routinely, it has been observed that in most instances of failure of prophylaxis the volume of foeto-maternal transfusion has been quite small or not detectable. In some of these mothers there might have been delayed appearance of foetal cells in the maternal circulation consequent on absorption from the peritoneal cavity but it is likely that this only applies to a proportion. Thus inadequate dosage of anti-D is unlikely as the explanation in most instances of failure. More likely is that a primary immune response has been initiated during the weeks prior to delivery.

Because of this, trials of antepartum therapy with anti-D are being conducted in some countries. Table 6 shows some recent results from Canadian and Australian trials.* Although in the Canadian trial three control mothers had developed antibody by delivery, presumably there was passive antibody at this time in some of the treated mothers, and this would make it very difficult to know whether any of these mothers had been actively immunized. These trials are inconclusive and it is going to take a very large series with follow-up through subsequent pregnancies before a final answer is possible. Should a reduction in the failure

* I am indebted to Dr. J. Bowman and Dr. M. G. Davey respectively for these data.

Table 6 Antepartum anti-D

Canadian trial
    300 μg anti-D at 28 and/or 34 weeks and postpartum
    Primiparæ—340 tested 6-9 months after delivery
                                  (Rh + infants)
          — None immunized
    324 mothers given postpartum anti-D only
          — 3 had antibody at delivery
          — no others immunized

Australian trial
    250 μg anti-D (×1 or ×2) in last weeks and postpartum
          — 364 tested 6 months after delivery
                            (Rh + infants)
          — Two had antibody — ? passive

rate be shown to result from this form of therapy it is still rather doubtful whether the practical problems involved will justify it as a routine measure.

Effect of Rh Prophylaxis on Disease Incidence and Mortality

The results of the clinical trials suggest that with the present wide application of Rh prophylaxis it should be possible to observe a progressive decline in the incidence of and the mortality from Rh haemolytic disease. The speed with which this decline occurs will depend on the efficiency of the prophylactic programme but also on the average family size and interval between successive births. Certain criteria may be affected by factors other than Rh prophylaxis. The crude incidence of Rh antibodies in a population is affected by the tendency in recent years to employ increasingly sensitive methods of detection. The use of phototherapy may lessen the frequency of exchange transfusion. It will probably therefore take several years before the full effect of the prophylactic programme can be assessed.

Hawes and Mordaunt (8) have produced some interesting data from California. Fig. 2 charts the infant death rate from Rh haemolytic disease in California, between 1947 and 1971. It is seen that there was a gradual decline in mortality over this period. There were thought to be two main reasons for this, one being limitation of family size with an increasing percentage of primiparous deliveries, and the other improved methods of diagnosis and management of the condition. In 1968 Rh prophylaxis was introduced on an increasingly wide scale. In 1970 it became a legal requirement in the State that all pregnant mothers be Rh typed and that all cases of Rh haemolytic disease be notified. It is therefore very likely that the data on incidence and mortality from the disease are now very accurate. The incidence of the disease fell from 4.1 cases per 1000 live births in the first quarter of 1970, to 2.9 in the corresponding quarter of 1972. The actual number of deaths attributed to the disease were 38 and 12 respectively during these two periods. The evidence strongly suggests that this very marked fall was largely due to the widespread use of anti-D gammaglobulin.

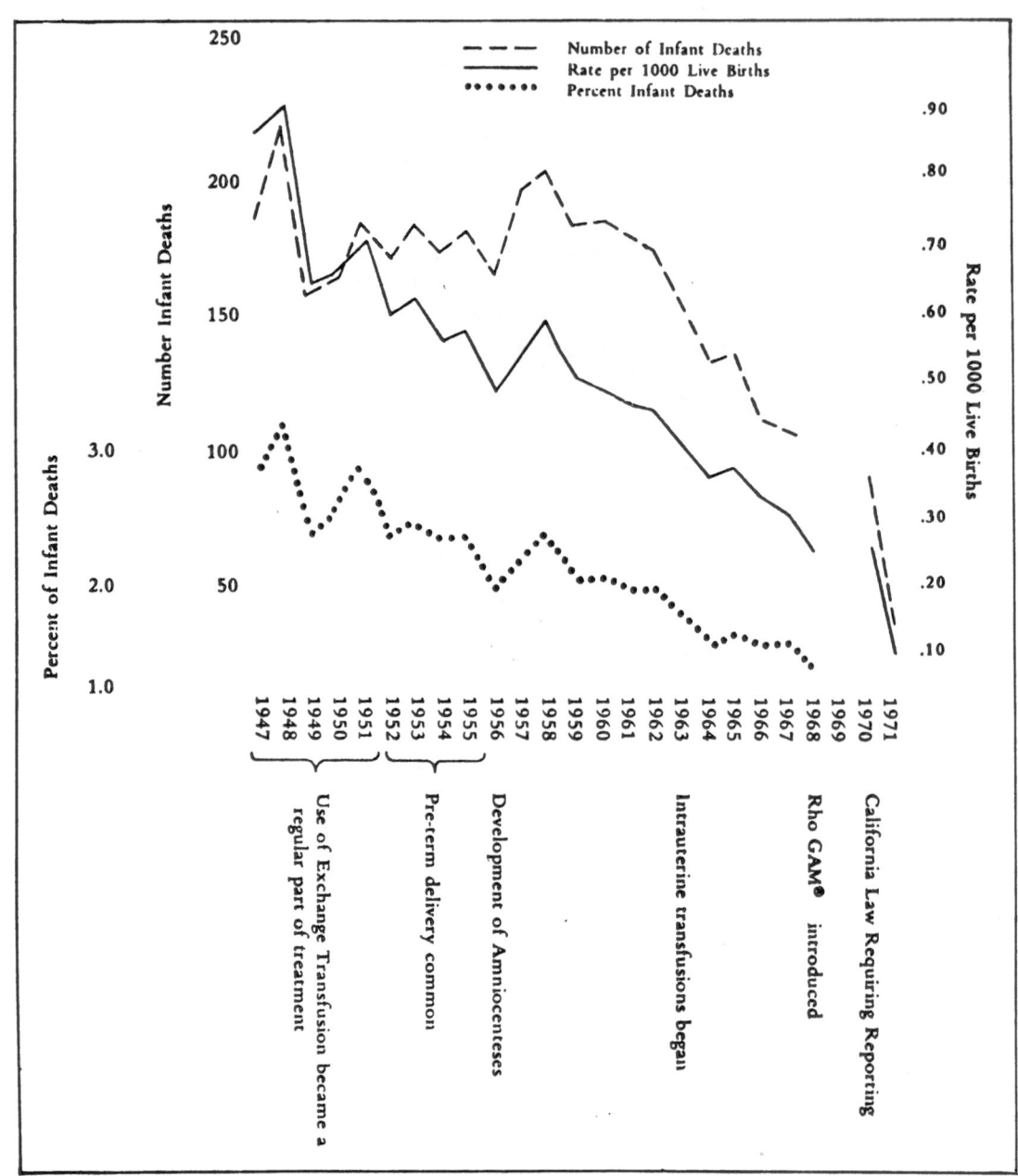

Fig. 2   Trends of infant death due to Rh haemolytic disease between 1947 and
1971. From Hawes and Mordaunt (8) by kind permission of the Authors.

Acknowledgments

I am grateful to many workers in the Rh field who have published data on
clinical trials which I have quoted. I wish to thank the Californian Medical
Association for permission to reproduce Fig. 2.

References

1. Hindemann, P. (1973). *Lancet, 1,* 46
2. Bishop, G. J. and Kreiger, V. I. (1970). *Med. J. Austral., 1,* 663
3. Schneider, J. (1972). *Z. Geburtsch. u. Perinat., 176,* 2
4. Eklund J. and Nevanlinna, H. R. (1973). *J. med. Genet., 10,* 1
5. Bowman, J. M. (1971). *J. Reprod. Med., 6,* 67
6. Bowman, J. M. (Personal communication), 1973
7. Hoppe, H. H. (1971). *Geburtsch. u. Frauenheilk, 6,* 493
8. Hawes, W. E. and Mordaunt, V. L. (1973). *Calif. Med., 118,* 28

Paper 48

48. Mollison, P. L. (1974). Rh and iso-immunisation. Summary of a workshop held at the 2nd International Congress of Immunology at Brighton, England, in July 1974. Chairman: C. A. Clarke Co-chairman. P. L. Mollison. *(Vox Sang* in press).

Commentary

Those who attended the Brighton workshop were chiefly interested in the preventive aspects of Rh HDN and the summaries of Professor Mollison's report show the lines of research which are being followed by workers in various parts of the world.

Rh and Isoimunization

Summary of a workshop held at the 2nd International Congress of Immunology at Brighton, England, in July 1974

CHAIRMAN: C. A. CLARKE
CO-CHAIRMAN: P. L. MOLLISON

(*Vox Sang;* in press)

It is generally accepted that some D-negative subjects are non-responders to D. In some series the incidence of non-responders has been as low as about 15% (F. Stratton) but in the largest and perhaps therefore the most instructive from this point of view the incidence has been 25-30%. By definition, a responder is a subject who produces serologically-detectable anti-D. However, the distinction between a responder and a non-responder can be made with a high degree of reliability by estimating the survival of D-positive red cells following a challenge (i.e. a second) injection of D-positive cells. In responders the red cells are destroyed at an accelerated rate from the time of the second injection onwards, indicating that some antibody has been made after the first injection, even when it cannot be detected serologically, whereas in non-responders the survival of a second injection of D-positive red cells and even of a sixth or seventh injection is normal.

Non-responsiveness to D does not seem to depend on the dose of D-positive red cells (at least over the range of about 1 to 100 ml red cells). By analogy with responsiveness to antigens in mice, it is to be expected that responsiveness to D is genetically determined and, again by analogy with findings in mice, that responsiveness may be linked to histocompatibility antigens. However, at a recent Workshop in Hungary no evidence was obtained of any relationship between responsiveness to D and HL-A group although, incidentally, there was a definite negative correlation between responsiveness to D and the level of some bacterial antibodies (Vox Sang.,1974, **26**, 470).

C. Stern reported that he had looked for a relationship between rosette formation and responsiveness to D-positive red cells. The results had proved impossible to interpret and this in his opinion was due to the large number of different antigens on red cells. He thought that no progress could be made with the approach until purified D antigen was available.

The possibility that some non-responders to D may in fact be weak D-positives was raised by W. Pollack, who had been able to elute anti-D from the red cells of two subjects who had originally been considered to be D-negative and who had failed to respond to D.

When D-negative women become immunized to D as a result of pregnancy with a D-positive fetus, they occasionally form anti-D by the time of delivery. However, this is unusual and it is much commoner for them to develop serologically-detectable antibody for the first time only 3-6 months after delivery. The reason for this timing seems to be mainly that relatively large transplacental haemorrhages occur for the most part at the time of delivery; it is possible that a contributory factor is a diminished responsiveness to primary immunization by fetal antigens during pregnancy. According to R. Finn, lymphocytes from pregnant women have a diminished response to stimulation by phytohaemagglutinin, indicating that there are significant changes in the immunological response of pregnant women.

It is difficult to prove that pregnancies which terminate at three months are capable of initiating primary Rh immunization although some observers maintain that spontaneous abortions cause primary immunization in 3-4% of D-negative women. In a series from Hungary (referred to by S. Hollán) in which 156 women whose pregnancies were terminated at three months and who were not given an injection of anti-D were followed to the end of a second full-term pregnancy with a D-positive infant, 6 (i.e. 3.8%) were found to have anti-D in their serum. Since the incidence of demonstrable anti-D at the end of first full-term D-positive pregnancies in women not known to have had a previous abortion is only about 1%, this finding certainly supports the idea that spontaneous abortions can initiate primary Rh immunization.

In a series of women treated with an injection of 50 μg of anti-D following termination of pregnancy at three months, the incidence of anti-D in the serum 3-6 months later was only 0.25% (S. Hollán, quoting I. Simonovits). This figure is difficult to interpret in the absence of a really satisfactory control series but is perhaps slightly suggestive of a beneficial effect of treatment. In any case, it is the general opinion at present that anti-D should be given prophylactically to D-negative women following abortion until or unless convincing evidence is produced that the treatment is unnecessary.

When anti-D is given by intramuscular injection to D-negative women immediately after delivery of their first D-positive infant, the proportion who become actively immunized, as shown by the presence of serologically-detectable anti-D in their plasma six months after delivery, is about 0.1% according to H. R. Nevanlinna. If these women are followed through a subsequent pregnancy with a D-positive infant, the proportion with anti-D rises to 0.8%. Since Nevanlinna also finds that 0.3% of D-negative women have anti-D in their plasma at the time of their first delivery, the over-all incidence of D-negative women who become immunized despite treatment is of the order of 1.2%. This figure is very similar to that recorded in a recent dose trial conducted by the MRC in the U.K. in which the overall failure rate in women given 50, 100 or 200 g anti-D after the end of a first pregnancy was about 1.4% (i.e. at the end of a subsequent pregnancy with a D-positive infant).

On the other hand, according to W. Pollack, no failures at all have been observed at the Columbia Presbyterian Medical Center in New York where 300 μg anti-D has been given intramuscularly at the time of delivery to all previously unimmunized D-negative women over the past few years.

In view of these discrepant findings, it is difficult to assess the value of giving anti-D during pregnancy, as has been done in Winnipeg over the last few years with apparent complete success, and it is also difficult to assess the value of giving anti-D intravenously at the time of delivery, as has been done for the past few years both in Hamburg and in Hanover. The potential advantage of giving anti-D intravenously rather than intramuscularly is simply that, for any given dose, higher plasma levels are reached and, moreover, when given intravenously, the antibody is immediately available in the circulation whereas, when given intramuscularly, the rate of uptake into the circulation is variable and relatively slow. H. Deicher suggested that it may also be important for anti-D to reach the lymphatic system as early as possible in certain cases in which red cells are spilt into the peritoneal cavity (for example, at Caesarean section), and may then enter the lymphatic glands at a very early stage. Whether the attainment of a relatively high plasma level of anti-D for a short period at the time when D-positive red cells are reaching the lymphatic system is important remains uncertain.

Some evidence about the effect of administering anti-D some considerable time after injecting D-positive red cells was provided by Diana Samson who had found that when anti-D was injected as long as two weeks after an injection of D-positive red cells, primary immunization appeared to be completely suppressed in about half the responders.

One circumstance in which it is advantageous to give anti-D intravenously rather than intramuscularly is after inadvertent transfusion of relatively large amounts of D-positive blood, since an injection of a large amount of anti-D immunoglobulin intramuscularly is painful. In relation to the suppression of Rh immunization following large amounts of red cells, W. Pollack said that his data suggested that the percentage of responders to D fell when passive anti-D was given with D-positive cells and he speculated that when the dose of anti-D given reached about 3000 μg, the incidence of responders to D might fall to less than 1 in 1000.

A strange consequence of Rh immunization, observed in only a small proportion of subjects, is the development of a positive direct antiglobulin test. B. Chown, in reviewing the cases in which this had occurred, said that in some of them at least the autoantibody appeared to be anti-LW.

Perhaps the most interesting observation presented at the Workshop was that reported by J. C. Woodrow which indicated that the suppression brought about by anti-D was not antigen-specific. Thirty-two D-negative, K-negative recipients had been given an injection of 1 ml of D-positive, K-positive red cells together with 16 μg of IgG anti-K. The red cells had been cleared within 24 hours, almost entirely to the spleen. Only one subject had made antibody. By contrast, of 33 control subjects given red cells without antibody, 7 out of 33 had developed anti-D; after a further injection, 2 out of 17 controls had developed anti-D but none out of 21 subjects given anti-K.* The findings, therefore, strongly suggest that rapid clearance of D-positive red cells from the circulation somehow inhibits primary Rh immunization. An observation in line with this was reported by H. Weitzel; in a splenectomised subject given in 4 ml of D-positive red cells together with 300 μg anti-D, the red cells were cleared from the circulation only slowly ($T_{\frac{1}{2}}$ ^{50}Cr 14.5 days) and anti-D was found in the subject's plasma four months later.

An unexpected finding was reported by H. Deicher. An $F(ab')_2$ preparation from IgG anti-D had been found to produce clearance of D-positive red cells at a rate similar to that of IgG anti-D, 50 μg of the preparation causing complete clearance of 1.5-2.0 ml of fetal blood within 24 hours. The preparation of $F(ab')_2$ was slightly contaminated (less than 5%) with IgG anti-D but it appeared that the amount of IgG anti-D present was far too small to account for the effects observed.

P. L. Mollison (co-chairman).
Professor P. L. Mollison, MRC Experimental Haematology Unit,
St. Mary's Hospital Medical School, London W2 1PG (England).

* Later information. 11 controls have now developed anti-D as compared with 1 subject given anti-Kell. (Ed.)

Further References
and Addresses

It has been impossible to include in this survey more than a small proportion of the literature relating to the topic. There is therefore appended a list of additional papers, or addresses of people working in the field and who have contributed significantly. These have been selected to include workers from many different parts of the world.

The list deals principally with the prophylactic section as this is an area of great interest at the present time.

REFERENCES

Alter, A. A. and Haut, I. H. (1971). Preventing maternal sensitization to Rh antigen. Legal implications. *New York State Journal of Medicine*, Oct. 1st, 2326-7

Alvey, P. J., Carroll, R. and Wilkes, C. (1968). Prevention of Rhesus immunisation. *J. Irish Med. Ass.*, 61, 311

Bartsch, F. K., Sandberg, L. and Unander, M. (1971). Prevention of Rh immunisation in Sweden, Atti del Convegno sui problemi attuali della malattia emolitica del neonato. Geneva. Ed: G. Sansone e F. Dambrosio, p. 111

Börner, P., Deicher, H., Hoppe, H. H., Hitschhold, H., Holtz, S. and Seifert, A. (1969). Prophylaxe der Rhesus-Sensibilisierung durch intravenöse Gabe von Immunoglobulin G anti-D. I. Klinische Ergebnisse und Untersuchungen zur anti-D.
Geburtsh. u. Frauenheilk. 29, 203

Börner, P., Deicher, H., Ghani, G., Geldmacher, H., Kayser, D., Kahnt, R., Klang, D., Klaus, H., Marks, V. and Nehawandian, O. A. (1971). Prophylaxis der Rhesus-Sensibilisierung durch intravenöse Gabe von Immunoglobulin anti-D. II. Generelle Prophylaxe mit niedrigen, dem Ausmass der fetomaternalen Transfusion angepassten Dosen von IgG-anti-D. *Geburtsh. u. Frauenheilk*, 31. J., H. 10, 911-923

Bowman, J. M. (1970). Prevention of haemolytic disease of the newborn. Annotation. *Brit. J. Haematol.*, 19, 653

Clarke, C. A. and McConnell, R. B. (1972). *Prevention of Rh Haemolytic Disease.* Springfield, Illinois, USA: Charles C. Thomas

Davey, M. G. (1968). The effectiveness of anti-Rh (D) immunoglobulin. Paper given at World Medical Association Symposium on 'The Conquest of Rh Haemolytic Disease', (Glebe, Australia: Australasian Medical Publishing).

Dudok de Wit, C., Borst-Eilers, E., de Weerdt, Ch. M. V. and Kloosterman, G. (1968). Prevention of Rhesus immunisation. A controlled clinical trial with a comparatively low dose of anti-D gammaglobulin. *Brit. Med. J.*, iv, 477

Eklund, J. and Nevanlinna, H. R. (1973). Rh prevention: a report and analysis of a national programme. *J. Med. Genet.*, 10, 1-7

Goti Iturriaga, J. L. (1968). La enfermedad Rh hemolitica en Vizcaya. Posibilidades actuales de su prevencion. *Gaceta Medica del Norte*, 18, 1-15

Hamilton, E. G. (1970). High-titer anti-D plasma for the prevention of Rh immunization. *Obstet. Gynec.*, 36, 331-340 (Paper 31 is relevant)

Jouvenceaux, A., Adenot, N., Berthoux F. and Revol, L. (1968). Gammaglobuline anti-D lyophilisée intra-veineuse pour la prévention de l'immunisation anti-Rh. *Proc. XI Int. Cong. Microbiol. Standardisation, Milan*

Makarov, V. S., Minakova, L. V., Dravert, E. D., Kozbinykh, L. F. and Kochetov, L. N. (1971). Pathogenesis of haemolytic disease. *Akusherstvo i Ginekologiia (Mosk)*, 47, 41-4 (In Russian; English Summary)

Moulinier, J. and Mesnier, F. (1969). Paper given at XII Int. Cong. Blood Transfusion, Moscow, on white cell antibodies in relation to Rh haemolytic disease (see Proceedings)

Nathenson, G. (1971). Development of Gm antibodies following injection of anti-Rh gammaglobulin. *Transfusion*, 11, 302-6

Petrov-Maslakov, M. A., Vasilieva, Z. F., Matveyeva, O. F., Balasanyan, I. G., Sorina, L. I. and Prigarnova, T. K. (1971). Prophylaxis of maternal Rh sensitization by means of anti-D immunoglobulin. *Archivum immunologiae et Therapiae Experimentalis*, 19, 343-347

Proceedings XIIth Int. Cong. Blood Transfusion, Moscow, 1969. (This contains many relevant references and addresses)

Queenan, J. T., Smith B. B., Haber, J. M., Jeffery, J. and Gadow, H. C. (1969). Irregular antibodies in the obstetric patient. *Obstet. Gynec.*, 14, 767-771

Queenan, J. T. (1971). Editor. *The Rh Problem: Clinical Obstetrics and Gynecology*, pp 491-652. (Contributors: J. T. Queenan, J. G. Robertson, C. R. Whitfield, H. Gordon, W. A. Bowes, Jnr., R. F. Friesen, J. F. Lucey, V. J. Freda, C. A. Clarke, W. Q. Ascari and J. G. Gorman). Harper and Row: New York.

Roberts, G. F. (1957). *Comparative aspects of haemolytic disease of the newborn*, p. 199. (Heineman Medical Books Ltd., London)

Robertson, J. G. (1968). Experience with Rh immunoglobulin in Edinburgh (Scotland). *Transfusion*, 8, 149-150

Schellong, G. and Grimm, W. (1970). Anti-D Behandlung nach Falschtransfusion: Verhütung der Rh Sensibilisierung. (Treatment with anti-D after a mismatched transfusion: prevention of Rh-sensitization.) *Deutsch. Med. Woch.*, 95, 2555-9. (In German; English summary)

Schneider, J. (1972). Die Prophylaxe der Rhesus-Sensibilisierung mit anti-D, zehn Jahre nach Beginn der ersten Untersuchungen. *Z. Geburtsh. u. Perinat.*, 176, 2-17

Speiser, P. (1971). IgG anti-D Prophylaxe. *Wiener Med. Woch.*, 615-7. (In German)

Spensieri, S., Carnevale, A. E. and Caldana, P. L. (1968). Rh iso-immunisation and transplacental transfer of foetal erythrocytes. *Monit. Obstet. Gynec. Endocr. Metabol.*, 39, (6 suppl.) 889-906

Tovey, G. H., Darke, C. C. and Fraser, L. D. (1970). Significance of HL-A cytotoxic antibodies in Rh haemolytic disease. *Lancet*, i, 1234-5

Tovey, L. A. D. (1972). The use of anti-D gammaglobulin for the prevention of Rh immunisation. *J. Obst. and Gynaec. British Commonwealth*, 79, 107-12

Woodrow, J. C. (1970). *Rh Immunisation and its Prevention*. Series; Haematologica Vol. III, 3 (Copenhagen: Munksgaard)

World Health Organisation (1971). Prevention of Rh sensitisation. Technical report series no. 468. (This also contains sources of information and addresses of those engaged in the work)

ADDRESSES

Archer, Dr Gordon, Australian Red Cross Society Blood Transfusion Service, 1 York Street, Sydney, NSW 2000, Australia

Bartsch, Dr F. K., Dept. of Obstetrics and Gynaecology, Ostra Sjukhuset and Blood Transfusion Centre, Sahgrenska Sjukhuset, Gothenburg Sweden

Biering, Dr G. M. D., Consultant in Paediatrics, Landspitalinn-Maternity Clinic, Reykjavik, Iceland

Bowman, Dr J. M., Rh Laboratory, 735 Notre Dame Avenue, Winnipeg, Canada R3E OL8

Davey, Dr M. G., Australian Red Cross Society, Western Australian Division, Blood Transfusion Service, 290 Wellington Street, Perth 6000, Western Australia

Hollán, Dr Susan, National Institute of Haematology and Blood Transfusion, Daróczi ut 24, Budapest XI, Hungary

Institute of Obstetrics and Gynecology, Moscow

Jennings, Dr A. R., 2801 Atlantic Avenue, Long Beach, California 90801, USA

Jouvenceaux, Dr A., Blood Transfusion Centre, Lyon, France

Persianinov, Professor, All-Union Scientific Research Institute of Obstetrics and Gynaecology, 2-6 Elanski, Moscow, USSR

Shapiro, Dr M., The South African Blood Transfusion Service, Cor. Klein and Esselen Streets, Hospital Hill, Johannesburg, South Africa. (Specialises in the use of anti-D given as plasma) (Paper 31 is relevant)

Sidelnikova, Dr Vera, All-Union Scientific Research Institute of Obstetrics and Gynaecology, 2-6 Elanski, Moscow, USSR

Snaedal, Dr G., Consultant in Obstetrics and Gynaecology, Landspitalinn-Maternity Clinic, Reykjavik, Iceland

Speiser, Dr P., Blood Group Serology Institute, University of Vienna

Index